Syncope Cases

Syncope Cases

EDITED BY

Roberto García-Civera,
Gonzalo Barón-Esquivias,
Jean-Jacques Blanc,
Michele Brignole,
Angel Moya i Mitjans,
Ricardo Ruiz-Granell
and Wouter Wieling

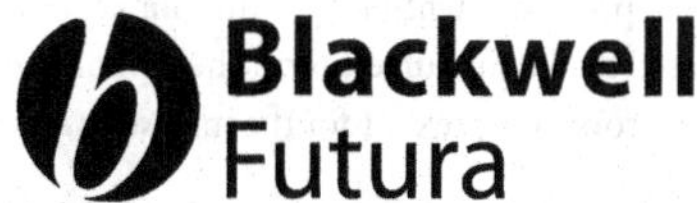

Blackwell Futura is an imprint of Blackwell Publishing
Blackwell Publishing, Inc., 350 Main Street, Malden, Massachusetts 02148-5020, USA
Blackwell Publishing Ltd, 9600 Garsington Road, Oxford OX4 2DQ, UK
Blackwell Science Asia Pty Ltd, 550 Swanston Street, Carlton, Victoria 3053, Australia

First published
1 2006

Library of Congress Cataloging-in-Publication Data

Syncope cases / edited by Roberto García-Civera . . . [*et al.*].
p. ; cm.
Includes bibliographical references.
ISBN-13: 978-1-4051-5109-2
ISBN-10: 1-4051-5109-9
1. Syncope (Pathology)—Case studies. I. García-Civera, Roberto.
[DNLM: 1. Syncope—diagnosis—Case Reports. 2. Cardiovascular Diseases—complications—Case Reports. 3. Syncope—complications —Case Reports. 4. Syncope—therapy—Case Reports. WB 182 S9916 2006]
RB150.S9S96 2006
616′.047—dc22

2005032202

ISBN-13: 978-1-4051-5109-2
ISBN-10: 1-4051-5109-9

A catalogue record for this title is available from the British Library

Commissioning Editor: Gina Almond
Development Editors: Vicki Donald and Beckie Brand
Book Development Assistant: Lauren Brindley

Set in 9/12pt Minion by Graphicraft Limited, Hong Kong

For further information on Blackwell Publishing, visit our website:
www.blackwellcardiology.com

The publisher's policy is to use permanent paper from mills that operate a sustainable forestry policy, and which has been manufactured from pulp processed using acid-free and elementary chlorine-free practices. Furthermore, the publisher ensures that the text paper and cover board used have met acceptable environmental accreditation standards.

Contents

Contributors

Editors

Gonzalo Barón Esquivias, MD
Cardiology Department
Hospital Universitario
Virgen del Rocío
Seville
Spain

Jean-Jacques Blanc, MD, FESC
Professor of Cardiology
Member, Task Force on Syncope, European Society of Cardiology
Chief, Department of Cardiology
University of Brest
Brest
France

Michele Brignole, MD, FESC
Chairman, Task Force on Syncope, European Society of Cardiology
Chief, Department of Cardiology
Ospedale Riuniti
Lavagna
Italy

Roberto García Civera, MD
Professor of Cardiology, Department of Medicine
Chief, Arrhythmology Section
Clinical University Hospital
University of Valencia
Valencia
Spain

Angel Moya i Mitjans, MD, FESC
Chief, Arrhythmology Section
Member, Task Force on Syncope, European Society of Cardiology
Vall d'Hebron General University Hospital
Barcelona
Spain

Ricardo Ruiz Granell, MD
Arrhythmia and Cardiac Pacing Unit
Clinical University Hospital
Valencia
Spain

Wouter Wieling, MD, PhD
Professor of Medicine in Syncope Unit
Department of Internal Medicine
Academic Medical Center
University of Amsterdam
The Netherlands

Contributors

P. Aguar Carrascosa, MD
Dr Peset University Hospital
Valencia
Spain

A. Aguilera, MD
Department of Cardiology
Virgen del Rocío University Hospital
Seville
Spain

C. Almodóvar, MD
Albacete General Hospital
Albacete
Spain

C. Alonso, MD
Cardiology Service
Vall d'Hebron General University Hospital
Barcelona
Spain

I. Anguera, MD
Departments of Cardiology and Internal Medicine
Corporació Sanitària
Parc Taulí Hospital
Sabadell
Spain

E. Arana, MD
Department of Cardiology
Virgen del Rocío University Hospital
Seville
Spain

M.F. Arkotxa, MD
Cardiology Service

Cruces Hospital
Bilbao
Spain

M. Atienzar, MD
General Hospital
Albacete
Spain

S.M. Ballesteros Pradas, MD
Department of Cardiology
Virgen del Rocío University Hospital
Seville
Spain

A. Bartoletti, MD
Syncope Center
Nuovo S. Giovanni di Dio Hospital
Florence
Italy

M.L. Blasco, MD
Intensive Care Unit
Clinical University Hospital
Valencia
Spain

M.C. Boer, BSc
Department of Medicine
Academic Medical Center
University of Amsterdam
Amsterdam
The Netherlands

N. Bottoni, MD
Unità Operativa di Cardiologia Interventistica
Azienda Ospedaliera S. Maria Nuova
Reggio Emilia
Italy

A. Carmona Ainat, MD
Clinical University Hospital
Zaragoza
Spain

P. Castellant, MD
University Hospital
Brest
France

M. Cazorla, MD
Departments of Cardiology and Internal Medicine
Corporació Sanitària
Parc Taulí Hospital
Sabadell
Spain

T. Cellai, MD
Geriatric and Cardiology Medicine Unit
University of Florence
Florence
Italy

R. Ceres, MD
General Hospital
Albacete
Spain

M. Cervantes, MD
Departments of Cardiology and Internal Medicine
Corporació Sanitària
Parc Taulí Hospital
Sabadell
Spain

O. Chapinal, MD
Departments of Cardiology and Internal Medicine
Corporació Sanitària
Parc Taulí Hospital
Sabadell
Spain

N. Colman, MD
Department of Cardiology
Academic Medical Center
University of Amsterdam
Amsterdam
The Netherlands

P. Cortelli, MD
Neurological Section
University of Modena and Reggio Emilia
Bologna
Italy

F. Croci, MD
Department of Cardiology and Arrhythmologic Center
Lavagna
Italy

B. Daga Calejero, MD
Clinical University Hospital
Zaragoza
Spain

J.H.A. Dambrink, MD
Department of Medicine
Academic Medical Center
University of Amsterdam
Amsterdam
The Netherlands

A. Del Rosso, MD
Cardiology Division
Ospedale S. Pietro Igneo
Fucecchio
Italy

A. Destrée-Vonk, MD
Department of Pediatrics
Academic Medical Center
University of Amsterdam
Amsterdam
The Netherlands

L.S. Díaz de la Llera, MD
Department of Cardiology
Virgen del Rocío University Hospital
Seville
Spain

J.G. van Dijk, MD
Department of Neurology and Clinical Neurophysiology
Leiden University Medical Center
Leiden
The Netherlands

N. van Dijk, MD
Department of Medicine
Academic Medical Center
University of Amsterdam
Amsterdam
The Netherlands

P. Donateo, MD
Department of Cardiology and Arrhythmologic Center
Lavagna
Italy

J. Enero, MD
General Hospital
Albacete
Spain

F. Errázquin Sáenz de Tejada, MD
Department of Cardiology
Virgen del Rocío University Hospital
Seville
Spain

P. Fabiani, MD
Syncope Center
Nuovo S. Giovanni di Dio Hospital
Florence
Italy

L. Facila, MD
Cardiology Service
Clinical University Hospital
Valencia
Spain

J. Fedriani, MD
General Hospital
Albacete
Spain

M. Fernández Quero, MD
Department of Cardiology
Virgen del Rocío University Hospital
Seville
Spain

A. Ferrero, MD
Cardiology Service
Clinical University Hospital
Valencia
Spain

G. Foglia-Manzillo, MD
Department of Cardiology
Ospedale Valduce
Como
Italy

J.A. Fournier Andray, MD, PhD, FESC
Chief of Interventional Cardiology Unit
Virgen del Rocío University Hospital
Seville
Spain

F. Gaita, MD
Divisione di Cardiologia
Ospedale Civile di Asti
Asti
Italy

S. Galán, MD
Corporació Sanitària
Parc Taulí Hospital
Sabadell
Spain

A. García Alberola, MD
Virgen de la Arrixaca University Hospital
Murcia
Spain

L. García Riesco, MD
Department of Cardiology
Virgen del Rocío University Hospital
Seville
Spain

J. García Sacristán, MD
General Hospital
Albacete
Spain

F. Giada, MD
Department of Cardiovascular Diseases
Umberto I Hospital
Mestre-Venice
Italy

M. Gil, MD
Departments of Cardiology and Internal Medicine
Corporació Sanitària
Parc Taulí Hospital
Sabadell
Spain

C. Giustetto, MD
Divisione di Cardiologia
Ospedale Civile di Asti
Asti
Italy

M. Gnoatto, MD
La Paz University Hospital
Madrid
Spain

C. Golzio, MD
Geriatric and Cardiology Medicine Unit
University of Florence
Florence
Italy

S. Gómez Moreno, MD
Department of Cardiology
Virgen del Rocío University Hospital
Seville
Spain

M. González Vasserot, MD
La Paz University Hospital
Madrid
Spain

A. Guisado, MD
Department of Cardiology
Virgen del Rocío University Hospital
Seville
Spain

J.R. Gumà, MD
Departments of Cardiology and Internal Medicine
Corporació Sanitària
Parc Taulí Hospital
Sabadell
Spain

G. Gusi, MD
Departments of Cardiology and Internal Medicine
Corporació Sanitària
Parc Taulí Hospital
Sabadell
Spain

E. Gutierrez Ibáñez, MD
Clinical University Hospital
Zaragoza
Spain

J.R. Halliwill, PhD
Department of Human Physiology
University of Oregon
Eugene, Oregon
USA

M.P.M. Harms, MD
Department of Medicine
University Medical Center
Groningen
The Netherlands

D.L. Jardine, FRACP, PhD
Department of General Medicine
Christchurch Hospital
Christchurch
New Zealand

M. Juez López, MD
Department of Cardiovascular Diseases
Clinical University Hospital
Valencia
Spain

J.M. Karemaker, MD
Department of Physiology
Academic Medical Center
University of Amsterdam
Amsterdam
The Netherlands

R.K. Khurana, MD
Division of Neurology
Union Memorial Hospital
Baltimore, Maryland
USA

R.A.M. Kortz, MD
Department of Cardiology
Flevoziekenhuis
Almere
The Netherlands

C.T.P. Krediet, MD
Department of Medicine
Academic Medical Center
University of Amsterdam
Amsterdam
The Netherlands

C. Lafuente, MD
General Hospital
Albacete
Spain

E. Lage Gallé, MD
Department of Cardiology
Virgen del Rocío University Hospital
Seville
Spain

A. Landi, MD
Geriatric and Cardiology Medicine Unit
University of Florence
Florence
Italy

J.W.M. Lenders, MD, PhD
Professor of Medicines
Department of Medicine
Radboud University Nijmegen Medical Center
Nijmegen
The Netherlands

A.M. van Leeuwen, MD
Department of Medicine
Academic Medical Center
University of Amsterdam
Amsterdam
The Netherlands

J.J. van Lieshout, MD, PhD
Department of Medicine
Academic Medical Center
University of Amsterdam
Amsterdam
The Netherlands

M. Linzer, MD
Professor of Medicine
Section of General Internal Medicine
University of Wisconsin
Madison, Wisconsin
USA

A. Llácer Escorihuela, MD
Cardiology Service
Clinical University Hospital
Valencia
Spain

G. Lolli, MD
Unità Operativa di Cardiologia Interventistica
Azienda Ospedaliera S. Maria Nuova
Reggio Emilia
Italy

F. López Pardo, MD
Department of Cardiology
Virgen del Rocío University Hospital
Seville
Spain

R. Maggi, MD
Department of Cardiology and Arrhythmologic Center
Lavagna
Italy

N. Malin, MD
Unit of Geriatric and Cardiology Medicine
University of Florence, Florence
Italy

A. Maraviglia, MD
Geriatric and Cardiology Medicine Unit
University of Florence
Florence
Italy

J.D. Martínez Alday, MD
Cardiology Service
Cruces Hospital
Bilbao
Spain

A. Martínez Brotons, MD
Cardiology Service
Clinical University Hospital
Valencia
Spain

J. Martínez León, MD
Department of Cardiovascular Diseases
Clinical University Hospital
Valencia
Spain

A. Martínez Martínez, MD
Department of Cardiology
Virgen del Rocío University Hospital
Seville
Spain

A. Martínez Rubio, MD
Departments of Cardiology and Internal Medicine
Corporació Sanitària
Parc Taulí Hospital
Sabadell
Spain

I. Martín González, MD
Department of Cardiovascular Diseases
Clinical University Hospital
Valencia
Spain

G. Masotti, MD
Geriatric and Cardiology Medicine Unit
University of Florence
Florence
Italy

C. Menozzi, MD
Unità Operativa di Cardiologia Interventistica
Azienda Ospedaliera S. Maria Nuova
Reggio Emilia
Italy

J.L. Merino, MD
La Paz University Hospital
Madrid
Spain

V. Montagud Balaguer, MD
Dr Peset University Hospital
Valencia
Spain

S. Morell Cabedo, MD
Cardiology Service
Clinical University Hospital
Valencia
Spain

J.I. Muñoz, MD
Department of Pediatrics
Clinical University Hospital
Valencia
Spain

J. Nicolás, MD
Cardiology Service
Beltvitge University Hospital
Barcelona
Spain

F. Nuñez, MD
Department of Pediatrics
Clinical University Hospital
Valencia
Spain

D. Oddone, MD
Department of Cardiology and Arrhythmologic Center
Lavagna
Italy

J.M. Ormaetxe, MD
Cardiology Service
Hospital de Basurto
Bilbao
Spain

M.D. Orriach, MD
Dr Peset University Hospital
Valencia
Spain

R.F.E. Pedretti, MD
Department of Cardiology
IRCCS Fondazione Salvatore Maugeri
Tradate
Italy

A. Pedrote Martínez, MD
Department of Cardiology
Virgen del Rocío University Hospital
Seville
Spain

R. Peinado, MD
La Paz University Hospital
Madrid
Spain

A. Peláez González, MD
Dr Peset University Hospital
Valencia
Spain

J. Pelegrín Díaz, MD
Clinical University Hospital
Zaragoza
Spain

E. Puggioni, MD
Department of Cardiology and Arrhythmologic Center
Lavagna
Italy

F. Quartieri, MD
Unità Operativa di Cardiologia Interventistica
Azienda Ospedaliera S. Maria Nuova
Reggio Emilia
Italy

A. Raviele, MD
Department of Cardiovascular Diseases
Umberto I Hospital
Mestre-Venice
Italy

C.A. Remme, MD
Department of Experimental Cardiology
Academic Medical Center
University of Amsterdam
Amsterdam
The Netherlands

G. Rodrigo Trallero, MD
Clinical University Hospital
Zaragoza
Spain

M.J. Rodríguez Puras, MD
Department of Cardiology
Virgen del Rocío University Hospital
Seville
Spain

N. Romero, MD
Department of Cardiology
Virgen del Rocío University Hospital
Seville
Spain

A. Roselló, MD
Cardiology Service
Clinical University Hospital
Valencia
Spain

X. Sabaté, MD
Cardiology Service
Beltvitge University Hospital
Barcelona
Spain

R. Sáez, MD
Cardiology Service
Cruces Hospital
Bilbao
Spain

J. Sagristá, MD
Cardiology Service
Vall d'Hebron General University Hospital
Barcelona
Spain

M. Sala, MD
Departments of Cardiology and Internal Medicine
Corporació Sanitària
Parc Taulí Hospital
Sabadell
Spain

A. Salvador Sanz, MD
Dr Peset University Hospital
Valencia
Spain

A. Sánchez González, MD
Department of Cardiology
Virgen del Rocío University Hospital
Seville
Spain

A. Sánchez Val, MD
Clinical University Hospital
Zaragoza
Spain

R. Sanjuán Mañez, MD
Intensive Care Unit
Clinical University Hospital
Valencia
Spain

M. Santarone, MD
Cardiology Department
Ospedale Valduce
Como
Italy

S. Sarzi Braga, MD
Department of Cardiology
IRCCS Fondazione Salvatore Maugeri
Tradate
Italy

F. Segura, MD
Departments of Cardiology and Internal Medicine
Corporació Sanitària
Parc Taulí Hospital
Sabadell
Spain

T.A. Simmers, MD
Amphia Hospital
Breda
The Netherlands

A. Solano, MD
Department of Cardiology and Arrhythmologic Center
Lavagna
Italy

H.J.L.M. Timmers, MD
Department of Medicine
Radboud University Nijmegen Medical Center
Nijmegen
The Netherlands

P. Tornos, MD
Cardiology Service
Vall d'Hebron General University Hospital
Barcelona
Spain

M.T. Tuzón Segarra, MD
Dr Peset University Hospital
Valencia
Spain

A. Ungar, MD
Geriatric and Cardiology Medicine Unit
University of Florence
Florence
Italy

B. Vaquerizo, MD
Dr Peset University Hospital
Valencia
Spain

S.C.J.M. Velzeboer, MD
Department of Medicine
Academic Medical Center
University of Amsterdam
Amsterdam
The Netherlands

M. Villa Gil-Ortega, MD
Department of Cardiology
Virgen del Rocío University Hospital
Seville
Spain

A.G.R. Visman, MD
Department of Cardiology
Beatrix Hospital
Gorinchem
The Netherlands

A.A.M. Wilde, MD
Professor of Cardiology
Department of Cardiology
Academic Medical Center
University of Amsterdam
Amsterdam
The Netherlands

Foreword

Syncope is one of the most common causes of transient loss of consciousness. Whatever its cause, syncope is a frightening experience and one that usually triggers a demand for prompt medical evaluation. In this setting, patients and their families are often quite alarmed, and seek help in order both to understand what has happened and to take steps to prevent recurrences. They are particularly worried about the implications of such spells for future health and economic well-being. Unfortunately, however, physicians often feel inadequately prepared to deal effectively with these concerns. They tend to be especially uncertain about whether they have investigated the problem properly, whether their diagnosis is accurate, and whether their advice is appropriate and up-to-date.

In terms of its relationship to the broad array of causes of transient loss of consciousness (TLOC), syncope encompasses those conditions in which loss of consciousness is caused by a period of self-limited inadequacy of cerebral perfusion (most often the result of a transient drop in blood pressure). It is this distinctive pathophysiology that distinguishes syncope from other disturbances of global cerebral dysfunction, such as:

- Epilepsy, in which TLOC is due to a primary electrical abnormality of the brain.
- Concussion, in which TLOC is due to cranial trauma.
- Intoxication, in which the reversible disturbance of consciousness has a toxic etiology.
- Psychogenic pseudosyncope (formerly erroneously termed "psychogenic syncope"), which is a condition of psychiatric origin in which TLOC does not really occur.

Given the frequency with which syncope occurs (estimated at 1–3% of all emergency department visits) and its potential for critical clinical implications (e.g., physical injury, driving restriction, loss of occupation, premature loss of independent living status), the development and fostering of a better understanding of strategies for optimal management of patients who have presumably suffered a syncope event is crucial. In recognition of this need, considerable recent attention has been directed toward identifying the most effective diagnostic techniques and treatments for patients with suspected syncope (e.g., the European Society of Cardiology Syncope Task Force clinical guidelines, published in 2001 and updated in 2004).

This volume, edited by seven prominent authorities on the management of syncope from four different countries and with 130 other contributors, provides a unique additional step in fostering a better understanding of the many factors that can cause syncope in humans, with the ultimate goal of facilitating the provision of more precise and cost-effective care for syncope patients.

In contrast to the somewhat tedious approach taken by most traditional textbooks and guideline statements, the authors of this volume have used a lively and easy-to-read case-study format—a teaching strategy with which medical practitioners are both comfortable and familiar. In essence, the reader encounters an array of realistic clinical scenarios, each described succinctly with pertinent illustrations. Examples of almost every cause of syncope are provided, ranging from various forms of neurally mediated reflex faints to both common and uncommon conditions known to be associated with real or seemingly real syncope events.

The uniform style of the case presentations is particularly pleasing, fostering easy reading and clarity of delivery. For good measure, appended to each case is a brief, focused, and expert editorial commentary. The latter feature is a novel one, providing the reader with a broader and easily understood context for the case as well as carefully selected pertinent citations from the literature.

The contributors to this volume represent a wide range of expertise from many different countries. All are experienced clinicians, and many are internationally recognized authorities in the evaluation and treatment of syncope. Cardiovascular medicine and physiology, internal medicine, and neuroscience and autonomic control are well represented. The result is a compendium of case studies suited to clinicians of all levels of experience and various specialties. The advanced trainee will find here a clinical experience that is otherwise unobtainable in one place; even many years of clinical practice would be insufficient. Similarly, family physicians, emergency-room doctors, and specialists in internal medicine, pediatrics, cardiology, and neurology will find the case studies to be enjoyable to read, enlightening, and immediately pertinent to improving their care of often very worrisome patients.

This volume is a valuable contribution to further education in this field. It is a contribution that should be widely read, and one that offers the possibility of markedly enhancing medical care for the syncope patient.

David G. Benditt, MD, FRCP(C), FACC, FHRS
Cardiac Arrhythmia Center, University of Minnesota Medical School
Minneapolis, Minnesota

Abbreviations

Terms for electrocardiographic deflections and patterns, and pacemaker codes, are not included.

ACC American College of Cardiology
ACE angiotensin-converting enzyme
AF atrial fibrillation
AICD automatic implantable cardioverter-defibrillator
AMI acute myocardial infarction
ARVC arrhythmogenic right ventricular cardiomyopathy
ARVD arrhythmogenic right ventricular dysplasia
ATP adenosine triphosphate
AV atrioventricular
AVB atrioventricular block
AVNRT atrioventricular nodal reentry tachycardia
BBB bundle-branch block
BBR VT bundle-branch reentry ventricular tachycardia
cAMP cyclic adenosine monophosphate
CI cardiac index
CKMB creatine kinase, myocardial-bound
CPVT catecholaminergic polymorphic ventricular tachycardia
CSH carotid sinus hypersensitivity
CSM carotid sinus massage
CSS carotid sinus syndrome
CT computed tomography
DC direct current
EAD early afterdepolarization
ECG electrocardiogram, electrocardiography
EEG electroencephalogram, electroencephalography
EPS electrophysiological study
HCM hypertrophic cardiomyopathy
5-HIAA 5-hydroxyindoleacetic acid
HIV human immunodeficiency virus
HUT head-up tilt (test)
ICD implantable cardioverter-defibrillator
ICOPER International Cooperative Pulmonary Embolism Registry
ICU intensive-care unit; intensive coronary unit
ILR implantable loop recorder
^{123}I-MIBG ^{123}iodinated metaiodobenzylguanidine
IRAD International Registry of Aortic Dissection
ISSUE International Study of Syncope of Uncertain Etiology
LASIK laser *in-situ* keratomileusis
LBBB left bundle-branch block
LQTS long QT syndrome
LVEF left ventricular ejection fraction
MD myotonic dystrophy
MRI magnetic resonance imaging
NIDCM nonischemic dilated cardiomyopathy
NYHA New York Heart Association (classification)
OCR oculocardiac reflex
PE pulmonary embolism
PEH post-exercise hypotension
POTS postural orthostatic tachycardia syndrome
PRA plasma renin activity
QSART quantitative sudomotor axon reflex test
RBBB right bundle-branch block
SI systolic index
SNRT sinus node recovery time
TdP *torsade de pointes*
TIMI Thrombolysis in Myocardial Infarction (classification)
TPRI total peripheral resistance index
TST thermoregulatory sweat test
VASIS Vasovagal Syncope International Study (classification)
VF ventricular fibrillation
VPS Vasovagal Pacemaker Study
VT ventricular tachycardia

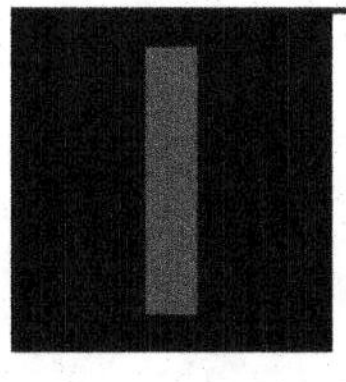

PART I
Neurally mediated (reflex) syncope

Clinical presentation

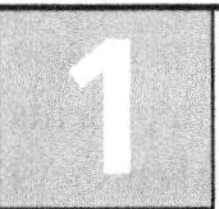

CASE 1
Vasovagal fainting in children and teenagers

W. Wieling

Case report

A 14-year-old boy was referred to our syncope unit for analysis of an unexplained episode of transient loss of consciousness. The episode occurred while the boy had been standing still after running during a soccer competition game. The patient denied experiencing any prodromal symptoms. The duration of the loss of consciousness was short (< 1 min).

Table 1.1 Classification of reflex syncope based on triggers.

Reflex-mediated
Vasovagal syncope
• Emotionally induced—e.g., venipunctures, immunizations, sight of blood) (central type)
• Orthostatically induced (peripheral type)
Ocular syncope
Gastrointestinal
• Swallow syncope
• Esophageal stimulation
• Gastrointestinal tract instrumentation
• Rectal/vaginal examination
• Defecation syncope
Urogenital
• (Post-)micturition syncope
• Urogenital tract instrumentation
• Pulmonary airway instrumentation
Mechanical/hydraulic factors
Initial orthostatic hypotension
Increased intrathoracic pressure: cough and sneeze syncope
• Wind instrument player's syncope
• Weight lifter's syncope
• Mess trick and fainting lark
• Stretch syncope

The patient's general health was excellent. Evaluations by two pediatricians, a pediatric cardiologist and a pediatric neurologist, including several electrocardiograms, an echocardiogram, a 24-h Holter recording, an exercise test, and blood examinations, were unremarkable. The patient was advised to refrain from playing soccer.

Additional history-taking revealed that three additional episodes of transient loss of consciousness had occurred—one while he had been standing still on a warm day during a vacation with his parents in Paris while a street artist was making a drawing of him. The other episodes also occurred when he was standing motionless while a friend of his mother was giving him a haircut. During these episodes, he was reported to be pale and sweating. Nausea was present during one of the episodes.

On the basis of this history, reflex vasovagal syncope was diagnosed. The mechanisms underlying the episodes were explained to the patient and his parents. The young patient and his parents were reassured and informed about lifestyle measures. The boy started to play soccer again, and no further syncopal episodes occurred.

Comment

By far the most common cause of transient loss of consciousness in young patients is a reflex syncopal event, particularly vasovagal fainting [1,2]. A variety of triggers have been identified (Table 1.1).

Two clinical scenarios in particular are known to provoke vasovagal fainting in young patients. First and foremost are situations that increase the pooling of venous blood below the heart, such as long periods

Table 1.2 Typical premonitory symptoms for reflex syncope.

- Lightheadedness, dizziness
- Palpitations
- Weakness
- Dimming or blurred vision
- Fading hearing, tinnitus
- Nausea, epigastric distress
- Feeling warm or cold
- Facial pallor
- Sweating, dilated pupils

of standing motionless, particularly in combination with elevated ambient temperatures. Young patients often experience prodromal signs and symptoms when a spontaneous vasovagal syncope is imminent (Table 1.2) [1,2]. These prodromes are reported to be more intense than those in elderly patients, perhaps related to more robust autonomic control. However, some young patients have little or no prodromal symptoms or do not recognize them, as during the first episode in this patient. The collapse occurs without warning. The second scenario is syncope at the time of distressing emotional situations or pain, which also appears to be more common in the young. A typical example is an event when a blood sample is being taken. Other emotional triggers reported in young patients include having the hair cut or brushed (as in this case), eye examinations or manipulation, dental procedures, or watching television programs about medical matters or animal biology [1–4].

The clinical presentation of vasovagal syncope may vary widely both within and among young patients [1,2]. The trigger may be emotional for one event and postural for another. Vasovagal episodes may also occur without an identifiable trigger, even in patients who are sitting. Apparently benign vasovagal episodes may also occur during normal daily exercises such as playing, walking, or cycling and even during strenuous exercise. However, when syncope occurs during exercise, a cardiac cause such as a long QT syndrome or catecholaminergic ventricular tachycardia should always be excluded [1,2].

It is important to consider all episodes and not just one unexplained event. When there is a history of typical vasovagal syncope for some of the episodes, the atypical presentations are very likely to be of vasovagal origin as well [1,2]. Events that occur when the patient is supine, in the absence of an emotional stimulus, are unlikely to be vasovagal, but vasovagal syncope during sleep has been described [5]. Additional reflex syncopal events that are typical of young patients include initial orthostatic hypotension (see Case 42), adolescent stretch syncope [6], postural tachycardia syndrome, and the fainting lark (see Case 45). "Stretch" syncope may occur during stretching with the neck hyperextended while standing. It is reported to occur in teenage boys with a familial tendency to faint. It has been attributed to the effects of straining (which decreases systemic blood pressure) in combination with decreased cerebral blood flow caused by mechanical compression of the vertebral arteries [6].

The incidence of syncope coming to medical attention appears to be clearly increased in two age groups—the young and the old (Fig. 1.1) [1,7].

A peak in the incidence occurs around the age of 15 years, with girls having more than twice the incidence among boys [8].

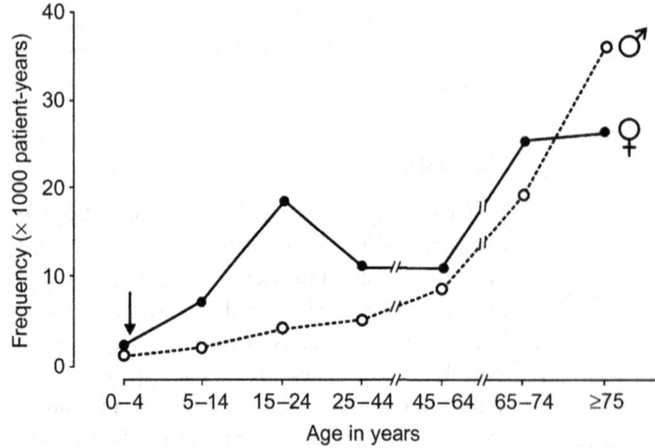

Figure 1.1 Frequency of the symptom of fainting as the reason for presentation in general practices in the Netherlands. The data are drawn from the General Practitioners' Transition Project, which includes an analysis of 93 297 patient-years. The arrow around 1 year is to indicate that a small peak occurs between 6 and 18 months (breath-holding spells). (Reproduced with permission from [11].)

Syncope is an infrequent occurrence in adults. The incidence of syncope progressively increases over the age of about 40 years to become high in the older age groups. A lower peak occurs in older infants and toddlers, most commonly referred to as "breath-holding spells" [2].

The incidence of syncope in young patients coming to medical attention varies from approximately 0.5 to three cases per 1000 (0.05–0.3%) [9]. Syncopal events that do not reach medical attention occur much more frequently. In fact, the recently published results of a survey of students with an average age of 20 demonstrated that about 20% of the men and 50% of the women reported having experienced at least one syncopal episode [8]. By comparison, the prevalence of epileptic seizures in a similar age group is approximately five per 1000 (0.5%) [10], and cardiac syncope (i.e., cardiac arrhythmias or structural heart disease) is much less common [1,7].

References

1 Wieling W, Ganzeboom KS, Saul JP. Reflex syncope in children and adolescents. *Heart* 2004; **90**: 1094–9.

2 Stephenson JBP, McLeod KA. Reflex anoxic seizures. In: David TJ, ed. *Recent Advances in Pediatrics*. Churchill Livingstone, Edinburgh, 2000: 18.

3 Lewis DW, Frank LM. Hair-grooming syncope seizures. *Pediatrics* 1993; **91**: 836–8.

4 Hall DM. Non-epileptic television syncope. *Br Med J* 1978; **ii**: 205.

5 Krediet CT, Jardine DL, Cortelli P, Visman AG, Wieling W. Vasovagal syncope interrupting sleep? *Heart* 2004; **90**: e25.

6 Pelekanos JT, Dooley JM, Camfield PR, Finley J. Stretch syncope in adolescence. *Neurology* 1990; **40**: 705–7.

7 Colman N, Nahm K, Ganzeboom KS, *et al.* Epidemiology of reflex syncope. *Clin Auton Res* 2004; **14** (Suppl 1): 9–17.

8 Ganzeboom KS, Colman N, Reitsma JB, Shen WK, Wieling W. Prevalence and triggers of syncope in medical students. *Am J Cardiol* 2003; **91**: 1006–8.

9 Driscoll DJ, Jacobsen SJ, Porter CJ, Wollan PC. Syncope in children and adolescents. *J Am Coll Cardiol* 1997; **29**: 1039–45.

10 Wallace H, Shorvon S, Tallis R. Age-specific incidence and prevalence rates of treated epilepsy in an unselected population of 2 052 922 and age-specific fertility rates of women with epilepsy. *Lancet* 1998; **352**: 1970–3.

11 Wieling W, Ganzeboom KS, Krediet CTP, Grundmeijer HGLM, Wilde AA, van Dijk JG [Initial diagnostic strategy in the case of transient loss of consciousness: the importance of the medical history] *Ned Tijdschr Geneesk* 2003; **147**: 849–54.

2

CASE 2

Typical vasovagal syncope (blood/injury phobia)

R. García Civera, R. Ruiz Granell, S. Morell Cabedo, A. Llácer Escorihuela

Case report

A 27-year-old man attended the outpatient clinic due to a history of recurrent episodes of syncope and presyncope since the age of 7. All of the episodes had been triggered by seeing blood or by being given an injection. The patient had a normal physical examination and a normal electrocardiogram (ECG) (Fig. 2.1).

The patient's ECG was monitored continuously while venous blood was being taken (for analytical purposes) while he was in the recumbent position. A syncopal episode developed during the blood sampling, and the sequence of electrocardiographic events was as follows (Fig. 2.1):

1 When the patient saw the needle, there was a slight increase in the sinus heart rate.

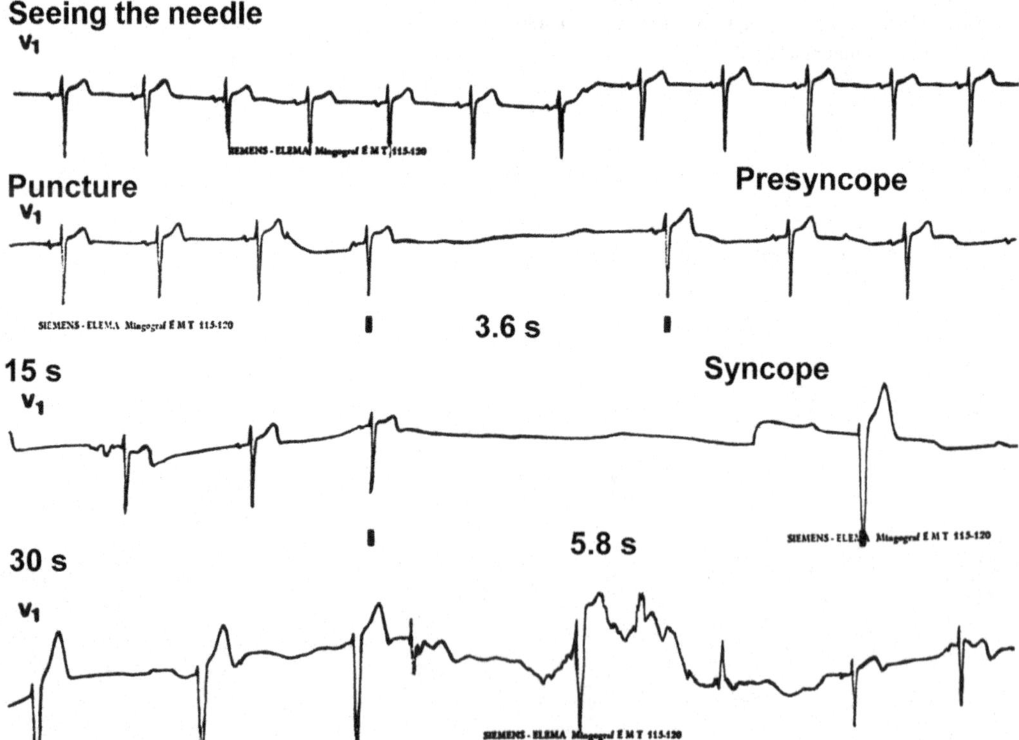

Figure 2.1 Electrocardiogram during blood sampling.

2 During the puncture procedure, sinus bradycardia progressing to a sinus pause of 3.6 s was observed. The patient was pale and complained of gastrointestinal discomfort and blurring vision.
3 Fifteen seconds after the puncture, the patient lost consciousness, coinciding with a sinus pause of 5.8 s that resolved with a ventricular escape beat, followed by a ventricular escape rhythm.
4 Unconsciousness lasted 15 s, with a bradycardic sinus rhythm during recovery.

Comment

This is a typical case of vasovagal syncope in a patient with blood/injury phobia. A phobia is defined as a marked and persistent fear of clearly discernible, circumscribed objects or situations. In the specific blood/injury phobia, the fear can be triggered by seeing blood, by an injury, by being given an injection, or by other invasive medical procedures [1]. Characteristically, the phobic response in these cases is manifested by syncope or presyncope [2].

In the classical description of the vasovagal syncope, Lewis considered emotional stress, pain, seeing blood, and several medical procedures as representing typical triggers [3]. When these triggers are present, the diagnosis of vasovagal syncope is made and no further clinical investigations are required.

Accurso *et al.* [4] carried out tilt-table tests on a group of patients with typical blood/injury phobia and on a control group. During tilting, 82% of the blood-phobic patients and 9% of the control individuals experienced syncope or presyncope ($P = 0.001$). The authors concluded that patients with syncope related to blood/injury phobia have an underlying autonomic dysregulation predisposing them to neurally mediated syncope, even in the absence of any blood or injury stimulus.

The management of patients with blood/injury phobia is complex. The most useful measure is of course to avoid the triggers, but this is not always possible. Several psychosomatic and biofeedback techniques have been proposed for the treatment of these patients [5,6].

References

1 American Psychiatric Association. Specific phobia. In: American Psychiatric Association Task Force on DSM-IV, eds. *Diagnostic and Statistical Manual for Mental Disorders: DSM-IV*, 4th ed. American Psychiatric Association, Washington DC, 1994: 403–11.
2 Thyer BA, Himle J, Curtis GC. Blood–injury–illness phobia: a review. *J Clin Psychol* 1985; **41**: 451–9.
3 Lewis T. Vasovagal syncope and the carotid sinus mechanism. *Br Med J* 1932; **i**: 873–6.
4 Accurso V, Winnicki M, Shamsuzzaman AS, Wenzel A, Johnson AK, Somers VK. Predisposition to vasovagal syncope in subjects with blood/injury phobia. *Circulation* 2001; **104**: 903–7.
5 Kozak M, Montgomery G. Behavioural treatment of recurrent injury-scene-elicited fainting. *Behav Psychother* 1981; **3**: 316–21.
6 Van Dijk N, Velzeboer SC, Destrée-Vonk A, Linzer M, Wieling W. Psychological treatment of malignant vasovagal syncope due to blood phobia. *Pacing Clin Electrophysiol* 2001; **24**: 122–4.

3

CASE 3

Reflex syncope in older adults

W. Wieling

Case report

A 62-year-old woman lawyer was referred by her general practitioner to the emergency department at our hospital after a fall resulting in a head wound [1]. On the day of the fall, she was up early and was having breakfast standing in the kitchen. The next thing she could remember was that she was on the floor bleeding from a head wound. She knew where she was and was able to stand up easily. However, in the standing position she passed out again. On regaining consciousness, she contacted her general practitioner and was transported by ambulance to the hospital. In the emergency department, no obvious explanation for the loss of consciousness could be found. The physical examination showed a head wound. The electrocardiogram (ECG) was normal. The patient told the attending physician that at the age of 30 she had been evaluated by a neurologist due to "dizziness" and headaches. Because of abnormalities on electroencephalography (EEG) suggesting epilepsy, she had been treated with phenytoin for several years.

The patient was admitted to the neurology department. An EEG showed irregularities over the temporal lobe. Phenytoin was restarted. However, the diagnosis of epilepsy was revised because of the rapid reorientation on regaining consciousness. The patient was discharged and referred to the cardiology outpatient department. Echocardiography, a 24-h Holter recording, and exercise testing were normal, and the patient was referred to the syncope unit. Additional history-taking revealed numerous fainting episodes in her youth, triggered by blood sampling and visits to the dentist. Standing in line for prolonged periods and hot showers were also triggers for fainting. Because of her fainting tendency, she had decided not to pursue a medical career. A week before the last episode of loss of consciousness, she had returned from a tiring journey in India, where she had suffered from episodes of diarrhea. Back home, she was still suffering from the long journey and the jet lag. She had hardly slept the night before the fall. The clinical diagnosis that a vasovagal faint was a very likely cause of the loss of consciousness was confirmed by a positive tilt-table test [1].

Comment

Epilepsy was considered in this patient because she had been treated previously with anti-epileptics and had sustained a head wound. In addition, the EEG showed abnormalities. A diagnosis of a vasovagal faint was not considered, since an obvious trigger and prodromal symptoms for fainting were lacking. However, it is important to realize that the clinical presentation of reflex syncope changes with age [2]. Reflex syncope during distressing emotional situations or pain is less common in the elderly, whereas situational and vasovagal orthostatic syncopes (micturition, defecation, cough syncope, etc.) are more common in the elderly. Classical carotid sinus syndrome only occurs in older patients [2]. It is not unusual for an older patient to experience atypical episodes of vasovagal syncope after the patient has suffered from typical vasovagal syncope at a younger age [3–5]. A history of syncope for many years (often decades), as in this patient, is typical in reflex syncope and helpful in establishing a likely cause of syncope [2].

A complete lack of warning symptoms is reported by some patients during apparent vasovagal episodes in daily life, but is rare during tilt-table testing [6]. The discrepancy may be accounted for by patients' unfamiliarity with subtle prodromal symptoms and perhaps a tendency to ignore these symptoms when engaged in other activities. Prodromal symptoms are less frequently reported by older patients, possibly due to greater susceptibility to retrograde amnesia, a lesser degree of autonomic activation, or less sensitivity to the sometimes subtle symptoms [2,4,5,7].

Orthostatic and postprandial hypotension and cardiac causes of syncope are more frequent in the elderly. This can be attributed to diminished efficiency of cardiovascular regulatory systems, the effects of multiple medications predisposing to syncope, and increased prevalence of organic disease (structural heart disease, cardiac arrhythmias, carotid sinus syndrome). Multiple potential coexisting causes of syncope are often present in the elderly, and the medical history may be less reliable than in the young. For example, syncope may be reported as a fall [8].

Acknowledgment

Parts of this case were previously published in Colman *et al.* [1]. We are grateful to the *Nederlands Tijdschrift voor Geneeskunde* for granting permission to reprint.

References

1 Colman N, Vermeulen M, Wieling W. [A patient with an unexplained loss of consciousness: a case for the neurologist or the cardiologist? In Dutch.] *Ned Tijdschr Geneeskd* 2003; **147**: 841–3.

2 Colman N, Nahm K, van Dijk JG, Reitsma JB, Wieling W, Kaufmann H. Diagnostic value of history taking in reflex syncope. *Clin Auton Res* 2004; **14** (Suppl 1): 37–44.

3 Cosin Aguilar J, Solaz Minguez J, García-Civera R, Ruíz Granell R. Epidemiologia del sincope. In: García-Civera R, Sanjuan Manez R, Cosin Aguilar J, Lopez Merino V, eds. *Sincope*. Editorial MCR, Barcelona, 1989: 53–71.

4 Fitzpatrick A, Sutton R. Tilting towards a diagnosis in recurrent unexplained syncope. *Lancet* 1989; **333**: 658–660.

5 Sutton R, Petersen ME. The clinical spectrum of neurocardiogenic syncope. *J Cardiovasc Electrophysiol* 1995; **6**: 569–76.

6 Alboni P, Dinelli M, Gruppillo P, *et al.* Hemodynamic changes early in prodromal symptoms of vasovagal syncope. *Europace* 2002; **4**: 333–8.

7 Benke T, Hochleitner M, Bauer G. Aura phenomena during syncope. *Eur Neurol* 1997; **37**: 28–32.

8 Colman N, Nahm K, van Dijk JG, Reitsma JB, Wieling W, Kaufmann H. Diagnostic value of history taking in reflex syncope. *Clin Auton Res* 2004; **14** (Suppl 1): 1/37–1/44.

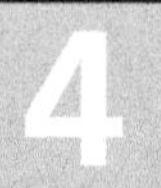

CASE 4

Transient loss of consciousness with muscle jerks: syncope or epilepsy?

W. Wieling, C.A. Remme, J.G. van Dijk

Case report

A 35-year-old otherwise healthy engineer was referred to the syncope unit for analysis of an episode of loss of consciousness, which had occurred during a return flight from a week-long holiday in Turkey. Before boarding the airplane at midnight, the patient felt tired and was continuously yawning without any other specific complaints. Once seated in the aircraft, he fell asleep almost immediately. After approximately 30 min of sleep, he retrieved an item from the overhead compartment without problems and quickly fell asleep again. About 1 h later, he woke up feeling weak and extremely thirsty, and decided to have a soft drink. The patient's partner, a cardiology resident, was woken by the sound of the drink can falling to the floor. She saw a tonic posture with the arms extended and the head and neck held backwards. The posture resembled the one people assume during stretching. After this, his arms jerked for about a minute, and he then became completely flaccid. His pulse was very slow and weak and he was breathing superficially. Before he could be transferred from his chair to the aisle, he regained consciousness. The duration of the period of unconsciousness was short (< 3 min). On regaining consciousness, he was well orientated but complained of tiredness, weakness and slowness in thinking and speech. There was no sign of urinary incontinence or tongue-biting. When he tried to stand up and walk a few steps, he collapsed again, with sensations of feeling very weak and inert, but without losing consciousness. After a few minutes, he was able to stand up and walk by himself. On examination, his pulse was approximately 40–45 beats/min (regular) with a blood pressure of 100/60 mmHg. He complained of muscle pain in his arms and shoulders, blurred vision, tiredness, and cold sweats. These symptoms gradually disappeared during the following 2 h after he had drunk three or four glasses of water with sugar. On arrival at the airport, he was checked by ambulance personnel and found to have a normal heart rate, blood pressure and blood glucose level. Physical and neurological examinations and electrocardiography (ECG) analysis at the Emergency Department of the Academic Medical Center in Amsterdam showed no abnormalities, and he was referred to the syncope unit.

The patient denied having had any earlier episodes of loss of consciousness. However, during visits to hospitals and while watching television programs with surgical scenes he had sometimes had a tendency to feel weak. He was not taking any medication. Based on the premonitory symptoms of feeling weak, prolonged motionless sitting, the documentation of a very slow and weak pulse during the episode, the tendency to faint again after regaining consciousness, and the previous sensations of near-faints during hospital encounters, a clinical diagnosis of vasovagal syncope was made. The patient was reassured. Specific instructions for future travel by airplane were given. Since the episode occurred, the patient has traveled by plane on several occasions without any problems.

Comment

The differential diagnosis in a patient with a transient loss of consciousness accompanied by muscle jerks includes an epileptic seizure and an episode of convulsive syncope. In the present case, the short duration of unconsciousness and rapid reorientation after regaining consciousness makes an epileptic seizure highly unlikely. An underlying cardiac abnormality is also unlikely, since the patient had no cardiac history and both the physical examination and the ECG were normal. This case report therefore points in the direction of convulsive vasovagal syncope. Vasovagal episodes are the most common in-flight medical events [1]. In addition to prolonged motionless sitting, mild hypoxia occurring during air travel may predispose towards syncope. The cabin pressure in commercial aircraft, usually adjusted to the equivalent of an altitude of 1500–2500 m above sea level, may be involved. Even mild hypoxia predisposes to vasovagal faints. It appears that hypoxic syncope results from the superimposed vasodilator effects of hypoxia on the cardiovascular system [2].

Jerky movements mimicking an epileptic seizure may occur during syncope. The circumstances determining whether they do or do not appear are not well known. In clinical practice, there is a clear tendency for jerks to appear following prolonged asystole of at least 10–14 s or a prolonged period of very low blood pressure. In the fainting lark, an experimentally induced syncope with a very abrupt cessation of cerebral perfusion (see Case 45), the jerky movements appeared almost as soon as the subject hit the ground. The "anoxic threshold" for myoclonic jerks is lower in children than in adults, and it is lowest in early childhood [3,4]. In contrast to clonic movements in epilepsy, jerks in syncope are usually not rhythmic, not synchronous in the extremities, and less coarse in comparison with those observed in epilepsy. In addition, in syncope the jerky movements never occur before falling, whereas in epilepsy they may occur before falling [5,6]. In a typical tonic–clonic epileptic seizure, however, the fall is due to the stiff tonic phase, and the clonic movements occur afterwards. The myoclonic activity is presumably due to a lack of inhibition from higher centers, but the site of origin remains unknown [5].

The prevalence of myoclonic jerks in patients with syncope is not well known. In a prospective study, Newman and Graves documented tetany, clonic movements, and twitching in 46% of 178 blood donors having a vasovagal reaction [7]. In the fainting lark, myoclonic jerks occurred in 90%. These vastly differing percentages suggest that the occurrence of jerky movements depends on the way in which hypoperfusion affects cerebral perfusion, but which factors are involved is unknown.

Urinary incontinence is uncommon in reflex syncope, but does occur, as does fecal incontinence. Incontinence cannot be used as a discriminating factor between epilepsy and syncope [8,9].

Typical symptoms and signs of epilepsy are tongue-biting, a cyanotic facial color and an aura. Benbadis *et al.* compared 34 patients with epileptic seizures to 45 syncopal patients. Eight patients with documented epileptic seizures suffered a lateral tongue bite. The tongue was lacerated in only one of 45 patients with syncope, and this was at the tip, suggesting that lateral tongue-biting is highly specific (99%) for the diagnosis of epileptic seizures [10]. Consistent turning of the head to one side is also reported as a specific sign for epilepsy [9], but lateral deviation of the head was also observed in experimental syncope induced by ocular compression [11]. Emotional stress has been reported as a precipitating factor for both reflex syncope and epilepsy [12,13], but, in syncope, emotional factors may provoke—and thus occur immediately prior to—fainting, whereas stress in epilepsy appears to have a less immediate effect, in the sense that seizures may occur during a longer period of stress. Important symptoms that distinguish between reflex syncope and epilepsy are the duration of the loss of consciousness and postictal confusion. In the recovery phase of an episode of syncope, there is usually little or no confusion [8,9]. Finally, circumstances such as prolonged standing and autonomic symptoms such as cold sweat and nausea make epilepsy unlikely as the cause for the event [7]. Epileptic seizures usually do not have a clear trigger. They occur more randomly—e.g., in the standing, sitting, or supine positions.

The sensitivity and specificity of data from the medical history are compared in Table 4.1.

References

1 Gendreau MA, DeJohn C. Responding to medical events during commercial airline flights. *N Engl J Med* 2002; **346**: 1067–73.

2 Halliwill JR, Minson CT. Cardiovascular regulation during combined hypoxic and orthostatic stress: fainters vs. nonfainters. *J Appl Physiol* 2005; **98**: 1050–6.

3 Stephenson JBP. *Fits and Faints.* Blackwell Scientific/MacKeith Press, Oxford, 1990.

4 Stephenson JBP, McLeod KA. Reflex anoxic seizures. In: David TJ, ed. *Recent Advances in Pediatrics.* Churchill Livingstone, Edinburgh, 2000: 18.

5 Gastaut H. Syncopes: generalized anoxic cerebral seizures.

Table 4.1 Diagnostic accuracy of specific items from the patient's history.

	Hoefnagels et al. *[8]*			*Sheldon* et al. *[9]*		
	Sensitivity	*Specificity*	*LR+*	*Sensitivity*	*Specificity*	*LR+*
Factors strongly suggesting epilepsy						
Tongue-biting	0.41	0.94	7.3	0.45	0.97	16.5
Turning of the head	NR	NR	NR	0.43	0.97	13.5
Muscle pain	0.39	0.85	2.6	0.16	0.95	3.4
Duration of loss of consciousness (> 5 min)	0.68	0.55	1.5	NR	NR	NR
Cyanosis	0.29	0.98	16.9	0.33	0.94	5.8
Postictal confusion	0.85	0.83	5.0	0.94	0.69	3.0
Factors strongly suggesting syncope						
Prolonged sitting or standing	NR	NR	NR	0.40	0.98	20.4
Sweating prior to loss of consciousness	0.36	0.98	18.0	0.35	0.94	5.9
Nausea	0.28	0.98	14.0	0.28	0.94	4.7
History of presyncope	NR	NR	NR	0.73	0.73	2.6
Paleness	0.81	0.66	2.8	NR	NR	NR

LR+, likelihood ratio of a positive test result; NR, not reported.

In: Magnus O, de Haas AML, eds. *Handbook of Clinical Neurology*, vol. 15: *The Epilepsies*. North-Holland, Amsterdam, 1974: 815–36.

6 Lempert T, Bauer M, Schmidt D. Syncope: a videometric analysis of 56 episodes of transient cerebral hypoxia. *Ann Neurol* 1994; **36**: 233–237.

7 Newman BH, Graves S. A study of 178 consecutive vasovagal syncopal reactions from the perspective of safety. *Transfusion* 2001; **41**: 1475–9.

8 Hoefnagels WA, Padberg GW, Overweg J, van der Velde EA, Roos RA. Transient loss of consciousness: the value of the history for distinguishing seizure from syncope. *J Neurol* 1991; **238**: 39–43.

9 Sheldon R, Rose S, Ritchie D, *et al.* Historical criteria that distinguish syncope from seizures. *J Am Coll Cardiol* 2002; **40**: 142–8.

10 Benbadis SR, Wolgamuth BR, Goren H, Brener S, Fouad-Tarazi F. Value of tongue biting in the diagnosis of seizures. *Arch Intern Med* 1995; **155**: 2346–9.

11 Gastaut H, Fischer-Williams M. Electro-encephalographic study of syncope: its difference from epilepsy. *Lancet* 1957; **ii**: 1018–25.

12 Friis ML, Lund M. Stress convulsions. *Arch Neurol* 1974; **31**: 155–9.

13 Van Lieshout JJ, Wieling W, Karemaker JM, Eckberg DL. The vasovagal response. *Clin Sci (Lond)* 1991; **81**: 575–586.

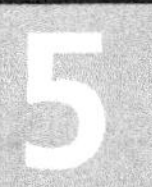

CASE 5
Tilt-induced syncope: mixed response

A. Moya i Mitjans, C. Alonso

Case report

A 64-year-old patient was sent for evaluation due to syncopal episodes. He reported having had several syncopal episodes during his youth, between the ages of 15 and 25. All of the episodes had occurred when he was in the standing position, and he had never had injury, seizure, or urinary incontinence. Afterwards, he had remained asymptomatic for several years.

Six months and 2 months previously, he had suffered two new syncopal episodes. He was in the standing position, there were no clear triggers, and he described the episode as being sudden and without any prodromal symptoms being recognized. There had been no witnesses during the two episodes, but the patient did not suffer any injuries or urinary incontinence.

The baseline physical examination was normal, there were no cardiac murmurs, and his arterial blood pressure was within the normal limits in the supine position as well as after resuming the standing position. The electrocardiogram (ECG) (Fig. 5.1) and chest radiograph were also normal. Because of the patient's age, echocardiography was carried out, but it did not show any abnormalities either.

A tilting test was indicated. The protocol was carried out without intravenous cannulation, and after 5 min in the supine position, the patient was tilted up to 60° for 20 min, without drugs (Fig. 5.2). There were no symptoms during this period, and the heart rate and arterial blood pressure were stable. After this, 400 μg of sublingual nitroglycerin was administered (Fig. 5.3). After nitroglycerin administration, the patient showed a transient sinus tachycardia followed by a rapid drop in heart rate to 58 beats/min and a fall in arterial blood pressure to 50 mmHg, with minimal prodromal symptoms, followed by loss of consciousness with seizures and recovery after he was placed in the Trendelenburg position (Fig. 5.4).

After recovery, the patient was asked if the induced episode reproduced the spontaneous symptoms, and he stated that the two episodes were similar, recognizing that minimal prodromic signs had been present in the spontaneous syncope.

The test was completed, and a diagnosis of neuromediated syncope with mixed response was made—type 1 in the Vasovagal Syncope International Study (VASIS) classification. The benign nature of the syncopal episodes was explained to the patient, and he was advised to increase water ingestion as well as to avoid long periods in the standing position.

Comment

This case illustrates a patient with a long-standing history of syncopal episodes that occurred with a biphasic presentation. The patient had had several syncopal episodes when he was young, and thereafter remained asymptomatic for several years until he had two further syncopal episodes. The episodes were relatively sudden, without typical triggers, although characteristically they both occurred when he was in the standing position, and the patient denied noticing any prodromal symptoms.

Since the baseline physical examination, ECG and echocardiogram were normal, it was considered that a cardiac etiology for syncope was unlikely. However, as the patient could not be diagnosed as having neuromediated syncope at the initial evaluation [1], due to the lack of triggers and typical prodromal symptoms, a tilt test was indicated. The patient was tilted up to 60°,

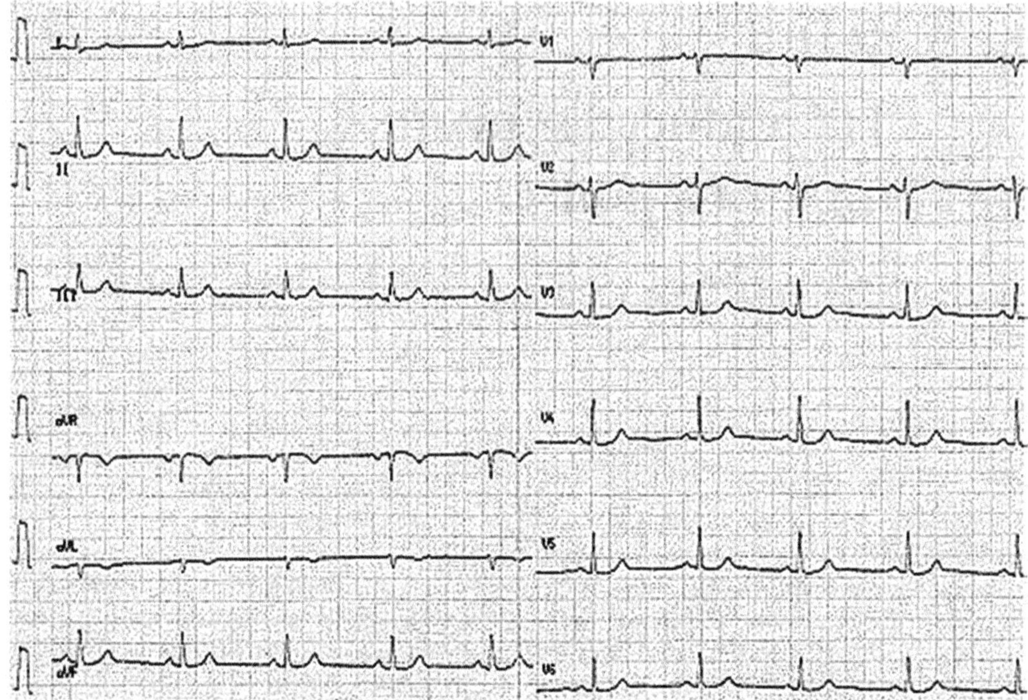

Figure 5.1 The baseline electrocardiogram, showing a normal sinus rhythm, with a PR interval of 180 ms, a normal QRS configuration and no abnormalities in the QRS complex.

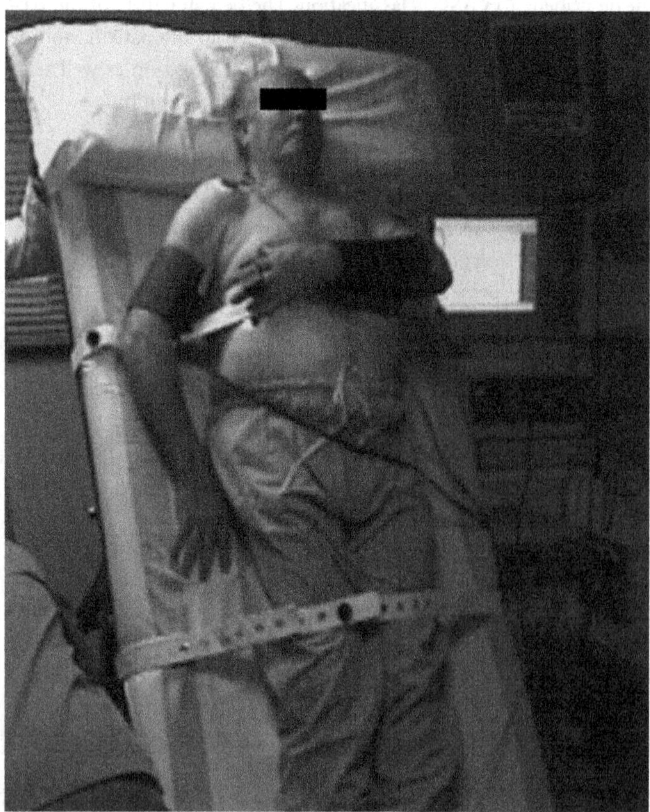

Figure 5.2 The patient was passively tilted up to 60°, with electrocardiographic monitoring as well as noninvasive arterial blood pressure measurement, in this case using the Task Force Monitor from CNSystems Medizintechnik Ltd. (Graz, Austria).

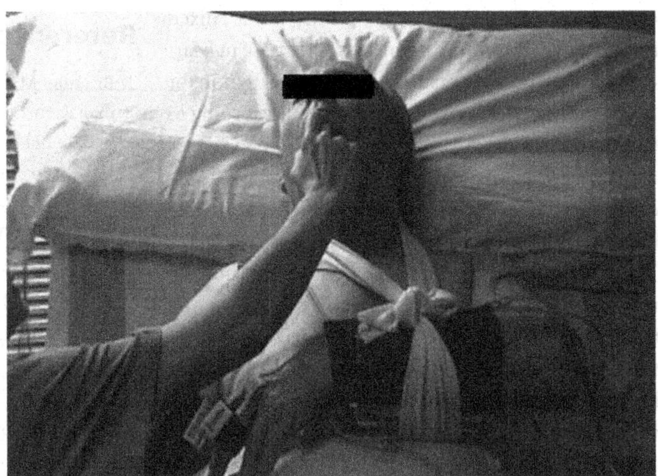

Figure 5.3 After an initial drug-free phase, 400 μg of sublingual nitroglycerin was administered, without returning the patient to the supine position.

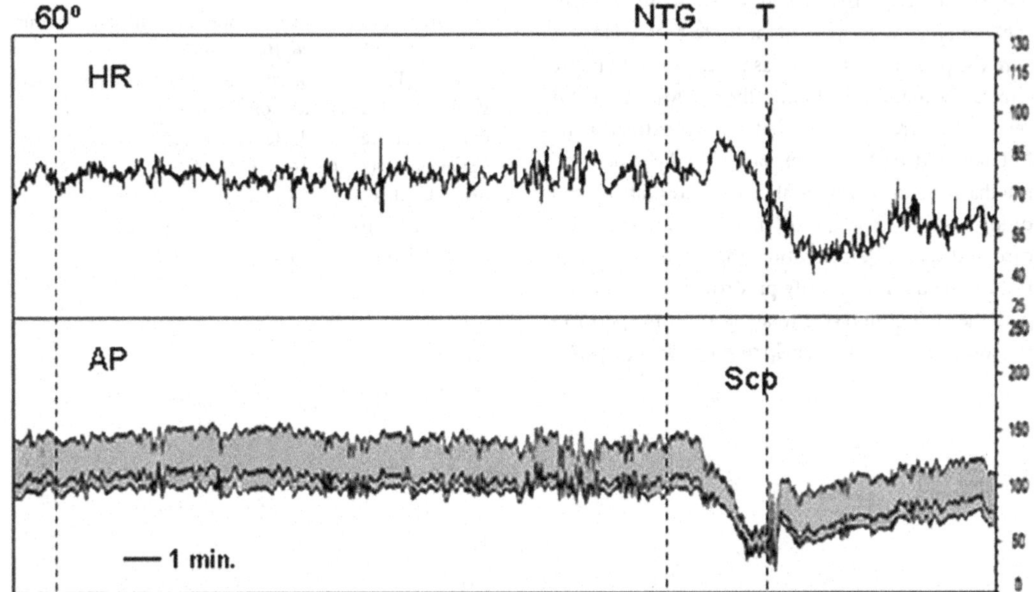

Figure 5.4 The heart rate trend (*top*) and arterial blood pressure (*bottom*). Immediately after tilting, a minimal increase in heart rate is observed. The patient remained stable during the initial 20-min drug-free phase.
A few minutes after the administration of sublingual nitroglycerin (NTG), there is a progressive decrease in the arterial blood pressure, initially with a marked increase in heart rate, followed by a decrease in both. The systolic arterial blood pressure falls to 55 mmHg and the heart rate falls to 50 beats/min. The patient lost consciousness with seizures (Scp) and was returned to the Trendelenburg position (T). After this, consciousness recovered and arterial blood pressure increased.

with a drug-free phase of 20 min, followed by the administration of 400 μg of nitroglycerin [2]. After nitroglycerin administration, the patient experienced a very fast drop in arterial blood pressure, decreasing to 70 mmHg, with a relative and simultaneous drop in heart rate to 53 beats/min, with development of syncope and seizures.

Positive responses to the tilt test have been classified according to the behavior and the temporal sequence of heart rate and arterial blood pressure [3]. The most common response has been classified as a mixed response (VASIS type 1), defined as a decrease in heart rate during syncope, but not to below 40 beats/min for 10 s, and absence of asystole. In addition, according to the current guidelines, a tilt test can be considered diagnostic when patients without structural heart disease have a positive response with syncope that reproduces the patient's spontaneous symptoms.

It is interesting to note that this patient initially reported that the syncopal episodes were sudden and that he did not recognize any prodromal signs. After the tilt test, in which minimal symptoms were elicited before syncope developed, the patient recognized that in fact he had had minimal prodromal signs during the spontaneous episodes.

In this patient, a positive response with reproduction of symptoms can be considered diagnostic, and as the patient recognized this response as reproducing the spontaneous symptoms, the tilt test served to reassure the patient. In fact, it has been shown that after clinical evaluation, including the tilt test, the recurrence rate decreases [4], so that no further treatment is initially needed. It can be explained to the patient that the diagnosis has been established and that the condition has a good prognosis, mainly due to the lack of cardiac disease [5]. In addition, the response to the tilt test can be used to identify prodromal signs that can help the patient in trying to avoid syncope, performing some maneuvers that help to avert syncope [6,7].

References

1 Brignole M, Alboni P, Benditt DG, *et al.* Guidelines on management (diagnosis and treatment) of syncope—update 2004. *Europace* 2004; **6**: 467–537.

2 Del Rosso A, Bartoletti A, Bartoli P, *et al.* Methodology of head-up tilt testing potentiated with sublingual nitroglycerin in unexplained syncope. *Am J Cardiol* 2000; **85**: 1007–11.

3 Brignole M, Menozzi C, Del Rosso A, *et al.* New classification of haemodynamics of vasovagal syncope: beyond the VASIS classification. Analysis of the presyncopal phase of the tilt test without and with nitroglycerin challenge. *Europace* 2000; **2**: 66–76.

4 Sheldon R, Rose S, Flanagan P, Koshman ML, Killam S. Risk factors for syncope recurrence after a positive tilt-table test in patients with syncope. *Circulation* 1996; **93**: 973–81.

5 Kapoor WN, Hanusa B. Is syncope a risk factor for poor outcomes? Comparison of patients with and without syncope. *Am J Med* 1996; **100**: 646–55.

6 Krediet CTP, van Dijk N, Linzer M, van Lieshout MJ, Wieling W. Management of vasovagal syncope: controlling or aborting faints by leg crossing and muscle tensing. *Circulation* 2002; **106**: 1684–9.

7 Brignole M, Croci F, Menozzi C, *et al.* Isometric arm counter-pressure maneuvers to abort impending vasovagal syncope. *J Am Coll Cardiol* 2002; **40**: 2053–9.

6

CASE 6

Tilt-induced syncope: cardioinhibitory response

G. Barón Esquivias, N. Romero, S. Gómez Moreno, A. Pedrote Martínez, A. Martínez Martínez, F. Errázquin Sáenz de Tejada

Case report

A 31-year-old woman, who is a fellow in the neurology department of our hospital, was woken up while on night duty to attend an emergency. While talking over the phone in an upright position, she felt sick and had syncope. She was attended by her colleagues, who verified that she had bradycardia and hypotension during the episode. In the following minutes, she suffered another syncopal attack, from which she recovered when she was placed in the Trendelenburg position.

Her medical history included two additional syncopal events during her youth. The results of a physical examination were normal. Neither electrocardiography (ECG), chest radiography, or echocardiography showed any abnormalities.

In our syncope study protocol, the tilt-table test is the next diagnostic step. After providing informed consent, the patient underwent a tilt-table test using the Westminster protocol, without infusion of any vasoactive substances. Before the test, a cannula was introduced into the right cephalic vein in accordance with the standard technique. During the test, a three-channel ECG was continuously recorded and non-invasive blood pressure monitoring was carried out every 2 min, or more often if symptoms developed.

After 10 min in the supine position, the patient was tilted to 60°. After 8 min without symptoms, she indicated that she felt "hot," "sick," and presyncopal. The ECG showed a rapidly progressive sinus bradycardia. The tilt was therefore modified from 60° to the Trendelenburg position. During this position change, which took 12 s, the patient suffered a sinus arrest, later asystole, and thereafter a prolonged hemodynamic derangement even during the observed low-nodal escape rhythm (Fig. 6.1). Cardiopulmonary resuscitation measures, including vigorous blows to the precordium, manual ventilation, and a 1-mg bolus of intravenous atropine, were necessary. Even during the electrocardiographically documented isolated bradycardic nodal escape rhythm, temporal hemodynamic compromise was evident up to 90 s later, when sinus tachycardia appeared. However, the patient completely recovered and was able to leave the laboratory walking without assistance.

After a few days and after receiving extensive information about the measures she could take to avert

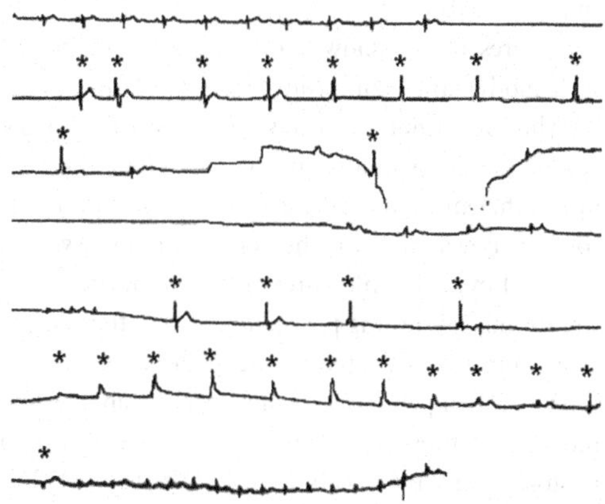

Figure 6.1 *Top*: The baseline electrocardiogram (ECG) before tilting. *Bottom*: Continuous ECG, starting with a bradycardic sinus rhythm, followed by asystole and occasionally occurring escape rhythm and beats (*) induced by vigorous blows to the precordium. The bradycardic arrhythmic events reverted to sinus tachycardia when the patient was returned to the Trendelenburg position and after administration of atropine.

syncope when feeling the first precursor symptoms, she returned to her usual activities without any specific medical treatment. At the time of writing, she had been asymptomatic for 24 months since the event described.

Comment

During vasovagal syncope induced by a head-up tilt test (HUT), vasodepressor, cardioinhibitory, or mixed responses can be observed. Two types of cardioinhibitory response are described in the Vasovagal Syncope International Study (VASIS) classification [1]:

Type 2a: cardioinhibition without asystole. The heart rate falls to a ventricular rate less than 40 beats/min for more than 10 s, but asystole of more than 3 s does not occur. The blood pressure falls before the heart rate does.

Type 2b: cardioinhibition with asystole. Asystole occurs for more than 3 s. The fall in blood pressure coincides with or occurs before the fall in heart rate.

A cardioinhibitory response is observed in 14–23% of positive responses, with slight differences in relation to the HUT protocol used [2]. The responses are usually sinus bradycardia, sinus arrest, sinoatrial block, and occasionally atrioventricular block. The prevalence of different bradycardic responses was studied by Pérez-Paredes *et al.*, who observed sinus arrest in 34 patients (8%) among 426 consecutive patients who underwent HUT [3].

The present case shows a dramatically long period of hemodynamic compromise (90 s). However, it also shows that not only can sinus arrest and asystole produce severe hemodynamic changes, but also that an insufficient bradycardic escape rhythm can occur, possibly alternating with hemodynamically asystolic periods. Emergency measures may therefore be necessary during this testing procedure, so that the test has to be conducted with appropriate medical supervision. Some 4–5% of patients who undergo tilt-table testing and 18% of those with abnormal HUTs develop an asystole of variable duration during the test [4]. The American College of Cardiology (ACC) Expert Committee recommends that if syncope occurs during the test, then tilting down should be fast and take 10–15 s [5]. The authors needed 12 s to change the patient's position. Because of the long-lasting hemodynamic compromise, we would suggest that the tilting-down time should ideally be even faster.

The authors' experience [4] suggests that the appearance of an asystole or long-lasting hemodynamic compromise during tilt-table testing does not necessarily imply a poorer prognosis. Today, a cardioinhibitory response during tilt-table testing should not definitively preclude treatment. However, an individualized approach and the provision of detailed information to the patient remain mandatory. In some selected patients, pacing might be considered until definitive and appropriate treatment is found. Unfortunately, the solution to vasovagal syncope is not clear. However, this long-lasting period of hemodynamic compromise in a patient who was later asymptomatic illustrates the complexity of an unresolved and frequent clinical problem.

References

1 Brignole M, Menozzi C, Del Rosso A, *et al.* New classification of hemodynamics of vasovagal syncope: beyond the VASIS classification. Analysis of the pre-syncopal phase of the tilt test without and with nitroglycerin challenge. *Europace* 2000; **2**: 66–76.

2 Barón-Esquivias G, Pedrote A, Cayuela A, Cabezón S, Morán JE, Errazquin F. Características clínicas y resultados del test de tabla basculante utilizando tres protocolos en 1661 pacientes con síncope. *Rev Esp Cardiol* 2003; **56**: 916–20.

3 Pérez-Paredes M, Barón-Esquivias G, Ruiz Ros JA, *et al.* Results of shortened head-up tilt testing potentiated with sublingual nitroglycerin in a large cohort of patients with unexplained syncope [abstract]. *Eur Heart J* 2002; **23** (Suppl): 286.

4 Barón-Esquivias G, Pedrote A, Cayuela A, *et al.* Long-term outcome of patients with asystole induced by head-up tilt test. *Eur Heart J* 2002; **23**: 483–9.

5 Benditt DG, Ferguson DW, Grubb BP, *et al.* Tilt table testing for assessing syncope. American College of Cardiology. *J Am Coll Cardiol* 1996; **28**: 263–75.

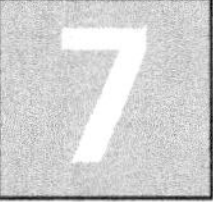

CASE 7

Tilt-induced syncope: purely vasodepressor response

A. Moya i Mitjans, C. Alonso

Case report

A 23-year-old woman was referred to the syncope unit due to recurrent syncopal episodes. She had no previously known cardiac disease, and no family history of syncope or sudden death. Her syncopal history had started 4 years before, and she had had five syncopal episodes during the previous 9 months. All of the episodes developed while she was standing; there were no clearly recognizable triggers, and the episodes were preceded by short prodromal symptoms. She had never had seizures or urinary incontinence. A mild cranial injury had taken place during one of the episodes.

The physical examination was normal, and there were no murmurs. The baseline arterial blood pressure was normal, and there were no abnormal changes when actively returning to an upright posture. The baseline electrocardiogram (ECG) showed a normal sinus rhythm at 70 beats/min, with normal PR and QT intervals and a normal QRS configuration.

Due to the recurrent nature of the episodes, the absence of structural heart disease, the occurrence of an injury during a syncopal episode, and the fact that the syncope was relatively sudden, a tilt test was indicated.

The tilt-test protocol was planned at 60° for 20 min without drug administration, followed by 400 μg of sublingual nitroglycerin. A continuous ECG was recorded, noninvasive arterial blood-pressure monitoring was carried out with a Finapres system (Finapres Medical Systems, Amsterdam, Netherlands), and both signals were recorded and displayed using the LabSystem (Bard Electrophysiology Division, Lowell, Massachusetts, USA). After tilting, the patient showed a marked increase in heart rate, and after 5 min, without drug administration, she described a very fast prodromal symptom that was followed by sudden loss of consciousness. At this point, the recording showed sinus tachycardia with progressive hypotension, followed by an abrupt drop in arterial blood pressure (Fig. 7.1). The patient was then tilted into the Trendelenburg position, and a slight decrease in her heart rate was observed. After this, consciousness and arterial blood pressure immediately recovered.

Due to the extremely sudden vasodepression, and to rule out potential measurement artifacts, a second tilt-table test was scheduled a week later. In the first few minutes and also during the drug-free phase, after minimal prodromal symptoms, the patient experienced a sudden loss of consciousness, which was followed by jerking movements, accompanied by a very fast drop in arterial blood pressure, with a minimal drop in heart rate (Fig. 7.2).

Comment

Positive responses to tilt testing have been classified in relation to the magnitude and timing of hypotension and bradycardia [1]. More recently, this classification has been modified to take account not only of the behavior of heart rate and arterial blood pressure during the syncopal response, but also during the presyncopal phase [2]. The most frequently observed response is a mixed response (type 1), followed by a cardioinhibitory response, most frequently type 2a. It has been reported that a purely vasodepressor response is usually associated with what is known as the dysautonomic vasovagal pattern in the presyncopal phase, which consists of a progressive fall in diastolic blood pressure that starts immediately after tilting.

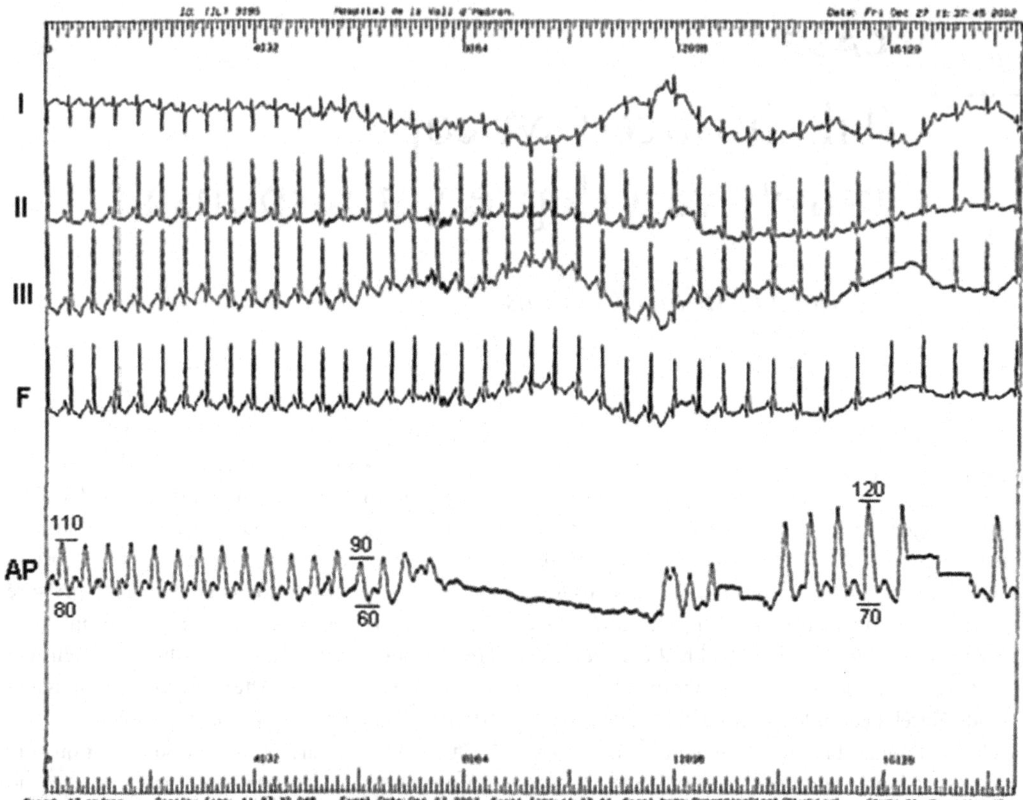

Figure 7.1 Progressive hypotension from 110 mmHg to 90 mmHg, with sinus tachycardia at 120 beats/min, followed by a sudden drop in arterial pressure (AP), which recovered after the patient was returned to the Trendelenburg position. It should be noted that the fall in arterial blood pressure is followed by a slight decrease in the heart rate.

In fact, although the response to the tilt test in this patient must be classified as a vasodepressor one (type 3), the arterial blood pressure during the first minute of tilting remained stable until rapid and progressive hypotension appeared. This suggests that the behavior of the presyncopal phase was more characteristic of a classic vasovagal response rather than a dysautonomic one. In addition, the patient had no clinical data suggestive of dysautonomia, as she had no hypotension or palpitations and only reported sudden syncopal episodes with complete recovery.

Tilt testing in this patient confirmed that sudden and severe hypotension without bradycardia was able to lead to a severe syncopal episode, as suggested by the injury during spontaneous syncope as well as the jerking movements during the second tilt-induced syncope.

The drop in arterial blood pressure observed in the first tilt test was so sudden that there were some doubts about the possibility of an artifact. The fact that the patient had lost consciousness simultaneously with the hypotension strongly suggested true hypotension. However, the authors decided to repeat the tilt test in order to confirm the mechanism. Although the drop in arterial blood pressure was not so sudden during the second tilt test a week later, the overall behavior was the same, and the response was again classified as a vasodepressor one.

Data regarding the reproducibility of the tilt test are not homogeneous, and the reproducibility of a positive response has ranged between 31% and 92% [3,4]. In addition, the reproducibility of the type of response has also been studied [5], and it has been shown to decrease over time and with repeated tilt tests. However, in this patient, in whom the tilt test was repeated 1 week later, it can be reasonably assumed that her syncopal episodes were mainly due to a severe vasodepressor response.

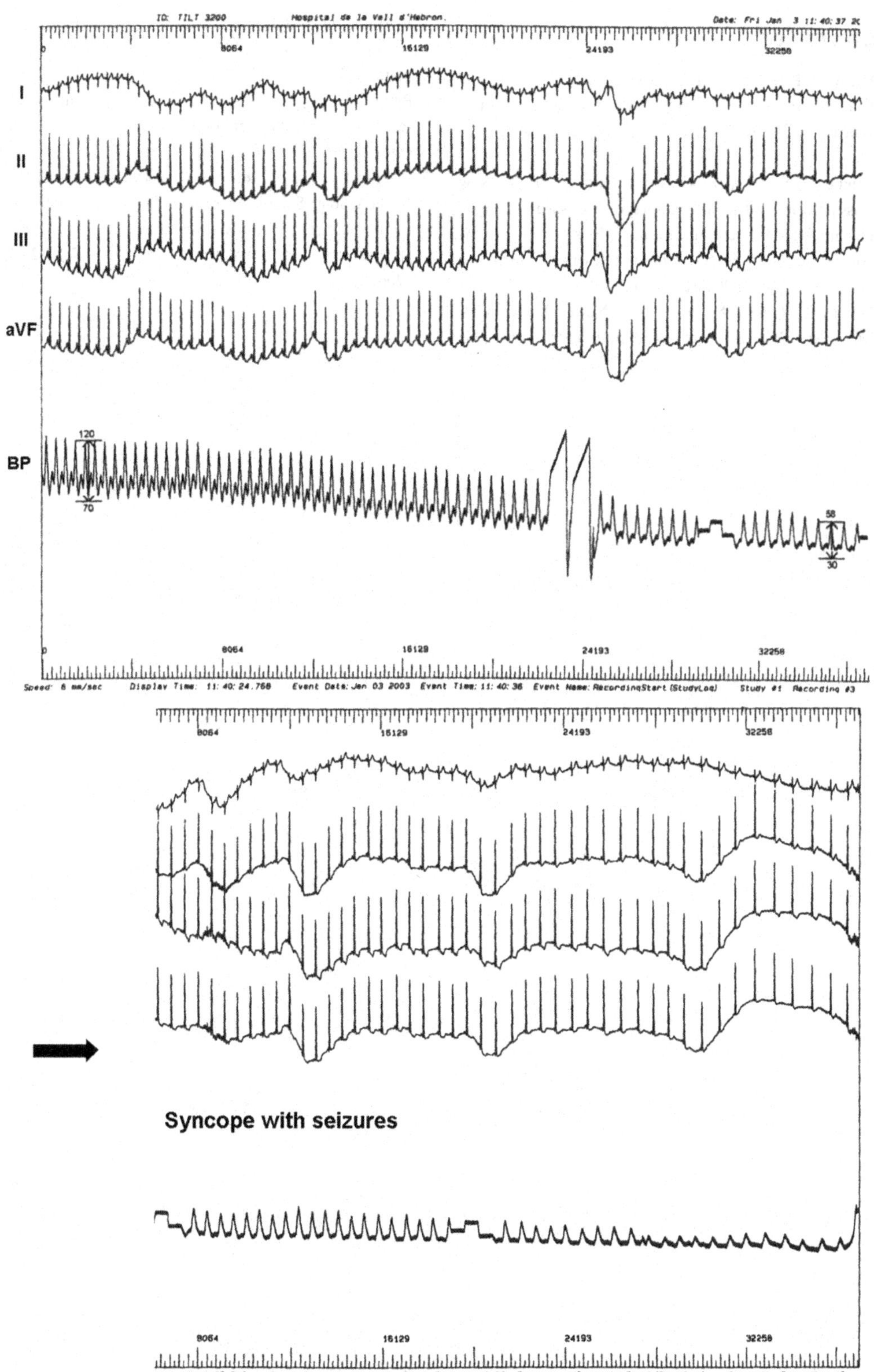

Figure 7.2 A second tilt test was carried out 1 week after the first, and the patient again showed a very fast and progressive decrease in arterial blood pressure (BP) in the drug-free phase, with a minimal decrease in heart rate that was accompanied by sudden syncope with seizures.

References

1 Sutton R, Petersen M, Brignole M, Raviele A, Menozzi C, Giani P. Proposed classification for tilt induced vasovagal syncope. *Eur J Cardiac Pacing Electrophysiol* 1992; **3**: 180–18.

2 Brignole M, Menozzi C, Del Rosso A *et al.* New classification of haemodynamics of vasovagal syncope: beyond the VASIS classification. Analysis of the pre-syncopal phase of the tilt test without and with nitroglycerin challenge. *Europace* 2000; **2**: 66–76.

3 Brooks R, Ruskin JN, Powell AC, Newell J, Garan H, McGovern BA. Prospective evaluation of day-to-day reproducibility of upright tilt-table testing in unexplained syncope. *Am J Cardiol* 1993; **71**: 1289–92.

4 Blanc JJ, Mansourati J, Maheu B, Boughaleb D, Genet L. Reproducibility of a positive passive upright tilt test at a seven-day interval in patients with syncope. *Am J Cardiol* 1993; **72**: 469–71.

5 Sagrista-Sauleda J, Romero B, Permanyer-Miralda G, Moya A, Soler-Soler J. Reproducibility of sequential head-up tilt testing in patients with recent syncope, normal ECG and no structural heart disease. *Eur Heart J* 2002; **23**: 1706–13.

CASE 8

Tilt-induced syncope: dysautonomic response

N. Bottoni, C. Menozzi, F. Quartieri, G. Lolli

Case report

A 69-year-old woman with arterial hypertension treated with calcium antagonists, and noninsulin-dependent diabetes mellitus, was referred to our institution due to two syncopal episodes during the previous year. The episodes had occurred when she was in the sitting position during the postprandial period; they were preceded for a few seconds by prodromes (weakness and epigastric discomfort), and were of short duration with a rapid recovery. Standard electrocardiography showed left ventricular hypertrophy, which was confirmed on two-dimensional echocardiography. Left ventricular systolic function was normal. A 24-h Holter recording was negative. She underwent neurally mediated tests. Carotid sinus massage in the upright position induced an asymptomatic sinus pause of 4 s, with a drop in systolic blood pressure of 50 mmHg. The tilting test induced syncope after nitroglycerin administration and was characterized by a peculiar hemodynamic pattern (Fig. 8.1). From the beginning of the tilt, while the heart rate showed a

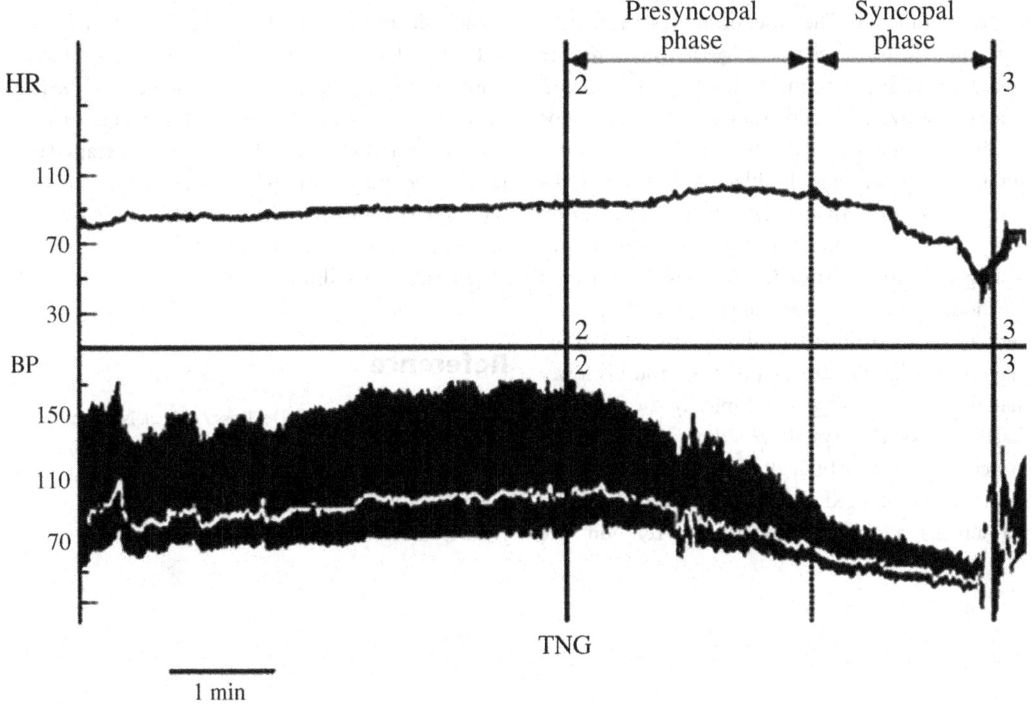

Figure 8.1 The head-up tilt test. BP, blood pressure; HR, heart rate; TNG, trinitroglycerin.

slight increase, blood pressure decreased slightly and progressively throughout the presyncopal and syncopal phases without a change in slope; since the systolic pressure declined more than the diastolic pressure, the pulse pressure also decreased. When the blood pressure reached a value of nearly 70 mmHg, a typical vasovagal reaction started, with slowing of the heart rate to a minimum of 42 beats/min together with a marked and abrupt fall in blood pressure. In accordance with the new Vasovagal Syncope International Study (VASIS) classification [1], this response was classified as type 1 mixed neurally mediated syncope with a dysautonomic pattern. It was suggested to the patient that she should increase her intake and wear compression stockings. No syncopal relapses occurred during a subsequent 10-month follow-up period.

Comment

On the basis of the modifications of blood pressure and heart rate preceding the syncope during the tilting test, the new VASIS classification [1] distinguishes three main patterns of syncope: classic, dysautonomic, and orthostatic intolerance. The patients with the classic pattern show a full compensatory reflex adaptation to the upright position, which suggests normal baroreflex function. The onset of the vasovagal reaction cannot be predicted by changes in blood pressure or heart rate, and the time of onset is very variable. Once the vasovagal reaction starts, it leads to syncope within a few minutes. Patients with the classic form are mainly young and healthy. Patients with the dysautonomic pattern are unable to achieve a steady-state reflex adaptation to the upright position, suggesting an impaired baroreflex response or impaired functioning of the target organs—the heart and peripheral vasculature. Accordingly, the value of the maximum heart rate reached by this group is lower than that in the classic group. Typically, the vasovagal reaction starts when systolic blood pressure decreases to a critical value of about 70–80 mmHg. It therefore seems that prolonged orthostatic hypotension may play a role as a trigger for the vasovagal reaction. The orthostatic intolerance pattern is similar to that in the dysautonomic group, but a clear vasovagal reaction does not appear.

Patients with dysautonomic syncope differ from those with classic syncope with regard to age, prevalence of structural heart disease, and the duration of syncopal episodes, but have a similar prevalence of a history of vasovagal or situational events. Patients with the dysautonomic pattern are mainly older, but the pattern may also occur in some younger individuals; many have associated diseases. The patients have a short history of syncope, and the episodes begin late in life, suggesting that they are due to the occurrence of some underlying neural dysfunction. Carotid sinus hypersensitivity is frequently present in these patients, suggesting that an impairment at some level of the carotid sinus baroreflex arc is also associated with the condition and, therefore, that a more complex autonomic dysfunction is present. For all these reasons, it is probable that dysautonomic syncope is due to a disease of autonomic function, which often starts late in the patient's life and is characterized by a compromised capability to adapt promptly to some external influences. Dysautonomic patients may benefit from the treatment usually administered for syndromes of autonomic dysfunction with orthostatic intolerance—namely, increasing blood volume (fludrocortisone), reducing blood volume in the lower limbs (compression stockings, sleeping with the head of the bed upright), or using alpha-stimulating agents such as midodrine and etilefrine. If preventive therapy fails, pacemakers may be useful in patients with the cardioinhibitory forms, particularly those with asystole, and when carotid sinus hypersensitivity may be associated with the condition.

Reference

1 Brignole M, Menozzi C, Del Rosso A, *et al.* New classification of hemodynamics of vasovagal syncope: beyond the VASIS classification. Analysis of the pre-syncopal phase of the tilt test without and with nitroglycerin challenge. *Europace* 2000; 2: 66–76.

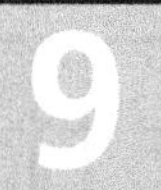

CASE 9

Tilt-induced syncope: chronotropic incompetence

F. Quartieri, C. Menozzi, N. Bottoni, G. Lolli

Case report

A 77-year-old man with arterial hypertension and normal left ventricular systolic function had had five syncopal episodes during the previous 3 years. The episodes occurred when he was in the sitting or standing position, with mild prodromes, and were of short duration with rapid recovery. Two episodes were situational and occurred after micturition. In one case only, a syncopal episode had been responsible for moderate cranial trauma. Other symptoms consisted of occasional fatigue and sporadic presyncope. He had been taking angiotensin-converting enzyme (ACE) inhibitors for arterial hypertension for 5 years. The standard electrocardiogram was normal, with moderate sinus bradycardia. A 24-h Holter recording showed a mean heart rate of 55 beats/min and no significant arrhythmias. Carotid sinus massage was negative in the supine position and induced a sinus pause of 5 s, symptomatic for presyncope in the upright position.

The tilt test induced a syncope after nitroglycerin challenge. A peculiar pattern was observed, characterized by a stable heart rate during the whole test, similar to the pre-tilting values, without increasing after nitroglycerin administration, and with a slow and progressive fall in blood pressure until the moment of the syncope (Fig. 9.1). Due to the evidence of moderate sinus bradycardia on the electrocardiogram, an electrophysiological study was carried out, which revealed a slight depression of the intrinsic sinus function.

A diagnosis of vasodepressive neurally mediated syncope with chronotropic incompetence was therefore made. The patient underwent dual-chamber pacemaker implantation and had no significant clinical events during a subsequent 18-month follow-up period.

Comment

In accordance with the new Vasovagal Syncope International Study (VASIS) classification [1], the syncope was classified as vasodepressive and neurally mediated, with chronotropic incompetence. Patients with this pattern show no increase in heart rate during the tilt test, with values similar to the baseline state (i.e., 10% from the rate before tilt) and with a slow and progressive decrease in diastolic and systolic blood pressure; both features are expressions of a coexistent autonomic dysfunction (dysautonomic pattern). The chronotropic incompetence is associated with older age; in one study, for example, this pattern was present in one-third of patients aged over 75 who were able to complete the tilt test [2]. Carotid sinus hypersensitivity is frequently present in these patients, suggesting that an impairment at some level of the carotid sinus baroreflex arc is also associated with the condition and, therefore, that a more complex autonomic dysfunction is present [1]. The coexistence in this patient of neuromediated syncope with chronotropic incompetence, cardioinhibitory carotid sinus hypersensitivity, and symptoms probably correlated with moderate sinus node dysfunction (inconstant fatigue) led the authors to implant a dual-chamber pacemaker.

References

1 Brignole M, Menozzi C, Del Rosso A, *et al.* New classification of hemodynamics of vasovagal syncope: beyond

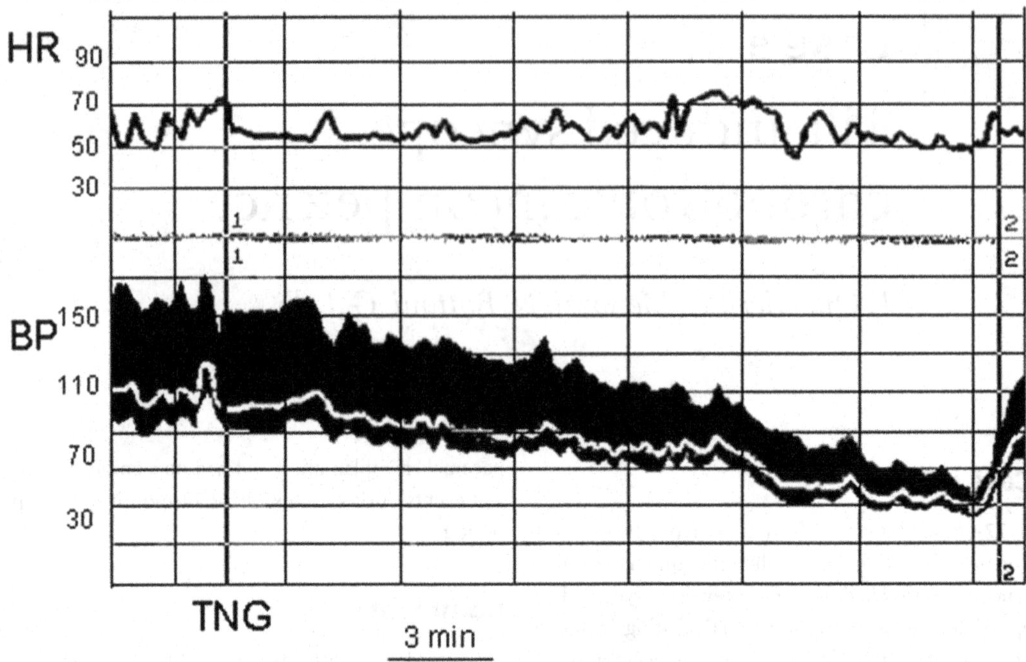

Figure 9.1 The head-up tilt table test. BP, blood pressure; HR, heart rate; TNG, trinitroglycerin.

the VASIS classification. Analysis of the pre-syncopal phase of the tilt test without and with nitroglycerin challenge. *Europace* 2000; **2**: 66–76.

2 Kurbaan AS, Franzen AC, Bowker TJ, *et al.* Usefulness of tilt test-induced patterns of heart rate and blood pressure using a two-stage protocol with glyceryl trinitrate provocation in patients with syncope of unknown origin. *Am J Cardiol* 1999; **84**: 665–70.

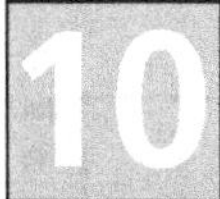

CASE 10

Syncope and postural orthostatic tachycardia syndrome

R. García Civera, R. Ruiz Granell, S. Morell Cabedo, R. Sanjuán Mañez

Case report

A 32-year-old woman was referred because of long-standing complaints of palpitations, near-fainting, and intolerance to effort. During the previous year, she had had three syncopal episodes and multiple pre-syncopal episodes. The symptoms developed during prolonged standing or during effort. Physical examination, electrocardiography, and echocardiography showed no abnormalities. In the supine position, the patient had a heart rate of 78 beats/min and blood pressure of 130/75 mmHg. After 3 min, the standing blood pressure was 130/80 mmHg and the heart rate was 125 beats/min. The 24-h electrocardiographic Holter tracing (Fig. 10.1) recorded a sinus rhythm, with the heart rate ranging from 47 to 175 beats/min. Multiple bouts of sinus tachycardia were recorded during the day, but not during the night. Standard laboratory measurements and thyroid hormones, urinary metanephrines, and vanillylmandelic acid were all within the normal ranges.

A tilt-table test, with nitroglycerin challenge and hemodynamic measurements, was carried out (Fig. 10.2). The figure shows the trends for heart rate, systolic index (SI), systolic, mean and diastolic blood pressures, and total peripheral resistance index (TPRI). With passive tilting to 60°, the heart rate rose progressively from 75 beats/min (standing) to 110,

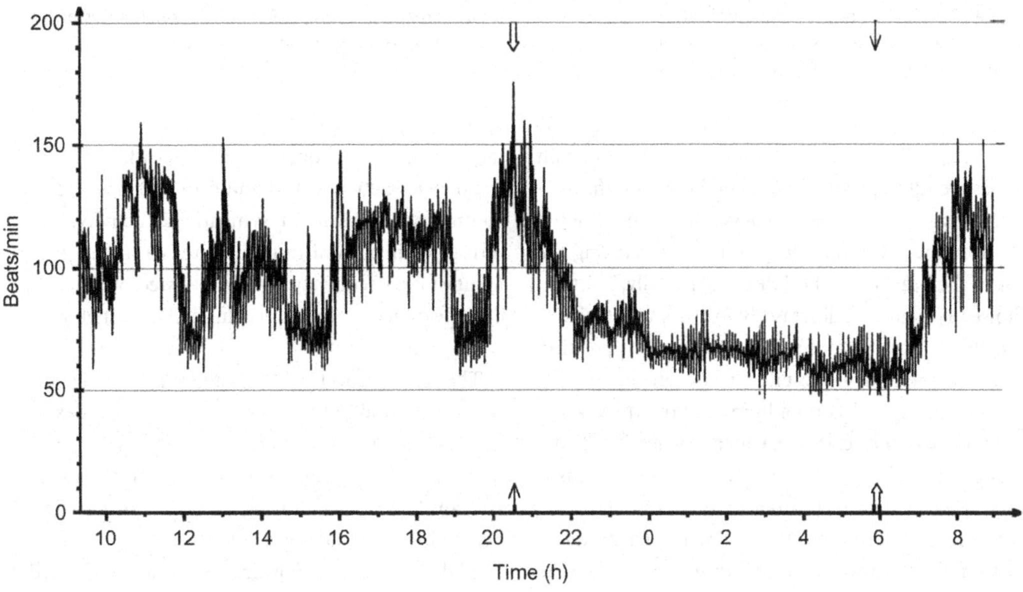

Figure 10.1 The heart rate trend during the 24-h Holter recording.

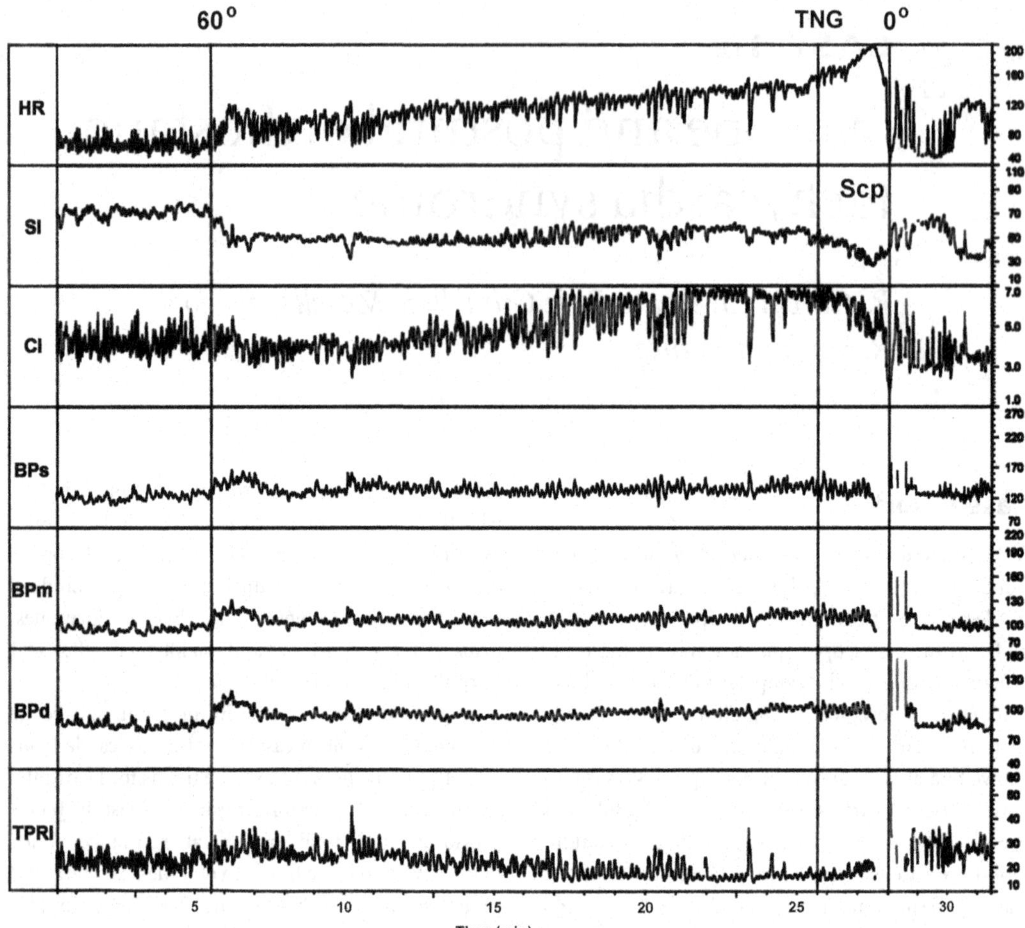

Figure 10.2 The hemodynamic trend during the tilt-table test. HR, heart rate; SI, systolic index; CI, cardiac index; BPs, systolic blood pressure; BPm, mean blood pressure; BPd, diastolic blood pressure; TPRI, total peripheral resistance index; TNG, trinitroglycerin; Scp, syncope.

120, 122, and 140 beats/min after 1, 5, 10, and 20 min of passive tilting, respectively. The SI fell significantly with tilting, reflecting the fall in venous return, but the cardiac index (CI) rose progressively, paralleling the rise in the heart rate. The TPRI rose initially, but then showed a progressive decrease. Blood pressure stabilized shortly after the patient reached the upright position and remained stable despite the progressive fall in TPRI. With nitroglycerin administration, there was a further rise in the heart rate, which reached 200 beats/min, and a fall in SI and CI, followed by a typical vasovagal reaction with an asystolic pause of 18 s.

Figure 10.3 shows the three-dimensional trend of diastolic blood pressure variability analysis during the tilt-table test. With tilting, there is a fast and continuous increase in low-frequency power (with a band of frequencies between 0.04 and 0.15 Hz), suggesting a continuous increase in sympathetic activity. With nitroglycerin administration, there is a further increment of low-frequency power, followed by an abrupt disappearance of the signal immediately before the syncope.

The response to the Valsalva maneuver (Fig. 10.4) showed mild abnormalities. The Valsalva index was normal (> 1.5), but an attenuated late phase II (consistent with a reduction in vasoconstrictive response) and an "overshoot" during phase IV (suggesting a hyperadrenergic state) were observed.

With a diagnosis of postural orthostatic tachycardia syndrome (POTS), the patient was referred to the

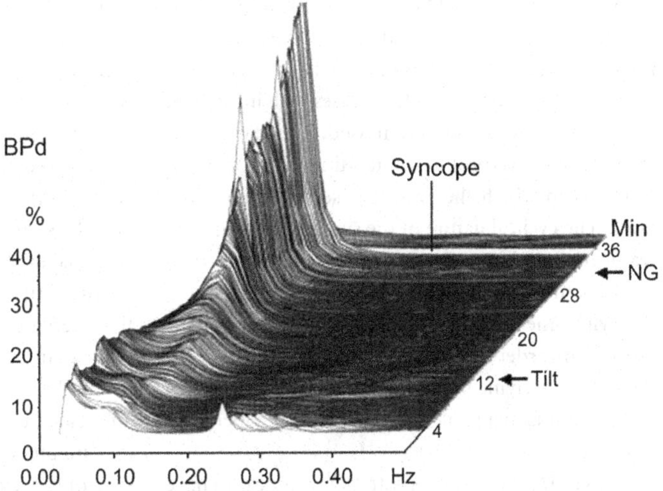

Figure 10.3 The three-dimensional trend in diastolic blood pressure variability during the tilt-table test. BPd, diastolic blood pressure; NG, nitroglycerin.

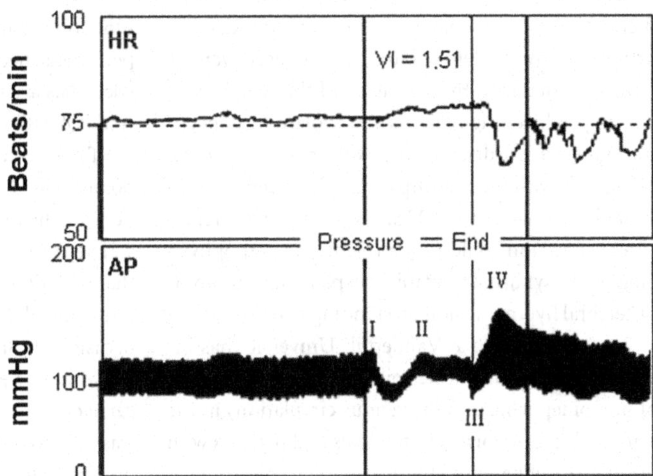

Figure 10.4 The response of the heart rate and blood pressure to the Valsalva maneuver. HR, heart rate; AP, arterial pressure.

neurology service for further evaluation, and a final diagnosis of partial dysautonomic disease with sympathetic denervation of the legs was made. Treatment with increasing intake of fluids and salt, fludrocortisone, and low doses of propranolol was initiated. During follow-up, syncope did not recur and other signs of orthostatic intolerance improved.

Comment

The postural orthostatic tachycardia syndrome (POTS) is characterized by persistent symptoms of orthostatic intolerance such as light-headedness, nausea, palpitations, weakness, and fatigue in the upright position, associated with an increase in heart rate of more than 30 beats/min from the supine to the upright position or with a heart rate > 120 beats/min within 10 min of head-up tilting. Characteristically, there is no significant hypotension with tilting or in the upright position [1–4]. Some patients also have syncope [5,6], but this is not a prerequisite for the diagnosis of POTS.

This syndrome has also been referred to as idiopathic orthostatic intolerance, chronic orthostatic intolerance, and idiopathic orthostatic tachycardia, and it has features in common with the mitral-valve prolapse syndrome, the hyperdynamic beta-adrenergic circulatory state, vasoregulatory asthenia, and chronic fatigue syndrome.

Most patients with POTS are young women [2], and in some cases there is an antecedent viral infection before the start of the symptoms. The clinical tolerance is variable and ranges from cases with infrequent symptoms or symptoms only in conditions of increased orthostatic stress (prolonged standing, exertion, heat) to others in which the patient is seriously incapacitated. The cyclical nature of the symptoms is another feature of POTS [2].

The pathophysiology of POTS is poorly understood; the syndrome probably represents a heterogeneous group of disorders with similar clinical characteristics. Possible underlying pathophysiologies include partial dysautonomia, hypovolemia, or a primary hyperadrenergic state.

A large group of patients with POTS appear to have a "partial dysautonomia" characterized by sympathetic denervation of the legs [7–9]. In the upright posture, there is excessive pooling of blood in the legs [9], orthostatic hypovolemia [10], and reduced venous return. Secondarily, the activation of the sympathetic system produces high plasma catecholamine concentrations (tachycardia, tremor). A decrease in cerebral blood flow with the head-up tilt test has been demonstrated in patients with POTS, suggesting that cerebral vasoconstriction could play a role in the pathophysiology of the syndrome and might explain the symptoms of cerebral hypoperfusion on standing [11,12].

Recently, a group at Vanderbilt University has investigated norepinephrine spillover (the rate of entry of norepinephrine into the venous circulation) in the arms and legs of normal individuals and patients with POTS. At the baseline, the plasma concentration of norepinephrine in the femoral vein was lower in patients than in controls. In response to stimulation of sympathetic activation, the norepinephrine spillover in the arms increased to a similar extent in the two groups, but increases in the legs were smaller in patients with POTS. This result argues in favor of the "partial dysautonomia" theory as the cause of POTS [8].

Some patients with POTS may have a component of beta-receptor supersensitivity [13]. It is not yet clear whether this supersensitivity is primary or due to secondary denervation supersensitivity.

The tilt-table test is a good tool for detecting patients with POTS. In a recent study [5], POTS was detected in 4.6% of 260 patients referred for the tilt test due to syncope of unknown cause. The tilt test was positive (syncope induction) in 50% of the cases, with half of the patients showing a cardioinhibitory response. In the study by Sandroni *et al.* [6], a fall instead of an increase in total peripheral resistance during tilting was the most consistent finding predictive of syncope appearing in POTS patients.

Complete evaluation of these patients requires further autonomic tests. The Valsalva maneuver is a global test of autonomic function. The Valsalva index (the maximal to minimal heart rate ratio) is usually normal, but it is possible to detect some anomalies in the arterial pressure response, such as a reduction of more than 50% in the pulse amplitude during early phase II (hypovolemia, reduced venous return), an attenuated or absent recovery of blood pressure during late phase II (suggesting a deficiency in vasoconstrictor capacity), and an "overshoot" during phase IV (suggesting a hyperadrenergic state) [2].

Autonomic tests that explore the sudomotor function are important for detecting the existence of peripheral neuropathy [14,15]. The most frequently used tests are the quantitative sudomotor axon reflex test (QSART) and the thermoregulatory sweat test (TST). According to Low *et al.* [15], these tests make it possible to demonstrate the presence of peripheral neuropathy in 50–60% of POTS cases.

The treatment of patients with POTS is similar to that of patients with autonomic failure. Beta-blockers can control tachycardia and palpitations, but may occasionally increase fatigability [15]. In a study in which radiofrequency ablation of the sinus node was carried out, aggravation of the orthostatic symptoms was observed during the follow-up [16]. Other treatments, including volume loading (by increasing salt and fluid administration), leg compression garments, fludrocortisone, or vasoconstrictors, would probably be beneficial, but the long-term effects of these measures have not been assessed.

References

1 Schondorf R, Low PA. Idiopathic postural orthostatic tachycardia syndrome: an attenuated form of acute pandysautonomia? *Neurology* 1993; **43**: 132–7.

2 Low PA, Opfer-Gehrking TL, Textor SC, *et al.* Postural tachycardia syndrome (POTS) *Neurology* 1995; **45** (Suppl 5): S19–S25.

3 Grubb BP, Kosinski DJ, Bohem H, *et al.* The postural orthostatic tachycardia syndrome: a neurocardiogenic variant identified during head-up tilt table testing. *Pacing Clin Electrophysiol* 1997; **20**: 2205–12.

4 Karas B, Grubb BP, Boehm K, Kip K. The postural orthostatic tachycardia syndrome: a potentially treatable cause of chronic fatigue, exercise intolerance, and cognitive impairment in adolescents. *Pacing Clin Electrophysiol* 2000; **23**: 344–51.

5 Folino AF, Buja GF, Russo G, Ilceto S. Prevalence of postural orthostatic tachycardia syndrome in patients with unexplained syncope: clinical presentation and tilt tests results [abstract]. *Europace* 2003; **4** (B6): A04-3.

6 Sandroni P, Opfer-Gehrking TL, Benarroch EE, Shen WK, Low PA. Certain cardiovascular indices predict syncope in the postural tachycardia syndrome. *Clin Auton Res* 1996; **6**: 225–31.

7 Streeten DH. Pathogenesis of hyperadrenergic orthostatic hypotension: evidence of disordered venous innervation exclusively in the lower limbs. *J Clin Invest* 1990: **86**: 1582–8.

8 Jacob G, Costa F, Shannon JR, *et al.* The neuropathic postural tachycardia syndrome. *N Engl J Med* 2000; **343**: 1008–14.

9 Streeten DH, Anderson GH, Richardson R, Thomas FD. Abnormal orthostatic changes in blood pressure and heart rate in subjects with intact sympathetic nervous function: evidence of excessive venous pooling. *J Lab Clin Med* 1988; **111**: 326–35.

10 Jacob G, Ertl AC, Shannon JR, Robertson RM, Robertson D. Idiopathic orthostatic tachycardia: the role of dynamic orthostatic hypovolemia and norepinephrine [abstract]. *Circulation* 1996; **94** (Suppl I): I-627.

11 Novak V, Spies J, Novak P, *et al.* Hypocapnia and cerebral hypoperfusion in orthostatic intolerance. *Stroke* 1998; **2**: 1876–81.

12 Hermosillo AG, Jauregui-Renaud K, Kostine A, Marquez MF, Lara JL, Cardenas M. Comparative study of cerebral blood flow between postural tachycardia and neurocardiogenic syncope during head-up tilt test. *Europace* 2002; **4**: 369–74.

13 Grubb BP. The postural tachycardia syndrome: etiology, diagnosis and treatment. In: Raviele A, ed. *Cardiac Arrhythmias 2001: Proceedings of the 7th International Workshop on Cardiac Arrhythmias, Venice, 7–10 October 2001*. Springer, Milan, 2002: 43–9.

14 Low PA. Laboratory evaluation of autonomic function. In: Low PA, ed. *Clinical Autonomic Disorders*, 2nd ed. Lippincott-Raven, Philadelphia, 1997: 179–208.

15 Low PA, Schondorf R, Novak V, Sandroni P, Opfer-Gehrking TL, Novak P. Postural tachycardia syndrome. In: Low PA, ed. *Clinical Autonomic Disorders*, 2nd ed. Lippincott-Raven, Philadelphia, 1997: 681–97.

16 Shen WK, Low PA, Jahangir A, *et al.* Is sinus node modification appropriate for inappropriate sinus tachycardia with features of postural tachycardia syndrome? *Pacing Clin Electrophysiol* 2001; **24**: 217–30.

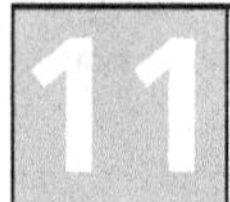

CASE 11

Electroencephalography recordings during syncope

J.G. van Dijk, W. Wieling

Case report

Tilt-table results from a 14-year-old girl with recurrent vasovagal syncope were examined. The period shown lasted 30 s and occurred 5 min after tilting. Blood pressure had already gradually dropped to 70/50 mmHg, and the heart rate had slowed to 51 beats/min when asystole set in, lasting for 11 s. After about 7 s of asystole, the electroencephalogram (EEG) changed from a normal alpha rhythm to slow large delta waves, which lasted for about 4 s. Consciousness was lost. Then the EEG was flat for 7 s. The tilt table was returned to the horizontal position in this period. The resumption of cortical activity started 9 s after the first heart beat following asystole. The EEG then changed in the reverse order. Some myoclonic jerks were observed, and can be recognized in the electrocardiogram (ECG) channel.

Figure 11.1 shows only four EEG channels (right frontal and occipital, left frontal and occipital). The ECG shows some movement artifacts. Blood pressure was measured with a Finapres device (FMS Finapres Medical Systems B.V., Amsterdam, Netherlands).

Comment

During syncope, the EEG in this patient showed progressive slowing with an increase in amplitude, followed by a sudden reduction of brain-wave amplitude, resulting in a "flat" EEG. The end of syncope was accompanied by changes in the reverse order, giving rise to a typical "slow–flat–slow" pattern. Myoclonic jerks occurred during the slow and flat stages of the EEG. These findings are in agreement with observations following eyeball pressure and carotid sinus massage to induce abrupt onset asystolic syncope ([1–6], review in [6]). Asystole lasting 3–6 s produces no EEG abnormalities and almost no clinical symptoms, except possibly unclear thinking. However, after 7–13 s of asystole, slow waves (theta and delta) appear, followed by abrupt flattening. This change is accompanied by rapid clouding and then complete loss of consciousness. With asystole longer than 10–14 s, myoclonic jerks can be observed, sometimes followed by a generalized tonic spasm in extension and even opisthotonus, while on the EEG there is cortical silence [1–6]. EEG findings during presyncope and syncope induced by tilt-table testing [7] show similar but more variable patterns than syncope induced by the fainting lark and eyeball pressure. The slower fall in systemic blood pressure during vasovagal syncope may be involved.

It is postulated that the myoclonic activity during a prolonged syncopal episode originates from the reticular formation; a release phenomenon from lower brainstem neurons no longer suppressed by higher centers is suggested [3]. However, it is not known why this activity sometimes appears and sometimes does not. Cerebral hypoxia has potent epileptogenic effects, and hyperventilation (causing cerebral vasoconstriction) is therefore routinely used to activate epileptic discharges during EEG recordings [8]. Nevertheless, only a few EEG-documented epileptic seizures developing from syncope have been reported. Almost all of the cases involve young children; only one adult case has been reported [6].

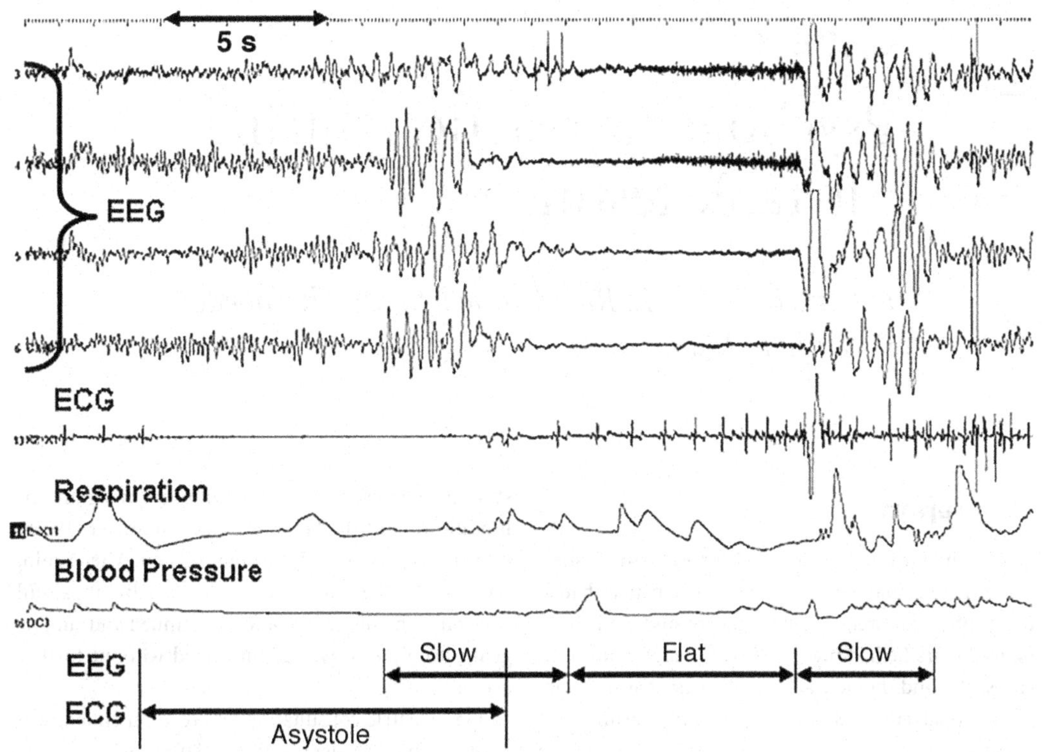

Figure 11.1 Only four electroencephalography (EEG) channels are shown, to facilitate inspection. Respiration was measured with a strain gauge and blood pressure with a Finapres device. It should be noted that the EEG responds to asystole with a highly specific "slow–flat–slow" pattern of changes, appearing with a delay after the onset of asystole. ECG, electrocardiography.

References

1 Lempert T, Bauer M, Schmidt D. Syncope: a videometric analysis of 56 episodes of transient cerebral hypoxia. *Ann Neurol* 1994; **36**: 233–7.

2 Gastaut H, Fischer-Williams M. Electro-encephalographic study of syncope: its difference from epilepsy. *Lancet* 1957; ii: 1018–25.

3 Gastaut H. Syncopes: generalized anoxic cerebral seizures. In: Magnus O, de Haas AML, eds. *Handbook of Clinical Neurology*, vol. 15: *The Epilepsies*. North-Holland, Amsterdam, 1974: 815–36.

4 Stephenson JBP. *Fits and Faints*. Blackwell Scientific/ MacKeith Press, Oxford, 1990.

5 Stephenson JBP. Fainting and syncope. In: Maria BL, ed. *Current Management in Pediatric Neurology*, 2nd ed. Decker, Hamilton, Ontario, 2002: 345–51.

6 Brenner RP. Electroencephalography in syncope. *J Clin Neurophysiol* 1997; **14**: 197–209.

7 Sheldon RS, Koshman ML, Murphy WF. Electroencephalographic findings during presyncope and syncope induced by tilt table testing. *Can J Cardiol* 1998; **14**: 811–16.

8 Flink R, Pedersen B, Guekht AB, *et al.* Guidelines for the use of EEG methodology in the diagnosis of epilepsy. International League Against Epilepsy: commission report. Commission on European Affairs: Subcommission on European Guidelines. *Acta Neurol Scand* 2002; **106**: 1–7.

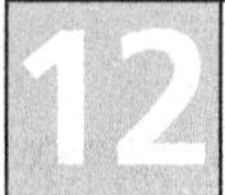

CASE 12

Psychogenic reaction during tilt-table testing

R. García Civera, R. Ruiz Granell, S. Morell Cabedo, R. Sanjuán Mañez

Case report

A 17-year-old boy was referred for evaluation after suffering multiple syncopal attacks. The patient had a congenital high-arched (ogival) palate, and in the previous 2 years he had presented with many symptoms (muscular and thoracic aches, weakness, nausea) and 19 syncopal episodes without triggers, warning, or trauma.

Multiple tests had been carried out because of the syncopal attacks (electrocardiography, echocardiography, Holter monitoring, cerebral magnetic resonance scanning, electroencephalography), but without diagnostic results. A previous tilt-table test without pharmacological challenge had also been negative. A year before admission, an electrophysiological study (EPS) had been carried out in another institution and a DDD pacemaker had been implanted because undetermined abnormal nodal conduction was found. The pacemaker implantation had not changed the frequency or characteristics of the syncopal episodes.

The results of physical examination, electrocardiography (ECG), carotid sinus massage, and orthostatic testing were normal. As the previous tilt test had been carried out without pharmacological challenge, a new tilt test with sublingual nitroglycerin provocation was scheduled. After the pacemaker had been programmed to VVI 30 beats/min, the patient was tilted to 60° and the heart rate and hemodynamic parameters were recorded using a Task Force Monitor (CNSystems Medizintechnik Ltd., Graz, Austria) (Fig. 12.1). After 18 min of passive tilting, the patient presented an apparent loss of consciousness (he suddenly shut his eyes, nodded off, and lay without responding to verbal stimuli). This event developed without any significant modification of the hemodynamic parameters (heart rate, blood pressure, cardiac output, etc). After 1 min, recovery of the patient was triggered by a painful stimulus. The tilt protocol was continued and sublingual nitroglycerin was administered without further events.

A psychiatric consultation was recommended, and a conversion disorder was the final diagnosis.

Comment

Psychogenic manifestations can be observed during the tilt-table test without significant hemodynamic changes [1–3]. These manifestations include apparent loss of consciousness, hypertonic states, convulsion, etc. This type of behavior during head-up tilt testing is most likely to be related to psychiatric disorders. In a study by Grubb *et al.* [1], there were no changes in the ECG or cerebral flux during these reactions. In addition, a psychogenic alteration was detected in all cases in the subsequent psychiatric evaluation.

The observed incidence of psychogenic reactions during tilt-table tests is 5.5% in adult patients [2] and 9% in children and adolescents between the ages of 7 and 18 [3].

According to van Dijk [4], there are three psychiatric disorders that resemble syncope: conversion reaction, factitious disorders, and malingering. In conversion disorders, patients show unexplained somatic symptoms, while psychological factors are also apparent. A "factitious disorder" means that the patient is intentionally pretending to be ill in order to assume the sick role. In "malingering," patients do the same, but in

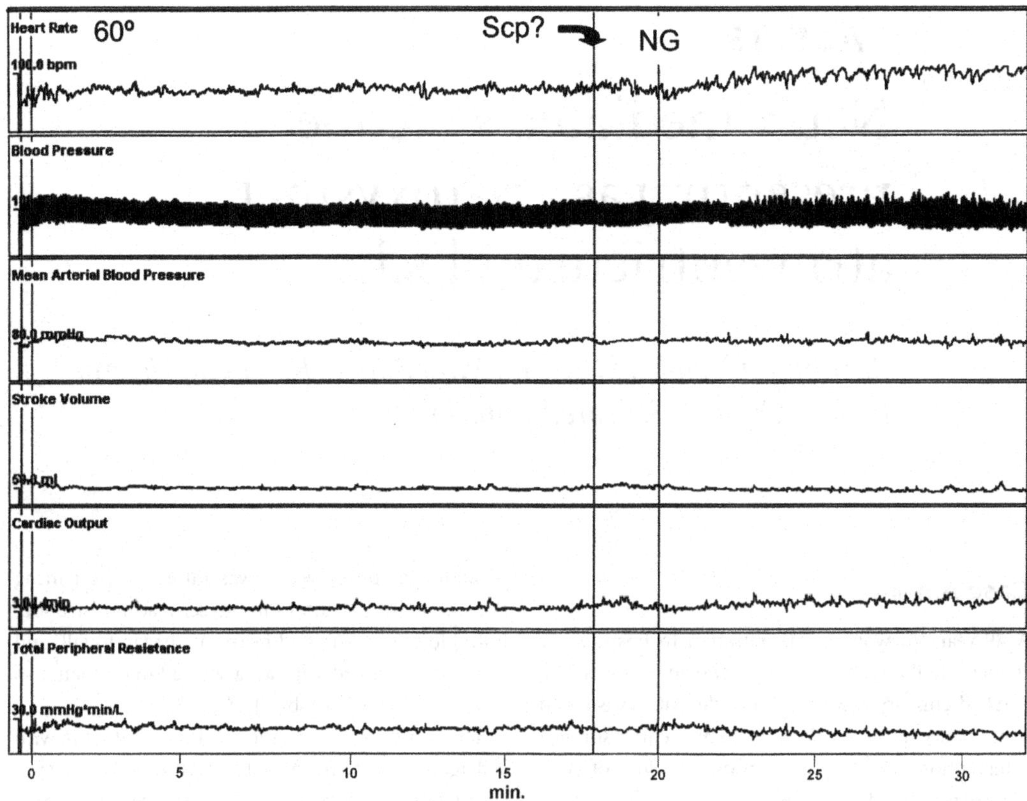

Figure 12.1 Task Force recordings during the tilt-table test. "Scp?" marks the moment of apparent loss of consciousness. NG, nitroglycerin.

order to gain some other advantage, such as avoiding a certain task or duty.

The most extreme case of psychiatric syncope is related to what is known as the Munchausen syndrome. This refers to a peculiar form of psychiatric illness in which patients go from hospital to hospital feigning serious medical illnesses. In a recent review of 58 published cases of Munchausen syndrome with cardiological complaints, syncope was the index symptom in three cases (5%) [5].

References

1 Grubb BP, Wolfe D, Gerard G. Syncope and seizures of psychogenic origin: identification with head up tilt testing. *Clin Cardiol* 1992; **15**: 834–42.

2 Petersen ME, Williams TR, Sutton R. Psychogenic syncope diagnosed by prolonged head-up tilt testing. *Q J Med* 1995; **88**: 209–13.

3 Kouakam C, Vaksmann G, Pachy E, Lacroix D, Rey C, Kacet S. Long-term follow-up of children and adolescents with syncope: predictor of syncope recurrence. *Eur Heart J* 2001; **17**: 1618–25.

4 van Dijk JG. Conditions that mimic syncope. In: Benditt D, Blanc JJ, Brignole M, Sutton R, eds. *The Evaluation and Treatment of Syncope.* Futura-Blackwell, Elmsford, New York, 2003: 184–200.

5 Metha NJ, Khan IA. Cardiac Munchausen syndrome. *Chest* 2002; **122**: 1649–53.

13

CASE 13

Neuromediated syncope presenting as a paroxysmal atrioventricular block

R. Sanjuán Mañez, L. Facila, M.L. Blasco, R. García Civera, R. Ruiz Granell, S. Morell Cabedo

Case report

A 49-year-old woman was admitted to hospital for transurethral resection of a vesical bladder mass. She had had a history of syncopal episodes with a vasovagal profile since the age of 17. After an uneventful surgical intervention, she had four episodes of loss of consciousness preceded by abdominal pain, discomfort, nausea, and vomiting during the convalescent period in the surgical ward. Myoclonic jerks were observed in one of the episodes. The episodes of unconsciousness were brief, with full recovery without sequelae. Electrocardiographic (ECG) monitoring of the last syncopal episode (Fig. 13.1) showed a paroxysmal complete atrioventricular (AV) block as the underlying rhythm. The patient was admitted to the intensive-care unit (ICU), where intravenous atropine was administered and a temporary pacemaker was inserted. The patient progressed satisfactorily in the ICU, with the sinus rhythm being maintained without new syncopal episodes. Cardiac investigations and ECG were normal.

Before discharge, a tilt-table test was carried out (Fig. 13.2). After an uneventful passive phase, 400 μg of sublingual nitroglycerin was administered. During the second minute after nitroglycerin administration, both blood pressure and heart rate began to fall, and syncope developed with an asystole longer than 15 s due to paroxysmal AV block (Fig. 13.3).

The patient was discharged without treatment, with a diagnosis of neuromediated cardioinhibitory syncope (Vasovagal Syncope International Study (VASIS) type 2b). She is still asymptomatic after a 2-year follow-up period.

Comment

The present case illustrates the possibility of paroxysmal AV block of neuromediated origin. The syncopal episodes were triggered by pain or discomfort after a urinary gallbladder intervention, and ECG monitoring during one of the episodes showed that the underlying rhythm was a paroxysmal AV block. Although arrhythmic syncope was considered, the clinical presentation of the syncopal episodes and the absence of intraventricular conduction defects in the basal ECG strongly suggested a neuromediated origin, and a tilt-table test

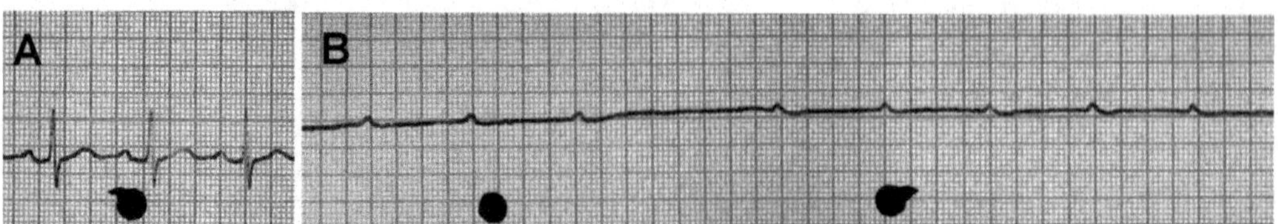

Figure 13.1 Electrocardiographic monitoring at baseline (A) and during a syncopal episode (B).

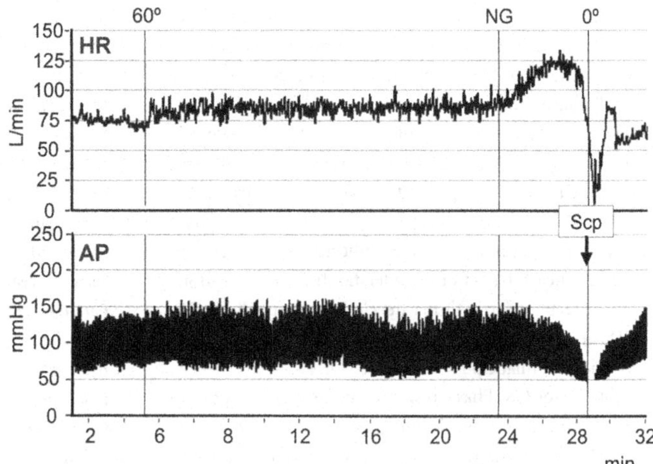

Figure 13.2 The head-up tilt-table test. HR, heart rate; AP, arterial pressure; NG, nitroglycerin; Scp, syncope.

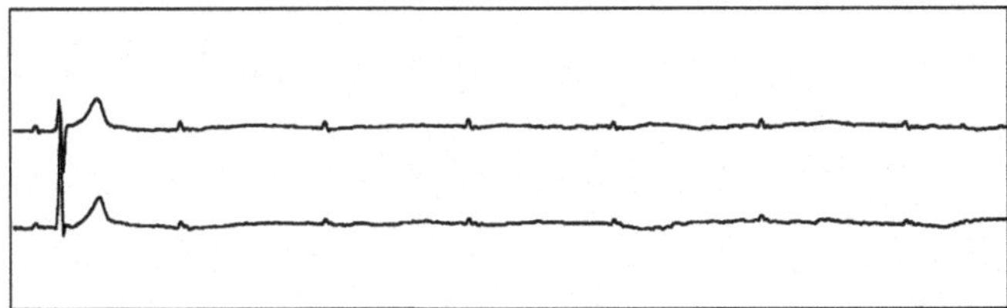

Figure 13.3 Asystole due to an atrioventricular block induced on tilting.

was conducted. During the test, the cardioinhibitory response due to the AV block was reproduced.

In the VASIS classification [1], a type 2b response (cardioinhibition with asystole) is considered to be present when "asystole occurs for more than 3 s and the blood-pressure fall coincides with or occurs before the heart-rate fall." The rhythm disturbance responsible for the asystole is not specified in the VASIS classification. The underlying heart rhythm is usually a prolonged sinus pause, but AV block occasionally supervenes. AV block during head-up tilt-table tests has been observed in 2.7% and 2.5% of positive cases in two series [2,3].

It is known that vagal discharge affects both the sinus node and AV node. However, it is not known why the vagal discharge can affect the AV node more in certain cases. Differences in the origin of the reflex, central integration, the intensity of the stimulus, the phase of the cardiac cycle, static and dynamic vagosympathetic interactions, or differences in neurohumoral responses could be responsible for the different types of cardiac response [4–7].

An adenosine triphosphate (ATP) test was not carried out in this case. The ATP test was initially introduced to identify vasovagal patients who were at high risk of a severe cardioinhibitory response [8]. Subsequent investigations suggested that the ATP test detects a special form of adenosine-sensitive AV block [9,10]. Although the patient populations identified by the ATP test and the head-up tilt-table test appear to be different [10], there is a certain amount of overlap, suggesting that a common pathophysiological mechanism is present.

In the present case, the usual therapeutic "reflex response" would be to implant a pacemaker. However, so far as we are aware, there have been no studies showing that this therapeutic approach is necessary or even better than a conventional strategy. A conservative attitude was chosen on this occasion, and the patient has remained asymptomatic during a 2-year follow-up period.

References

1 Brignole M, Menozzi C, Del Rosso A, *et al.* New classification of haemodynamics of vasovagal syncope: beyond the VASIS classification. Analysis of the presyncopal phase of the tilt test without and with nitroglycerin challenge. *Europace* 2000; 2: 66–76.

2 García Civera R, Sanjuán R, Ruíz R, *et al.* "Patrones" electrocardiográficos de cardioinhibición durantel las pruebas de basculación. Un estudio controlado con registros de Holter [abstract]. *Rev Esp Cardiol* 2001; **54** (Suppl 2): 133.

3 Del Rosso A, Bartoli P, Bartoletti A, *et al.* Shortened head-up tilt testing potentiated with sublingual nitroglycerin in patients with unexplained syncope. *Am Heart J* 1998; **135**: 564–70.

4 Zipes DP, Miyazaky T. The autonomic nervous system and the heart: basis to the understanding of interactions and effects on arrhythmia development. In: Zipes DP, Jalife J, eds. *Cardiac Electrophysiology: from Cell to Bedside.* Saunders, Philadelphia, 1990: 312–30.

5 Jalife J, Moe GK. Phasic responses of SA and AV nodes to vagal stimulation. In: Rosenbaum MB, Elizari MV, eds. *Frontiers of Cardiac Electrophysiology.* Nijhoff, Boston, 1983: 501–21.

6 Kawada T, Sugimachi M, Shishido T, *et al.* Simultaneous identification of static and dynamic vagosympathetic interactions in regulating heart rate. *Am J Physiol* 1999; **276**: R782–9.

7 Vanderheyden M, Goethals M, Nellens P, Andries E, Brugada P. Different humoral responses during head-up tilt testing among patients with neurocardiogenic syncope. *Am Heart J* 1998; **135**: 67–73.

8 Flammang D, Church T, Waynberger M, Chassing A, Antiel M. Can adenosine-5′-triphosphate be used to select treatment in severe vasovagal syndrome? *Circulation* 1997; **26**: 1201–8.

9 Brignole M, Gaggioli G, Menozzi C, *et al.* Adenosine-induced atrioventricular block in patients with unexplained syncope: the diagnostic value of ATP test. *Circulation* 1997; **96**: 3921–7.

10 Brignole M, Gaggioli G, Menozzi C, *et al.* Clinical features of adenosine sensitive syncope and tilt induced vasovagal syncope. *Heart* 2000; **83**: 24–8.

14

CASE 14

Multiple manifestations of the cardioinhibitory mechanism detected during prolonged electrocardiographic monitoring

C. Menozzi, N. Bottoni, F. Quartieri, G. Lolli

Case report

A 75-year-old man suffering from coronary artery disease who had undergone coronary bypass surgery 10 years earlier, with no previous myocardial infarction, no residual ischemia, and normal left ventricular systolic function, had had three syncopal episodes during the previous 2 years. Two syncopal episodes that had been witnessed occurred when he was in the sitting position, without prodromal symptoms or signs, were of short duration with rapid recovery, and the patient had amnesia following loss of consciousness. The third episode occurred while he was standing and was preceded for a few seconds by weakness and sweating. Apart from syncope, he was asymptomatic and felt well. He was not taking any medication except low-dose aspirin. Cardiac syncope was suspected, but a cardiological investigation, including standard electrocardiography, 24-h Holter monitoring, and a complete electrophysiological study, was negative.

As part of the reappraisal process, he underwent neurally mediated tests. Right carotid sinus massage in the upright position induced an asymptomatic sinus pause of 4 s. Tilt testing with nitroglycerin challenge induced syncope in association with marked hypotension and relative bradycardia at 65 beats/min. A diagnosis of neurally mediated syncope was therefore made.

An implantable loop recorder was inserted in December 2000 to assess the relative contribution of cardioinhibition and vasodepression before embarking on specific treatment. During the following 5 months, the patient remained free of clinical events, although he had 43 bradycardic episodes, mostly with long ventricular pauses (mean duration 8 ± 6 s) due to sinus arrest (Fig. 14.1), sinus bradycardia associated with atrioventricular (AV) block (Fig. 14.2), or paroxysmal atrial fibrillation with long ventricular pauses (Fig. 14.3). The episodes occurred at various times during the day, although they were more frequent during the night. At the end of this period, a dual-chamber permanent pacemaker was implanted. The patient has remained asymptomatic during the subsequent 11 months.

Comment

Typically, patients affected by neurally mediated syncope are event-free at the time of evaluation, and the opportunity to capture a spontaneous event during conventional diagnostic testing is rare. The natural history of these syndromes is therefore largely unknown. In one study [1], 74% of the patients affected by cardioinhibitory neurally mediated syncope had pauses > 3 s during a 15-month period of follow-up, but the vast majority of pauses with a duration of 3–6 s were asymptomatic.

The following issues of interest arise from this case report. The hidden (asymptomatic) part of the syndrome was largely predominant over the overt

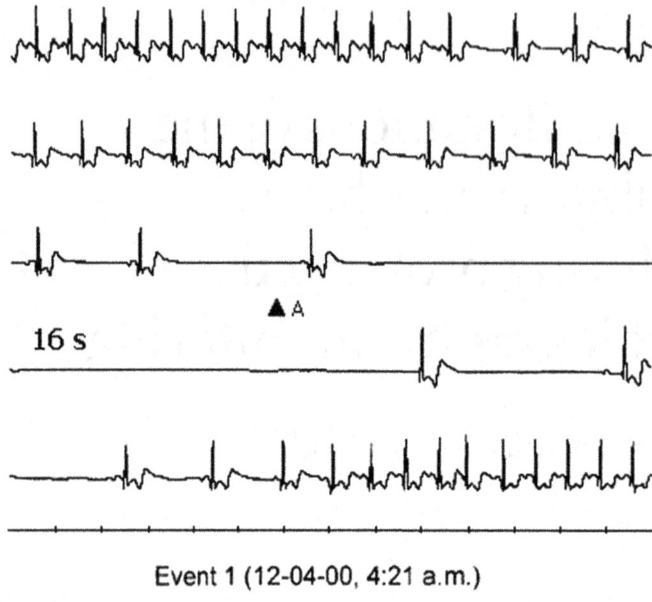

Figure 14.1 Implantable loop recorder tracing, showing sinus arrest. A, activation.

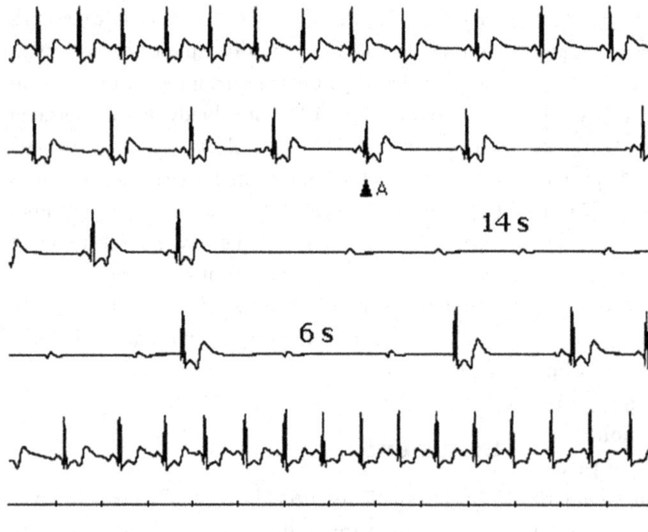

Figure 14.2 Implantable loop recorder tracing, showing an atrioventricular block. A, activation.

(symptomatic) part; this offers an explanation for the apparent paradox of a persistent disease (an abnormality of the autonomic nervous system) associated with an unpredictable clinical manifestation with a long period of absence of symptoms. The patient did not perceive symptoms, despite very prolonged ventricular pauses. A recent study [2] has shown that patients affected by neurally mediated syncope have mean asystolic periods of 17 s at the time of spontaneous syncope. The duration of asystole needed to cause syncope is thus much longer than is usually thought. The perception of symptoms may have been influenced by amnesia with loss of consciousness, which is observed in older adults in particular [3]. Moreover, although the episodes occurred at various times during the day, there is no information available

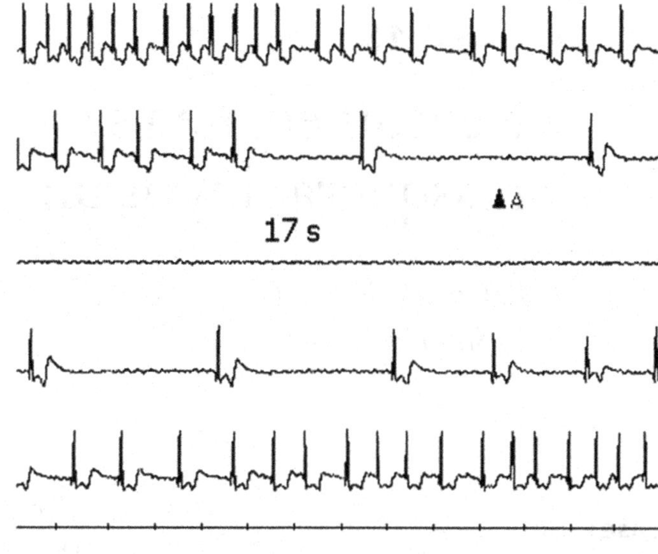

Figure 14.3 Implantable loop recorder tracing, showing atrial fibrillation with long ventricular pauses. A, activation.

about the circumstances (e.g., posture, activity, etc.) that might have influenced cerebral hypoperfusion during the event. A variety of rhythm disturbances were recorded—i.e., sinus arrest, AV block, and paroxysmal atrial fibrillation with long pauses; some episodes at the same time showed marked sinus bradycardia associated with AV block. Thus, the effect of an abnormal reflex on the cardiac target organ is variable over time. This observation definitely rules out a major role of intrinsic disease of the cardiac conduction system in the genesis of the episodes.

References

1 Menozzi C, Brignole M, Lolli G, *et al.* Follow-up of asystolic episodes in patients with cardioinhibitory, neurally mediated syncope and VVI pacemaker. *Am J Cardiol* 1993; **72**: 1152–5.

2 Moya A, Brignole M, Menozzi C, *et al.* The mechanism of syncope in patients with isolated syncope and in patients with tilt-positive syncope. *Circulation* 2001; **104**: 1261–7.

3 Kenny RA, Traynor G. Carotid sinus syndrome: clinical characteristics in elderly patients. *Age Ageing* 1991; **20**: 449–54.

15

CASE 15

Neuromediated syncope masquerading as unexplained falls

R. García Civera, R. Ruiz Granell, S. Morell Cabedo, R. Sanjuán Mañez

Case report

A 68-year-old woman was referred for cardiovascular evaluation from the neurology department after three unexplained falls in the previous month. The patient had mild hypertension, which was being treated with valsartan. The patient did not remember anything about the falls (she only remembered finding herself lying on the floor without apparent cause). She had suffered a shoulder fracture during the last fall.

The physical examination was normal. The electrocardiogram (ECG) showed a sinus rhythm at 80 beats /min, a PR interval of 0.18 s, and a QRS with normal morphology. Right and left carotid sinus massage was carried out with the patient in both the supine and upright positions (head-up tilt to 60°), with normal responses. Orthostatic stress tests were also normal. A two-dimensional echocardiogram and Doppler studies documented normal cardiac chambers and preserved ventricular function (left ventricular ejection fraction of 59%). A 24-h Holter recording showed a sinus rhythm between 57 and 147 beats/min (mean 80 beats/min) and occasional ventricular ectopic beats.

A tilt-table test with sublingual nitroglycerin challenge was carried out (Fig. 15.1). In the fifth minute after nitroglycerin administration, both blood pressure and heart rate fell and syncope occurred (positive tilt-table test, Vasovagal Syncope International Study classification type 1).

Vasovagal syncope with amnesia for the episode was suspected to be the cause of the falls. However, to obtain a symptom–rhythm correlation, a Reveal

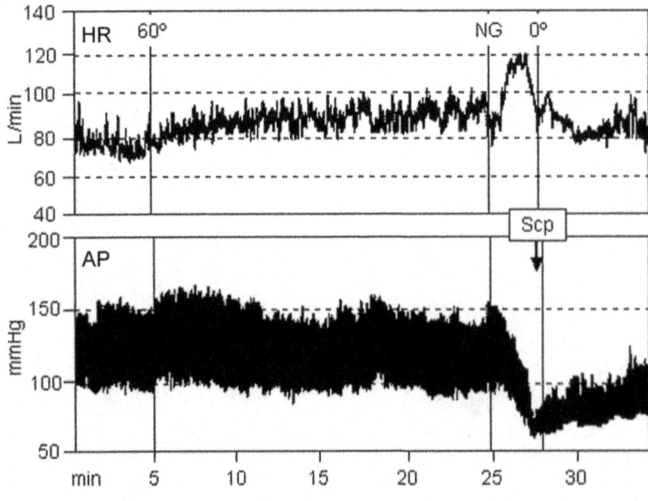

Figure 15.1 The head-up tilt test. HR, heart rate; AP, arterial pressure; NG, nitroglycerin; Scp, syncope.

implantable loop recorder (ILR) (Medtronic Inc., Minneapolis, Minnesota, USA) was implanted. The patient remained asymptomatic during an 8-month follow-up period after ILR implantation.

Comment

Falls are common in the elderly general population. Thirty percent of individuals over the age of 65 who live at home suffer falls each year [1], and 2–6% of the falls result in fractures. A significant proportion of falls after which the patients present to the emergency department are considered to be nonaccidental or unexplained falls. There is evidence of considerable overlap between unexplained falls, drop attacks, and syncope in elderly patients [2–6]. Cardiovascular syncope appears to be the principal cause of unexplained falls and drop attacks. Several studies by the Newcastle group have found a high prevalence of carotid sinus hypersensitivity (CSH) of the cardioinhibitory type among patients over the age of 50 presenting to an emergency room due to an unexplained fall [2–4], but falls can also be due to other causes such as orthostatic hypotension [3] or neuromediated syncope [6].

In the present case, the carotid sinus massage administered in both the supine and upright positions produced a normal response, excluding CSH as the cause of the falls. On the other hand, the positive response to the tilt-table test suggested that vasovagal syncope was the cause [3,6]. An ILR was implanted to obtain a symptom–rhythm correlation, but the patient remained asymptomatic during the 8-month follow-up period (suggesting a possible placebo effect of the Reveal device).

References

1 Tinetti ME, Speechley M, Ginter SF. Risk factors for falls among elderly patients living in the community. *N Engl J Med* 1988; **319**: 1701–7.

2 Shaw FS, Kenny RA. The overlap between falls and syncope in the elderly. *Postgrad Med J* 1997; **72**: 635–9.

3 Dey AB, Stout NR, Kenny RA. Cardiovascular syncope is the most common cause of drop attacks in the elderly. *Pacing Clin Electrophysiol* 1997; **20**: 818–9.

4 Richardson DA, Bexton RS, Shaw F, Kenny RA. Prevalence of cardioinhibitory carotid sinus hypersensitivity in patients over 50 years presenting to the accident and emergency department with unexplained and recurrent falls. *Pacing Clin Electrophysiol* 1997; **20**: 820–3.

5 Kenny RA, Richardson DA, Steen N, Bexton RS, Shaw F, Bond J. Carotid sinus syndrome: a modifiable risk factor for nonaccidental falls in older adults (SAFE PACE). *J Am Coll Cardiol* 2001; **38**: 1491–6.

6 Parry SW, Kenny RA. Vasovagal syncope masquerading as unexplained falls in an older patient. *Can J Cardiol* 2002; 7: 757–8.

16

CASE 16

Post-exercise vasovagal syncope

C.T.P. Krediet, A.A.M. Wilde, J.R. Halliwill, W. Wieling

Case report

A 28-year-old male firefighter in excellent general condition lost consciousness transiently after completing a routine check-up exercise test [1]. The episode occurred while he was sitting motionless on the bicycle ergometer after the test and his skinfold thickness was being measured. The patient was declared unfit for his job. The patient was referred to our syncope unit for further analysis of the episode.

The exercise test was repeated using continuous noninvasive blood-pressure monitoring. Figure 16.1 shows the original continuous blood pressure and instantaneous heart rate tracing.

After cycling at 175 W, the patient was asked to sit upright briefly and then stand for several minutes. As can be seen, his blood pressure and heart rate declined over several minutes in the upright position, leading to an eventual post-exertion vasovagal response with obvious bradycardia and hypotension. The subject was then placed in the supine position, and pressure subsequently recovered quickly. The patient recognized the symptoms. The exercise test was repeated once again. This time, the patient was told to keep moving after the test, and syncope did not occur. Post-exercise vasovagal syncope was diagnosed. The patient was reassured about the nature of his problem and was advised to avoid standing motionless after heavy exercise. Since his episodes occurred only during a predictable provocation—i.e., motionless sitting/standing—and he experienced clear preceding symptoms, we declared the patient fit for work as a

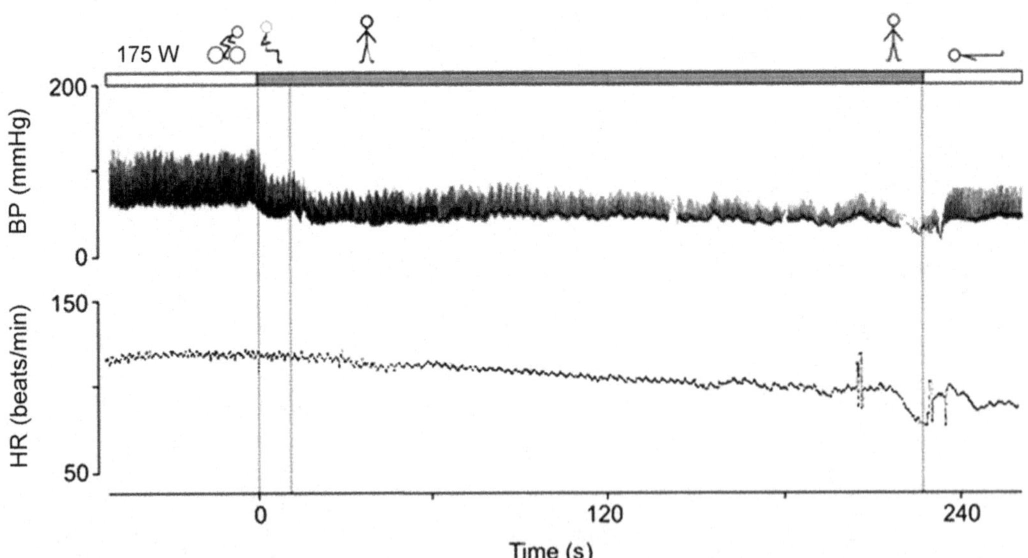

Figure 16.1 Instantaneous changes in heart rate and blood pressure in the fingers induced by free standing after submaximal bicycle exercise. BP, blood pressure; HR, heart rate.

firefighter. During a 5-year follow-up period, he has had no further episodes of syncope.

Comment

The majority of cases of syncope occurring after exercise fall into two related categories: firstly, an exaggerated form of the normal post-exercise hypotension response; and secondly, neurally mediated syncope (i.e., vasovagal reactions). It is probable that the former triggers the latter [1].

Post-exercise hypotension

During post-exercise hypotension (PEH), the mechanisms that regulate arterial pressure drive a modest but sustained reduction in arterial pressure. The cause of PEH is twofold, involving both neural and local vascular mechanisms [2,3]. In comparison with rest, PEH is characterized by a persistent drop in systemic vascular resistance that is not completely offset by increases in cardiac output [2,3]. The vasodilation that underlies PEH is not restricted to the sites of active skeletal muscles, but involves inactive regions as well. The associated rise in arterial blood inflow through the vasodilated regions contributes to an increase in venous pooling of blood.

During exercise, rhythmically contracting skeletal muscles in the lower part of the body reduce the degree of venous pooling by squeezing veins—in effect, pumping blood back to the heart. This phenomenon is known as the "muscle pump." This "pump" is absent during passive recovery from exercise. The increase in venous pooling, in conjunction with the loss of plasma volume associated with exercise, leads to a reduction in central venous pressure ($\approx$ 2 mmHg supine) and cardiac filling [3,4]. Despite this fall in cardiac preload, stroke volume is maintained due to the reduction in cardiac afterload and a probable increase in cardiac contractility [2,4]. The net result of these influences on the blood vessels and heart is that cardiac output is elevated (heart rate is higher with unchanged stroke volume). Thus, PEH is due to a persistent drop in systemic vascular resistance that is not completely offset by increases in cardiac output.

The main point is that PEH is common after moderate-intensity dynamic exercise. In general, this is a benign process, and in the majority of individuals PEH is insufficient to cause syncopal symptoms.

The magnitude of PEH can be exaggerated in the seated or standing positions (compared to supine) [2–5], and arterial pressure may fall to the level at which presyncopal signs or symptoms occur.

Neurally mediated syncope after exercise

It appears that the underlying mechanism for neurally mediated syncope occurring after the termination of exercise is similar to that of PEH. The sudden removal of the muscle-pump activity, decreasing cardiac preload, may be a trigger, along with a rapid return of vagal tone to the heart when exercise stops [1].

Characteristically, these events occur while the individual is standing motionless during the first 5–10 min after exercise [5,6]. Individuals rapidly recover in the supine position. It has been estimated that the incidence rate of neurally mediated syncope after routine treadmill testing may be in the order of 0.3–3.0% [7]. However, when treadmill testing is immediately followed by passive head-up tilt testing, this percentage can increase up to 50–70% [7,8]. Neurally mediated syncope after exercise is considered to be a benign occurrence [1].

In a tiny minority of cases of syncope during exercise and exertion, the vasovagal reaction is thought to be the underlying pathophysiological mechanism [1]. The way in which the reaction is triggered in these conditions remains to be elucidated [1,9]. Nausea is a commonly reported symptom before such episodes, and the following mechanisms may be involved:

- Supraphysiological stimulation of ventricular mechanoreceptors in the left ventricle, especially when cardiac filling is decreased at a high heart rate, is thought to be a trigger for vasovagal reactions (i.e., the Bezold–Jarisch hypothesis) [10]. Abrahamsson and Thoren reported the observation that this type of stimulation also leads to reflex gastric dilation and eventual vomiting in the cat [11]. However, many dispute the Bezold–Jarisch hypothesis, as evidence for the existence of ventricular mechanoreceptors in humans is lacking [10]. The newly discovered mechanoreceptors in the coronaries of the dog could provide an alternative explanation for the results that were once thought to demonstrate the existence of the ventricular mechanoreceptors [12].
- Using pancreatic polypeptide as a measure for vagal activity in humans, Holmqvist *et al.* showed that abdominal vagal activity increases during maximal exercise, reaching its highest values after exertion [13].

They suggest that high vagal outflow of this type may also cause nausea.

Although patients suffering from "vasovagal syncope during exercise" have been studied intensively, there are no objective observations of this type of loss of consciousness during exercise. This raises the question of whether this disease truly exists as a separate entity. If not, this form of syncope could actually be the same as vasovagal syncope occurring after exercise, only differing in the time between stopping and loss of consciousness. In cases in which this takes place within a certain amount of time, patients will be inclined to report that consciousness was lost during exercise, when in fact it happened shortly afterwards. The importance of detailed history-taking in these cases is beyond doubt.

Syncope related to exercise may be the first indication of a dangerous underlying cardiovascular condition. The aim of the initial diagnostic work-up in patients presenting with exercise-related syncope is to exclude such conditions.

Acknowledgment

Parts of this case were previously published in *Clinical Autonomic Research* [1]. We are grateful to Springer Verlag (Darmstadt, Germany) for permission to reprint.

References

1 Krediet CT, Wilde AA, Wieling W, Halliwill JR. Exercise related syncope: when it's not the heart. *Clin Auton Res* 2004; **14** (Suppl 1): 25–36.

2 Kenney MJ, Seals DR. Postexercise hypotension: key features, mechanisms, and clinical significance. *Hypertension* 1993; **22**: 653–64.

3 Halliwill JR. Mechanisms and clinical implications of post-exercise hypotension in humans. *Exerc Sport Sci Rev* 2001; **29**: 65–70.

4 Halliwill JR, Minson CT, Joyner MJ. Effect of systemic nitric oxide synthase inhibition on postexercise hypotension in humans. *J Appl Physiol* 2000; **89**: 1830–6.

5 Bjurstedt H, Rosenhamer G, Balldin U, Katkov V. Orthostatic reactions during recovery from exhaustive exercise of short duration. *Acta Physiol Scand* 1983; **119**: 25–31.

6 Tsutsumi E, Hara H. Syncope after running. *Br Med J* **1979; ii**: 1480.

7 Holtzhausen LM, Noakes TD. The prevalence and significance of post-exercise (postural) hypotension in ultramarathon runners. *Med Sci Sports Exerc* 1995; **27**: 1595–1601.

8 Sakaguchi S, Shultz JJ, Remole SC, Adler SW, Lurie KG, Benditt DG. Syncope associated with exercise: a manifestation of neurally mediated syncope. *Am J Cardiol* 1995; **75**: 476–81.

9 Krediet CT, Wilde AA, Halliwill JR, Wieling W. Syncope during exercise, documented with continuous blood pressure monitoring during ergometer testing. *Clin Auton Res* 2005; **15**: 59–62.

10 Hainsworth R. Syncope: what is the trigger? *Heart* 2003; **89**: 123–4.

11 Abrahamsson H, Thoren P. Vomiting and reflex vagal relaxation of the stomach elicited from heart receptors in the cat. *Acta Physiol Scand* 1973; **88**: 433–9.

12 Wright CI, Drinkhill MJ, Hainsworth R. Responses to stimulation of coronary and carotid baroreceptors and the coronary chemoreflex at different ventricular distending pressures in anaesthetised dogs. *Exp Physiol* 2001; **86**: 381–90.

13 Holmqvist N, Secher NH, Sander-Jensen K, Knigge U, Warberg J, Schwartz TW. Sympathoadrenal and parasympathetic responses to exercise. *J Sports Sci* 1986; **4**: 123–8.

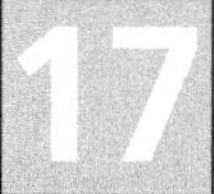

CASE 17

Post-exercise neuromediated syncope

R. García Civera, R. Ruiz Granell, S. Morell Cabedo, R. Sanjuán Mañez

Case report

A 26-year-old man who was a long-distance runner was referred for evaluation of syncope associated with effort. He had experienced two syncopal episodes after the end of two competitive races. He had no history of heart disease or hypertension, and the physical examination and electrocardiogram were normal. A two-dimensional echocardiogram study documented normal cardiac chambers with normal left ventricular function. On exercise testing, he tolerated a maximum Bruce protocol without any abnormal events.

A head-up tilt test was carried out using the Task Force Monitor (CNSystems Medizintechnik Ltd., Graz, Austria) (Fig. 17.1). At minute 16 of the passive tilting phase, peripheral resistance and blood pressure began to fall, and syncope developed 1 min later, with an asystolic pause of 20 s (Fig. 17.2). Figure 17.3 shows the trend of autonomic changes during the tilt test. With tilting to 60°, sympathetic tone rises slowly and then stabilizes while vagal tone falls. Shortly before the syncope, there is a mild decrease in sympathetic tone.

Empirical beta-blocker treatment was scheduled, and the patient was able to return to competitive activity without syncopal attacks.

Comment

Effort syncope is infrequent. In a study of 337 patients with syncope [1], 17 patients (5%) had syncope during

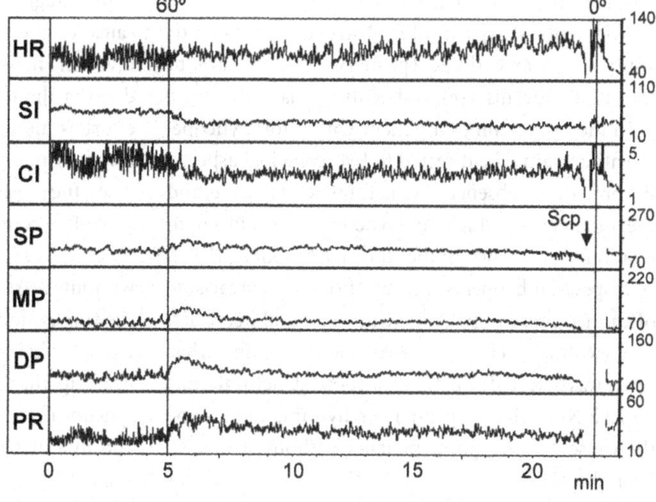

Figure 17.1 The hemodynamic trend during the head-up tilt-table test. HR, heart rate; SI, stroke index; CI, cardiac index; SP, systolic pressure; MP, mean pressure; DP, diastolic pressure; PR, peripheral resistance. Scp indicates the moment of syncope.

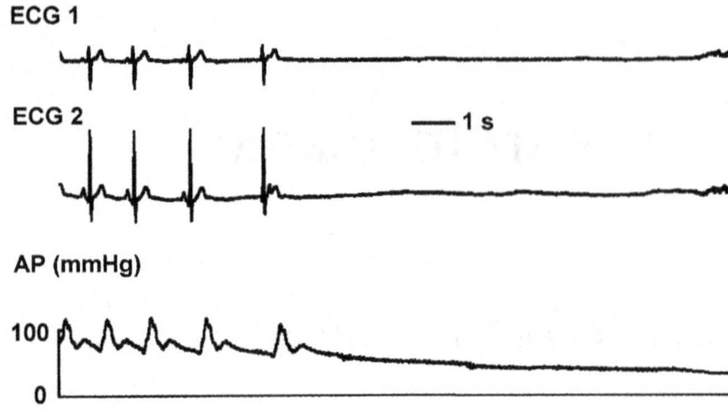

Figure 17.2 In minute 17 of passive tilting, syncope developed, with an asystolic pause of 20 s. ECG, electrocardiography; AP, arterial pressure.

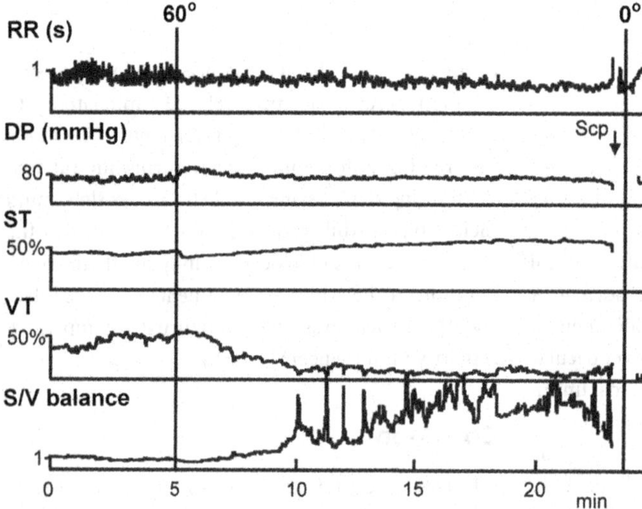

Figure 17.3 Autonomic changes during the head-up tilt test. RR, RR interval; DP, diastolic blood pressure; ST, sympathetic tone; VT, vagal tone; S/V balance, ratio between sympathetic and vagal tone. Scp indicates the moment of syncope.

effort and seven (3%) post-effort. There are three main mechanisms underlying effort syncope: obstructive (aortic stenosis, hypertrophic obstructive cardiomyopathy, etc.); arrhythmic (primary or secondary to structural heart disease); and neuromediated.

In the evaluation of a patient with effort syncope, attention should be directed to two principal aspects: the presence or absence of structural heart disease, and the moment at which the syncope is produced in relation to the effort. In the study by Alboni *et al.* [1], syncopes that happened during effort were invariably of cardiac cause in patients with structural heart disease (with a specificity of 96%), while a noncardiac cause was detected in patients without structural heart disease. Nevertheless, primary arrhythmia can also be the cause of syncope in patients without structural heart disease.

In patients with neuromediated syncope during effort, exaggerated vasodilation [2,3] appears to be the cause of the syncope, which generally has a course involving marked hypotension and without bradycardia. On the other hand, syncope that happens after effort is almost invariably due to a neuromediated mechanism or to autonomic failure [4], and, in these cases, the presence of hypotension with bradycardia or asystole is common.

Several recent reports have shown that, in patients without heart disease who have post-effort syncope, the conventional effort tests have poor sensitivity and reproducibility for inducing syncope [5,6]. Conversely, head-up tilt tests show a high rate of induction of syncope in these cases [7, 8]. In the general population and in athletes, the prognosis of post-effort syncope is good.

References

1 Alboni P, Brignole M, Menozzi C, *et al.* Diagnostic value of history in patients with syncope with or without heart disease. *J Am Coll Cardiol* 2001; **37**: 1921–8.
2 Sneddon J, Scalia G, Ward D, McKenna W, Camm AJ, Frenneaux M. Exercise induced vasodepressor syncope. *Br Heart J* 1994; **71**: 554–7.
3 Thomson HL, Atherton JJ, Khafagi FA, Frenneaux MP. Failure of reflex venoconstriction during exercise in patients with vasovagal syncope. *Circulation* 1996; **93**: 953–9.
4 Smith GPD, Mathias CJ. Postural hypotension enhanced by exercise in patients with chronic autonomic failure. *Q J Med* 1995; **88**: 251–6.
5 Calkins H, Seifert M, Morady F. Clinical presentation and long term follow-up of athletes with exercise-induced vasodepressor syncope. *Am Heart J* 1995; **129**: 1159–64.
6 Colivicchi F, Ammirati F, Biffi A, Verdile L, Pelliccia A, Santini M. Exercise-related syncope in young competitive athletes without evidence of structural heart disease: clinical presentation and long-term outcome. *Eur Heart J* 2002; **23**: 1125–30.
7 Grub BP, Temsy-Armos P, Samoil D, Wolfe D, Hahn H, Elliot L. Tilt table testing in the evaluation and management of athletes with recurrent exercise-induced syncope. *Med Sci Sports Exerc* 1993; **25**: 24–8.
8 Sakaguchi S, Schultz J, Remole S, Adler S, Lurie K, Benditt DG. Syncope associated with exercise: a manifestation of neurally-mediated syncope. *Am J Cardiol* 1995; **75**: 476–81.

18

CASE 18

Vasovagal syncope interrupting sleep

C.T.P. Krediet, D.L. Jardine, P. Cortelli, A.G.R. Visman, W. Wieling

Case report

A female patient had her first nocturnal syncopal episode at the age of 40. After having slept for a few hours, she woke up during the night aware of nausea, abdominal discomfort, and an urge to defecate. She lost consciousness while supine. She sweated profusely, but did not bite her tongue. Her husband observed transient myoclonic jerking. After this, similar episodes occurred regularly (at least one per month) and only at night. The syncopal episodes never lasted longer than 1 min and were atraumatic. She was incontinent of urine and feces on one occasion. A tilt test provoked a vasovagal reaction followed by 7 s of asystole and reproduced her nocturnal symptoms. Due to continuing symptoms, she underwent neurological investigations, and a typical nocturnal episode was recorded during constant electroencephalography (EEG) and electrocardiography (ECG) monitoring (Fig. 18.1).

The EEG was judged to be normal by two independent neurologists. However, the ECG showed pronounced bradycardia (36 beats/min) during the episode, with an atrioventricular node escape rhythm. When the patient was aged 44, a permanent dual-chamber pacemaker was implanted, and she reported less syncope but continuing episodes of nocturnal presyncope with abdominal discomfort [1].

Comment

At three syncope units worldwide, we have seen 13 patients (10 women) with nocturnal episodes similar to those in the present patient. They all gave a history of waking up at night with nausea and an urge to defecate. In some patients, syncope occurred in bed; in others, it happened immediately after they left the bed in an effort to reach the toilet. The syncope was of short duration and often accompanied by profuse sweating. After regaining consciousness, most patients felt very weak and could not remain upright, but were orientated. Bradycardia was documented in five patients. The frequency of attacks varied from weekly to annually, and there was no relation with menstruation or alcohol consumption. Three patients reported nightmares immediately before the episode. Some patients had learned to partly avert the episodes by remaining supine in bed. Nine patients also had daytime syncopal and presyncopal episodes associated with vasovagal symptoms.

Tilt-table testing was carried out in 11 patients and was positive in seven, with typical prodromal symptoms. A significant cardioinhibitory reaction (asystole > 3 s) was recorded in four of these seven patients. The possibility of organic cardiac or cerebral pathology as a cause of the episodes was excluded by appropriate additional testing. Interictal EEG in seven patients revealed epileptiform activity in one.

It was concluded that the patient in this report and all of the other patients described have nocturnal vasovagal syncope as the primary cause of their symptoms. Although the attacks start when the patient is supine, the associated symptoms described are typical of vasovagal syncope. These include nausea, sweating, light-headedness, abdominal discomfort, and weakness during the attack, followed by tiredness afterwards. Because the attacks occur at night in bed, epilepsy is often diagnosed, especially if muscle jerking is observed. However, it should be realized that tran-

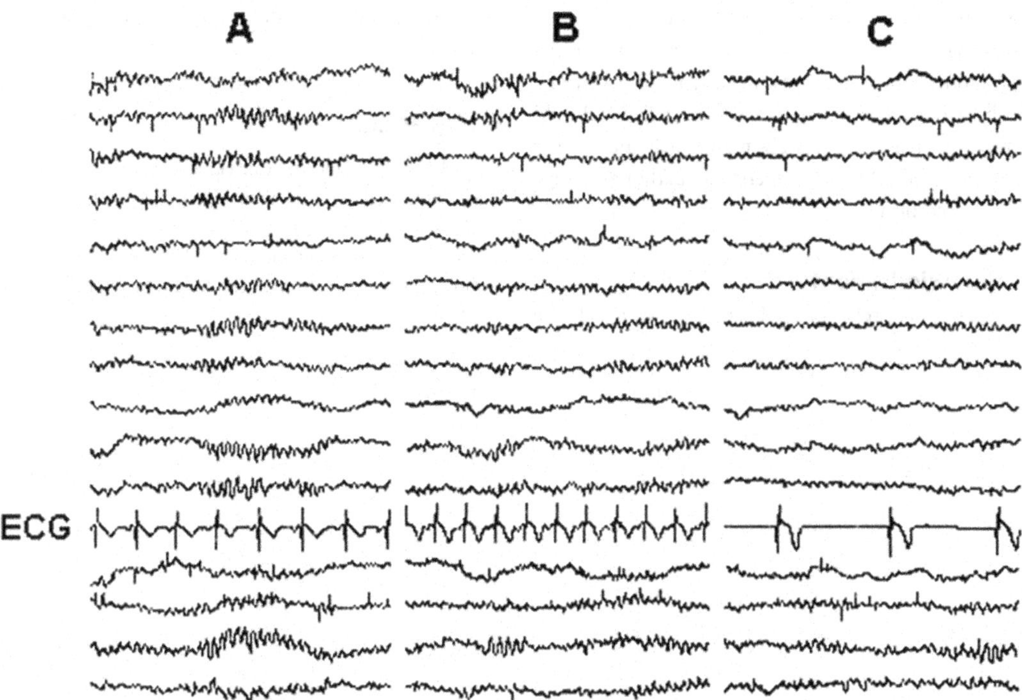

Figure 18.1 Simultaneous electroencephalography (EEG) and electrocardiography (ECG) recordings preceding and during a typical nocturnal episode. The arrangement consists of four sets of channels running anterior to posterior, with recording from the right parasagittal, left parasagittal, right temporal, and left temporal areas, respectively. **A.** Time 5:49 a.m., normal sleep EEG, heart rate 90 beats/min. **B.** Time 5:50 a.m., EEG unchanged, heart rate 126 beats/min. **C.** Time 5:52 a.m. (after calling for the nurse). The patient was lying supine in bed unable to move; the EEG was unchanged and the heart rate was 36 beats/min. The patient was pale and sweating profusely.

sient myoclonic jerking is more often a feature of cerebral hypoperfusion than epilepsy (see Case 11). Other more reliable features of epilepsy, including tongue-biting, postictal confusion, and hypersomnolence, are absent. On the basis of an algorithm derived from a study of patient-history criteria that distinguish syncope from seizures [2], all of our patients fulfilled the diagnostic criteria for vasovagal syncope with very high levels of certainty (> 90%). In addition, we have demonstrated a normal EEG during a typical nocturnal episode in one patient and normal interictal EEGs in 46% of the group.

The association with nightmares is suggestive of a central trigger similar to the mechanism proposed for vasovagal syncope associated with phobias. Syncope is occasionally triggered by bowel evacuation or colonoscopy, and has been induced reliably by inflating rectal balloons. Thus, the predominance of pronounced gastrointestinal symptoms associated with these attacks would suggest a gastrointestinal trigger mechanism. Because there was no association with the consumption of spicy food or alcohol, nor were there any symptoms of gastroenteritis, we consider that abdominal discomfort is more likely to be an effect of vagal overactivity, rather than the cause. The prominent cardioinhibitory response during tilt-table testing suggests a cardiovascular autonomic imbalance, which may also occur during sleep.

Based on these observations, we believe that patients who have nocturnal loss of consciousness and classical vasovagal prodromal symptoms should be considered to have true vasovagal syncope. A positive tilt-table test can support this diagnosis, as the test's sensitivity is low. Long QT and Brugada syndromes should be excluded by ECG. Mastocytosis should also sometimes be excluded.

Patients with nocturnal vasovagal syncope should not be treated with antiepileptic agents. If long-term outpatient ECG monitoring shows pronounced bradycardia or asystole, a pacemaker may improve the symptoms. However, as vasovagal syncope is believed to be a relatively benign condition, patients should initially be reassured and given an explanation of the known, but as yet poorly understood, pathophysiology of the condition.

Acknowledgment

This case was previously published in *Heart* [1]. We are grateful to the BMJ Publishing Group for permission to reprint.

References

1 Krediet CT, Jardine DL, Cortelli P, Visman AG, Wieling W. Vasovagal syncope interrupting sleep? *Heart* 2004; **90**: e25.
2 Sheldon R, Rose S, Ritchie D, *et al.* Historical criteria that distinguish syncope from seizures. *J Am Coll Cardiol* 2002; **40**: 142–8.

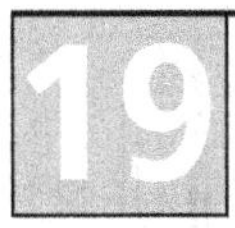

CASE 19
Syncope during pregnancy

A. Moya i Mitjans, C. Alonso

Case report

A 28-year-old woman with no history of previous diseases was sent to our syncope unit due to recurrent syncopal episodes. She reported that 5 years previously, during her first pregnancy, she had had multiple syncopal episodes. The first appeared in the 24th gestational week. All of the episodes were of sudden onset, always while she was standing, and on one occasion she suffered a nonsevere injury. After delivery, she had remained totally asymptomatic for 5 years until the new syncopal episode. Because of the new episode, she had suspected she was pregnant again, and a pregnancy test had proved positive. After this syncope, new syncopal episodes occurred, recurring at a rate of more than one a week. There were no clear triggers; the episodes had minimal prodromal symptoms, always occurred while she was standing, and she did not experience seizures, injury, or urinary incontinence.

The physical examination was normal, without cardiac murmurs. Her arterial blood pressure was 130/70 mmHg in the supine position and 110/79 mmHg after standing up. The baseline electrocardiogram was normal. Twenty-four-hour electrocardiographic monitoring was carried out, and there were no symptoms during the recording time. The trace showed a normal sinus rhythm with a mean heart rate of 103 beats/min, ranging between 59 and 169. An echocardiogram did not show any abnormalities.

Due to the recurrent syncope, a tilt test was carried out, which was positive at minute 13 during the drug-free phase, with a mixed response (Vasovagal Syncope International Study classification type 1) (Fig. 19.1).

The mechanism of syncope was explained to the patient, and advice was given on some general measures for avoiding it, such as increasing the fluid intake and avoiding prolonged standing. Despite these initial measures, the patient continued to have syncopal recurrences. As she had shown a trend toward sinus tachycardia in both the Holter recording and the tilt-table test, beta-blockers were initially indicated. She started with 25 mg of atenolol per day, subsequently increased to 50 mg, without any improvement. Beta-blocker administration was therefore stopped.

As the recurrences were still continuing, we suggested a short trial of tilt training. The first tilt in the program was also positive, with the same pattern as in the initial test, and on the second day, the patient had a spontaneous syncopal episode when she arrived at the syncope unit, immediately before the tilt test was conducted. As she was in the syncope unit, she was monitored, and severe hypotension with bradycardia was documented. The tilt training was therefore stopped. At this point the patient was in the 34th week of pregnancy. She was advised to avoid the standing position as much as possible, and delivery was advanced and took place in the 35th week without any complications.

After delivery, the patient had no further syncopal episodes, and she has been followed up for more than a year without any more symptoms. She has been advised not to become pregnant again.

Comment

Dizziness and syncope have been reported late in pregnancy in up to 10% of women [1]. The syncope usually occurs when patients adopt the supine or sitting position [2] and is relieved when they move to the left lateral position. This phenomenon has been related to inferior vena cava occlusion by the gravid uterus [2].

However, other mechanisms of syncope have also been recognized during pregnancy. Patients with a

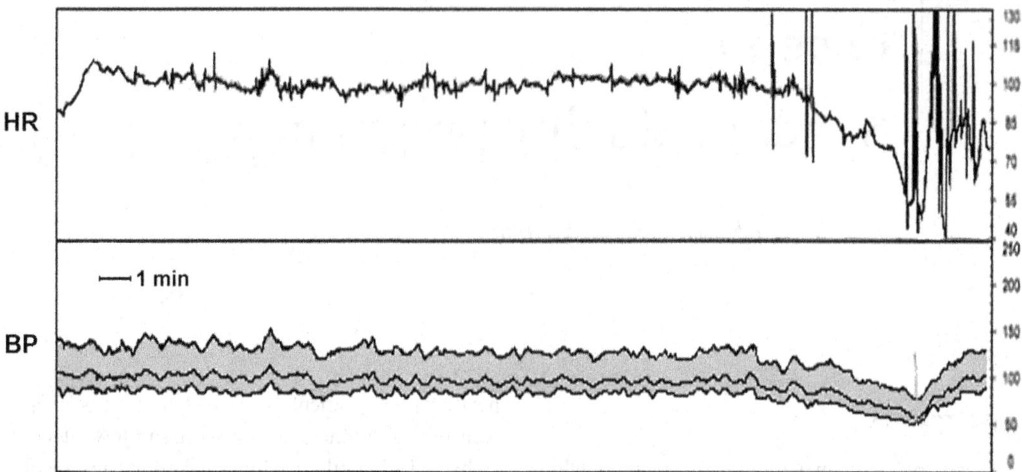

Figure 19.1 Response to the tilt test. At baseline, the resting heart rate was 80 beats/min. Immediately after tilting, the heart rate increased to 115 beats/min, and remained at approximately 100 beats/min during the first 10 min, after which arterial blood pressure and heart rate began to decrease progressively, with syncope, reproducing the spontaneous episodes. The patient was immediately switched to the Trendelenburg position, and she recovered consciousness with normalization of arterial blood pressure. HR, heart rate; BP, blood pressure.

long QT syndrome can have an increased risk of malignant ventricular arrhythmias during pregnancy, leading to syncopal episodes [3,4]. The development of new-onset ventricular tachycardias has also been described in patients without previous arrhythmias causing syncope [5,6]. It has also been reported that, in patients with complete atrioventricular (AV) block, syncopal symptoms can increase during pregnancy [7].

This is the second patient we have seen with syncopal episodes only during pregnancy. Both patients were characterized by the fact that syncopal episodes started early in the course of the pregnancy. This patient in particular first became aware of the pregnancy due to a recurrent episode of syncope. In these patients, none of the above mechanisms appears to be the cause of syncope, since the syncopal episodes started very early in their pregnancies and also always occurred when they were in the standing position, never when they were supine or sitting. In addition, syncope was induced by the tilt test, reproducing their syncopal episodes, and it was possible to record the arterial blood pressure and pulse during a spontaneous episode. Primary arrhythmia was therefore also excluded.

The mechanism of syncope cannot be clearly determined in this patient, but it may be suspected that the hormonal and volume changes that occur during pregnancy may favor the development of neuromediated syncope, as the syncopal episodes were easily reproducible with the tilt test, without any drug challenge.

Due to the high rate of recurrences, it was decided to provide treatment, and beta-blockers were selected as a first choice, as they have proved to be relatively safe during pregnancy. However, as in another report [8], they proved to be ineffective and were stopped. The decision to try tilt training [9] may be controversial for two reasons: firstly, the effectiveness of this has not been definitively proved; and secondly, there may be concerns regarding the provocation of additional syncopal episodes in a pregnant woman, since new anoxic episodes might be dangerous for the fetus. In this specific case, it was considered that, with repeat spontaneous episodes, there was not only a risk of further anoxic episodes for the fetus in any case, but also a risk of traumatic injury. Consequently, all efforts to stop the syncopal recurrences were considered to be justified. However, as the tilt training was ineffective, it was abandoned at the very start. Due to the high rate of recurrences, with a severe impact on the patient's quality of life and with the risk of traumatic injury to the fetus, it was decided to induce delivery in the 35th week of pregnancy. Since delivery, the patient has remained completely asymptomatic.

When new syncopal episodes appear during pregnancy, every effort should be made to rule out worsening of preexistent arrhythmia, as in patients with a long QT syndrome or a complete AV block, or the appearance of new-onset ventricular arrhythmias. In most cases, when syncope appears late in pregnancy and is related to the supine position, reasonable management consists of advising the patient to avoid this position.

References

1 Kunzel W. Vena cava occlusion syndrome: Cardiovascular parameters and uterine blood supply. *Fortschr Med* 1976; **94**: 949–53.

2 Huang MH, Roeske WR, Hu H, Indik JH, Marcius FI. Postural position and neurocardiogenic syncope in late pregnancy. *Am J Cardiol* 2003; **92**: 1252–3.

3 Rashba EJ, Zareba W, Moss AJ, *et al.* Influence of pregnancy on the risk of cardiac events in patients with hereditary long QT syndrome. *Circulation* 1998; **97**: 451–6.

4 McCurdy CM, Rutherford SE, Coddington CC. Syncope and sudden arrhythmic death complicating pregnancy: a case report of Romano–Ward syndrome. *J Reprod Med* 1993; **38**: 233–4.

5 Brodsky MA, Sato DA, Oster PD, Schmidt PL, Chesnie BM, Henry WL. Paroxysmal ventricular tachycardia with syncope during pregnancy. *Am J Cardiol* 1986; **58**: 563–4.

6 Brodsky M, Doria R, Allen B, Sato D, Thomas G, Sada M. New-onset ventricular tachycardia during pregnancy. *Am Heart J* 1992; **123**: 933–41.

7 Grand A, Huret JF, Farge C, Ferry M, Perret SP. [Auriculo-ventricular block and pregnancy; in French.] *Arch Mal Coeur Vaiss* 1981; **74**: 909–16.

8 Madrid AH, Ortega J, Rebollo JG, *et al.* Lack of efficacy of atenolol for the prevention of neurally mediated syncope in a highly symptomatic population: a prospective, double-blind, randomized and placebo-controlled study. *J Am Coll Cardiol* 2001; **37**: 554–9.

9 Reybrouck T, Heidbuchel H, Van De Werf F, Ector H. Long-term follow-up results of tilt training therapy in patients with recurrent neurocardiogenic syncope. *Pacing Clin Electrophysiol* 2002; **25**: 1441–6.

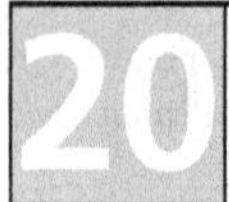

CASE 20

A pilot with vasovagal syncope: fit to fly?

N. van Dijk, N. Colman, J.H.A. Dambrink, W. Wieling

Case report

A 20-year-old commercial pilot was referred for evaluation. He had fainted during a briefing for a training session in the hypobaric room. During a subsequent medical examination by a neurologist and cardiologist, the patient collapsed twice while talking about the first episode. During the faints, he experienced lightheadedness, paleness, and sweating. In his youth, the patient had fainted once during mass in church. He also avoided watching surgical procedures on television. The patient had been grounded by the aeromedical service due to his faints [1].

The patient was referred for further examination and advice. The physical examination and electrocardiogram were normal. His blood pressure in the supine position was 130/70 mmHg and the heart rate was 75 beats/min. The patient showed a normal heart rate and blood pressure response to active standing. After 5 min of standing, the attending physician (W.W.) deliberately started talking about the first fainting episode. Within 1 min, the patient became lightheaded, experienced a warm feeling, looked pale, and was sweating. His heart rate dropped to 45 beats/min and his blood pressure fell from 160/85 mmHg to 80/45 mmHg. Lying down averted the ongoing vasovagal syncope (Fig. 20.1).

The patient recognized the symptoms. This confirmed the clinical diagnosis of emotionally induced vasovagal syncope. He was reassured about the nature of his problem and was advised to avoid provocative medical situations. While his episodes occurred only during predictable provocations and he experienced clear preceding symptoms, the chances of an episode occurring during flying were considered to be low. We therefore recommended that the patient should be declared fit to fly. During a 5-year follow-up period, he has had no episodes of syncope and has been working as a commercial pilot.

Comment

Vasovagal syncope is described as a benign condition, and the mortality of patients due to vasovagal spells is very low [2]. However, loss of consciousness in a critical situation such as driving or flying could lead to serious accidents. According to European criteria established by the Joint Aviation Authorities, pilots with loss of consciousness can only be declared fit to fly when there is no chance of recurrence, the cause of syncope is clear, and a neurological examination shows no abnormalities [3]. According to the United States Federal Aviation Administration, a first syncopal episode makes a pilot unfit to fly. Only if there is a clear and avoidable medical explanation for the episode can the pilot be declared fit to fly [4]. This criterion may be applicable to pilots suffering from vasovagal syncope induced by medical situations [1].

Whether a pilot with vasovagal syncope can be declared fit to fly depends on the possibility of recurrences during flying. To determine the risk, the vasovagal nature of the syncope has to be absolutely certain [5]. Secondly, the patient should have clear prodromal signs in order to ensure that precautions can be taken if symptoms develop. It is crucial for the patient to have an awareness of provocative situations, to allow precautions to be taken at an early stage [6]. The

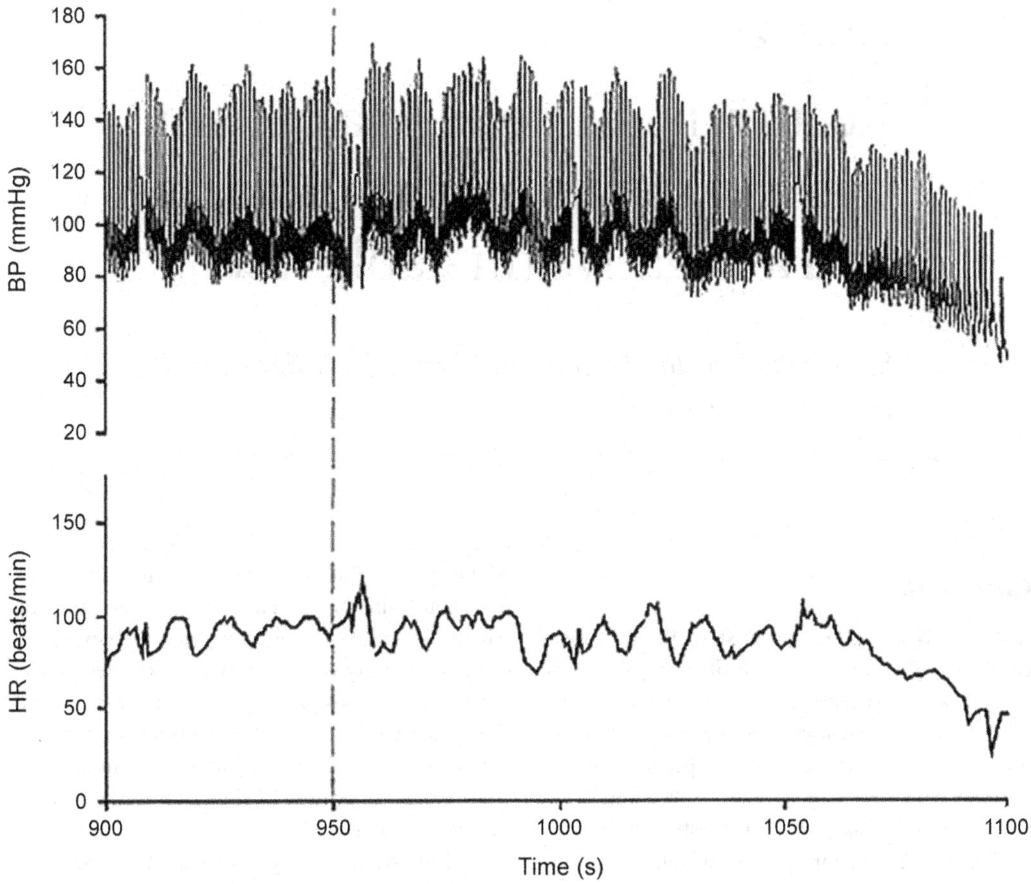

Figure 20.1 Continuous blood pressure and heart-rate recording. The line indicates the start of the emotional conversation. BP, blood pressure; HR, heart rate.

provoking factor should be avoidable during flying. A restriction to flying "as or with a co-pilot" during a certain observation period may be considered as an initial measure in resuming flying [6].

References

1 van Dijk N, Colman N, Dambrink JH, Wieling W. Pilots with vasovagal syncope: fit to fly? *Aviat Space Environ Med* 2003; **74**: 571–4.

2 Kapoor WN. Evaluation and outcome of patients with syncope. *Medicine (Baltimore)* 1990; **69**: 160–75.

3 Joint Aviation Authorities. *JAR-FCL Part 3: Flight Crew Licensing (Medical).* Joint Aviation Authorities, Hoofddorp, Netherlands, 2000.

4 Department of Transportation. Federal Aviation Administration. *Guide for Aviation Medical Examiners.* Federal Aviation Administration, Washington, DC, 1999: 24–5, 28a, 61–2.

5 Sutton R. Vasovagal syncope: prevalence and presentation. An algorithm of management in the aviation environment. *Eur Heart J Suppl* 1999; **1** (Suppl D): D109–13.

6 Joy M. Introduction and summary of principal conclusions of the Second European Workshop in Aviation Cardiology. *Eur Heart J Suppl* 1999; **1** (Suppl D): D1–12.

21

CASE 21

Recurrent syncope in a patient with no structural heart disease and a negative tilt-table test

S. Morell Cabedo, R. Sanjuán Mañez, R. Ruiz Granell, R. García Civera

Case report

A 42-year-old man was referred to the outpatient cardiology clinic for evaluation of syncopal attacks. He had had six syncopal episodes during the previous 2 years. Loss of consciousness occurred abruptly, without warning symptoms and with no specific triggers.

The physical examination, electrocardiogram (ECG), carotid sinus massage, orthostatic tests, and an echocardiogram were all normal. A 24-h Holter recording showed sinus rhythm (rate between 160 and 45 beats/min) over the whole period without arrhythmias or syncopal events. A tilt-table test with sublingual nitroglycerin challenge was carried out, also with negative results.

With the patient under local anesthesia, a Reveal implantable loop recorder (ILR) (Medtronic Inc., Minneapolis, Minnesota, USA) was implanted subcutaneously in the left parasternal region, and the patient and relatives were instructed to activate the device after every episode of syncope or presyncope. During the follow-up, an ILR-documented syncopal event occurred 2 months after implantation, with the data showing a 20-s asystolic pause as the cause of syncope (Fig. 21.1). Figure 21.2 shows the heart rate trend during the episode.

A diagnosis of vasovagal syncope of the cardioinhibitory type was made, and a DDDR pacemaker was implanted. After implantation of the pacemaker, the patient did not suffer any further syncopal episodes.

Comment

The patient described here had repeated syncopal

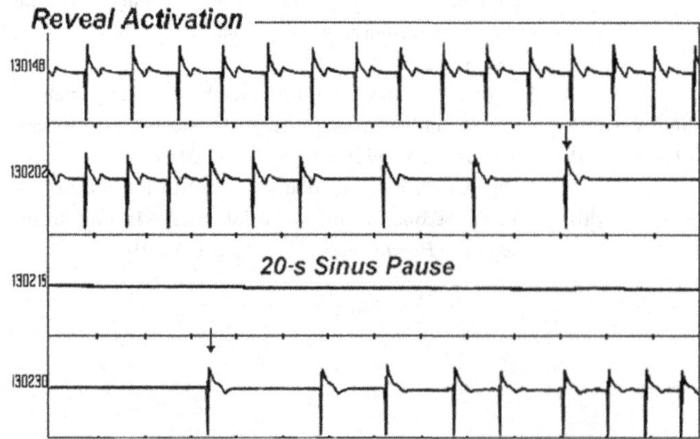

Figure 21.1 A 20-s sinus pause was detected during the syncopal event.

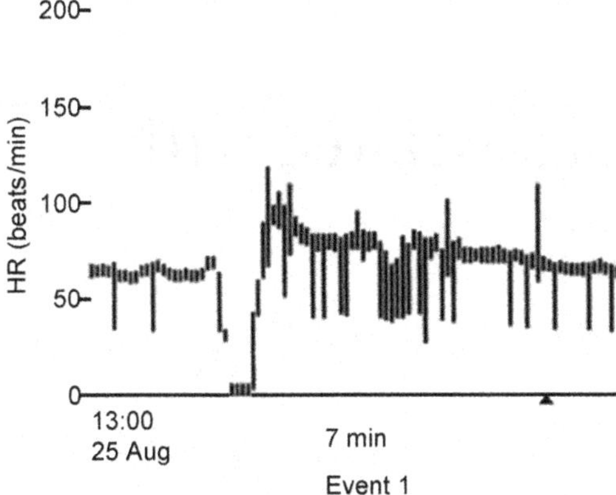

Figure 21.2 The heart rate (HR) trend during the syncopal episode.

attacks without typical triggers or warning symptoms; structural heart disease was ruled out by the initial work-up, and the baseline ECG was normal. In this type of patient, the tilt-table test with sublingual nitroglycerin challenge is frequently positive (in 70% of cases in a recent study [1]). However, the test was negative in this case.

How should one proceed in such cases? There is general agreement that electrophysiological studies are not a useful strategy in this group of patients [2], so there are two main possibilities—clinical follow-up [1] or follow-up with an ILR implant [3].

In the International Study of Syncope of Uncertain Etiology (ISSUE), an ILR was implanted in 82 patients with absence of structural heart disease, normal ECG findings, and negative tilt testing (isolated syncope). During a follow-up period of 3–15 months, syncope recurred in 28 of the patients (34%) and a bradycardic episode suggestive of neurally mediated syncope was recorded in 54% of the cases of recurrent syncope. The remaining patients had a normal sinus rhythm or sinus tachycardia during syncope. None of the patients died during the study period, and only one patient experienced severe injury due to a syncopal relapse [4]. The ISSUE results thus show that patients with isolated syncope have a good prognosis, a low rate of recurrence, and a neuromediated mechanism in most cases.

In the present case, an ILR was inserted and a cardioinhibitory response was detected during the follow-up. Because of the long asystolic pause, a DDDR pacemaker was implanted, and the patient has since remained free of symptoms. Pacemaker treatment in patients with vasovagal syncope and a marked cardioinhibitory component is controversial. The Vasovagal Pacemaker Study (VPS) [5] and the Vasovagal Syncope International Study (VASIS) [6] demonstrated the effectiveness of DDD with a rate drop response and of DDI with hysteresis pacemakers in patients with vasovagal syncope and a positive response to the tilt-table test. However, two randomized and placebo-controlled trials, the VPS-II trial [7] and the Synpace trial [8], were unable to demonstrate clearly the superiority of active pacing versus inactive pacing in patients with severe neuromediated syncope. Further studies are necessary to clarify the role of pacing in the treatment of vasovagal syncope.

References

1 Garcia-Civera R, Ruiz-Granell R, Morell-Cabedo S, *et al.* Selective use of diagnostic tests in patients with syncope of unknown cause. *J Am Coll Cardiol* 2003; **41**: 787–90.

2 Brignole M, Alboni P, Benditt DG, *et al.* Guidelines on management (diagnosis and treatment) of syncope: update 2004. Task Force on Syncope, European Society of Cardiology. *Europace* 2004; **6**: 467–537.

3 Krahn AD, Klein GJ, Yee R, *et al.* Randomized assessment of syncope trial: conventional diagnostic testing versus a prolonged monitoring strategy. *Circulation* 2001; **104**: 46–51.

4 Moya A, Brignole M, Menozzi C, *et al.* Mechanism of syncope in patients with isolated syncope and in patients with tilt-positive syncope. *Circulation* 2001; **104**: 1261–7.

5 Conolly S, Sheldon R, Roberts R, *et al.* The North American Vasovagal Pacemaker Study (VPS): a randomized trial of permanent cardiac pacing for the prevention of vasovagal syncope. *J Am Coll Cardiol* 1999; **33**: 16–20.

6 Sutton R, Brignole M, Menozzi C, *et al.* Dual-chamber pacing in the treatment of neurally mediated tilt-positive cardioinhibitory syncope: pacemaker versus no therapy: a multicenter randomized study. The Vasovagal Syncope International Study (VASIS) Investigators. *Circulation* 2000; **102**: 294–9.

7 Conolly S, Sheldon R, Thorpe K, *et al.* Pacemaker therapy for prevention of syncope in patients with recurrent severe vasovagal syncope. *J Am Med Assoc* 2003; **289**: 2224–9.

8 Raviele A, Giada F, Sutton R, *et al.* The vasovagal syncope and pacing (Synpace) trial: rationale and study design. *Europace* 2001; **3**: 336–41.

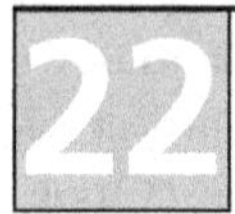

CASE 22

Swallow syncope associated with asystole

F. Giada, A. Raviele

Case report

A 23-year-old man was referred to the syncope unit because he had had three syncopal episodes and four presyncopes during the previous 18 months. The symptoms were always associated with swallowing, especially during the ingestion of large amounts of beverages or large boluses of solid food. In one case, syncope was associated with severe trauma. The patient had no risk factors; he did not smoke, drink alcohol, or use illicit drugs. The physical examination was normal. Electrocardiography, echocardiography, and tilt testing were negative.

Holter monitoring was then considered appropriate in order to obtain an electrocardiographic recording in the causative situation. During the monitoring period, the patient had two recurrences of presyncope, and prolonged sinus pauses were recorded (Fig. 22.1). An electrophysiological study demonstrated the absence of any intrinsic conduction system disease, with normal AH (77 ms) and HV (43 ms) intervals, normal SA node function (correct sinus recovery time

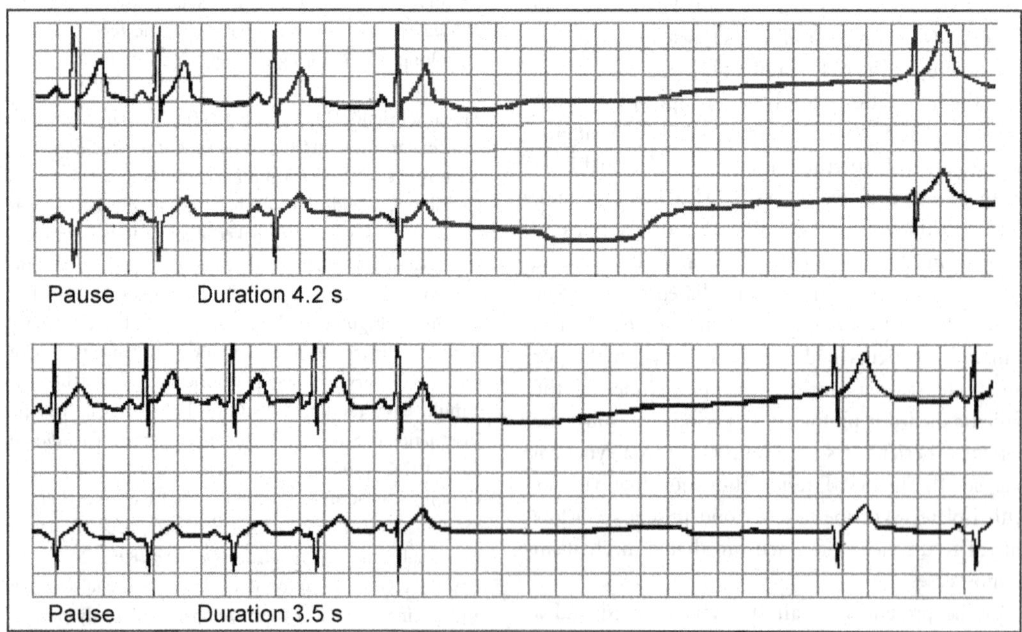

Figure 22.1 Electrocardiography tracings from Holter monitoring during two spontaneous episodes of presyncope, showing prolonged sinus pauses.

289 ms), and normal atrioventricular nodal function (Wenckebach point 170 beats/min).

Esophageal radiography and esophagogastroduodenoscopy showed only mild dysfunction of the lower esophageal sphincter, while dynamic esophageal pH-metry revealed clear signs of gastroesophageal reflux. The patient was treated with omeprazole (20 mg b.i.d), and remained asymptomatic during a 2-year follow-up period.

Comment

See Case 23 for comments and references on this case.

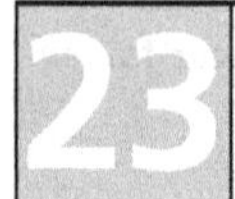

CASE 23

Swallow syncope presenting with atrioventricular block

J. García Sacristán, R. Sanjuán Mañez, R. García Civera

Case report

A 42-year-old man was referred for evaluation due to multiple episodes of presyncope and syncope triggered by deglutition. When he ate solid food, he experienced dizziness or loss of consciousness. He had previously been examined in the gastroenterology department, and a hiatus hernia was identified on an upper gastrointestinal barium examination. A Nissen fundoplication procedure was suggested, but the patient had declined the surgical intervention, and medical treatment was unable to control the syncopal episodes.

The findings of a cardiovascular examination, electrocardiography, and carotid sinus massage were normal. The 24-h Holter recording (Figs. 23.1, 23.2) revealed ventricular pauses related to paroxysmal atrioventricular (AV) block, coinciding with the time of the meals. A DDD pacemaker was implanted, and the patient suffered no further syncopal attacks.

Comments (Cases 22 and 23)

Swallowing is a rare cause of syncope [1]. The mechanism of swallowing syncope is a reflex originating in the mechanical receptors that innervate the esophagus. The triggers are usually eating of solid food or drinking of liquids, but in certain cases the trigger can be more selective (cold or hot liquids, carbonated beverages, etc.) Activation of the mechanoreceptors causes glossopharyngeal or vagal afferent stimulation, which leads to sympathetic withdrawal (resulting in peripheral vasodilation and hypotension) and vagal efferent stimulation (resulting in bradycardia, AV block, or asystole). The cardioinhibitory response appears to predominate in many of the cases and can be inhibited

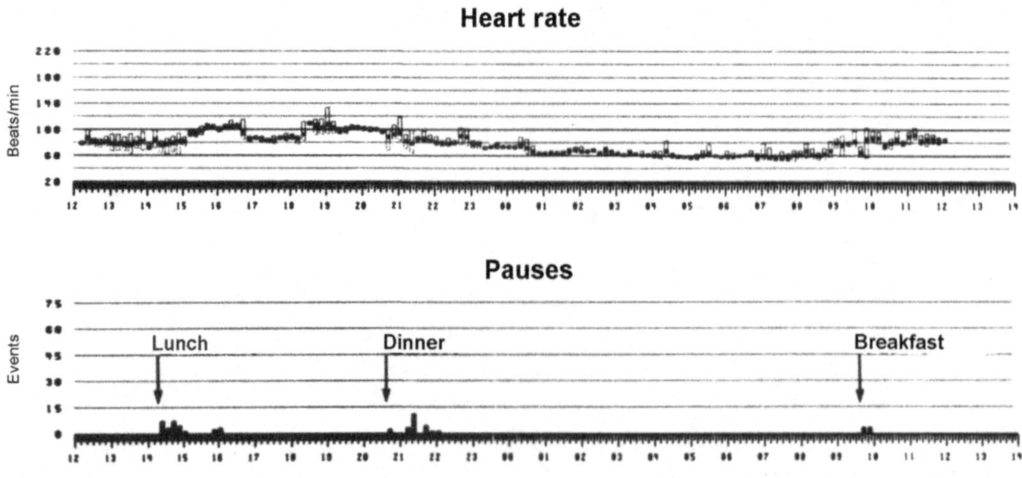

Figure 23.1 Holter monitoring, showing ventricular pauses coinciding with the time of meals.

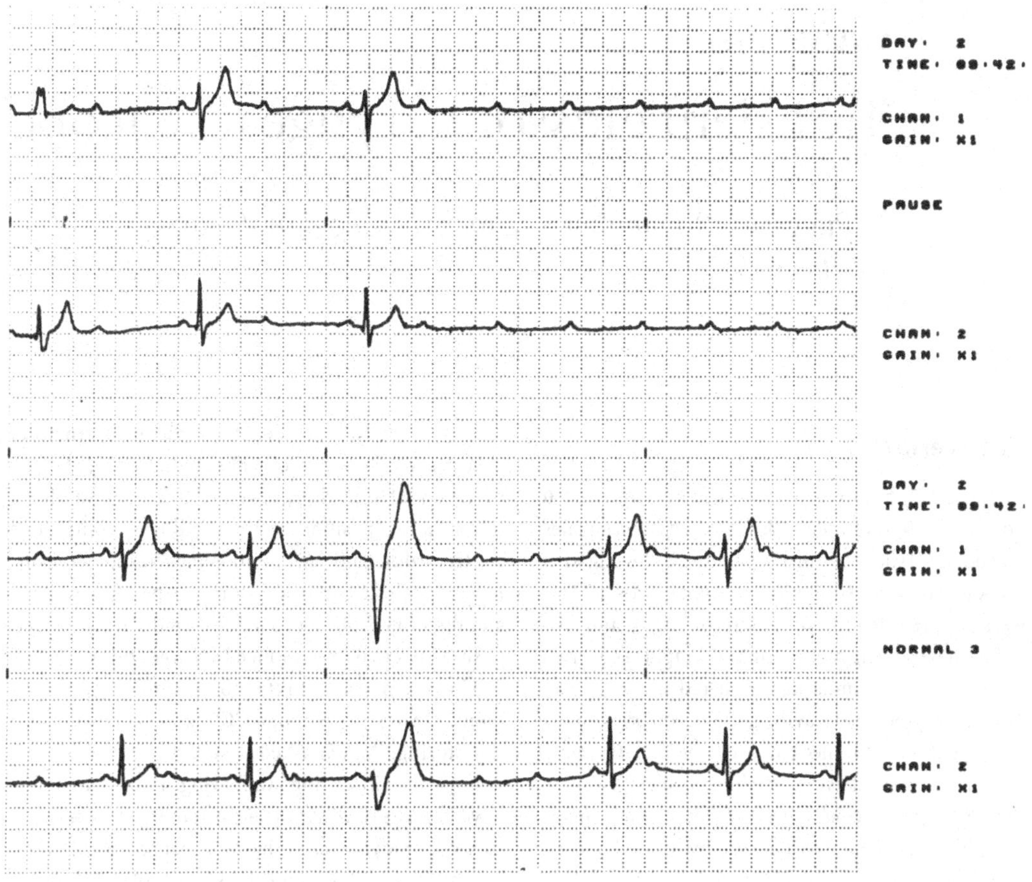

Figure 23.2 The ventricular pauses in Holter monitoring are related to high-grade paroxysmal atrioventricular block.

with atropine or corrected with pacemaker implantation [1]. However, cases of a pure vasodepressor response have also been described [2,3].

Swallow syncope may be associated with cardioactive drug therapy, myocardial infarction, and gastroesophageal disorders (e.g., esophageal diverticula, esophageal carcinoma, or hiatus hernia) [1]. Some patients are also found to have no etiology [4]. The two patients described here and in Case 22 had gastroesophageal disorders (gastroesophageal reflux and hiatus hernia) and cardioinhibitory responses (sinus arrest in one case and AV block in the other).

Swallowing syncope is a typical situational syncope and does not require complex diagnostic techniques other than those necessary to detect the possible gastroesophageal pathology and the underlying rhythm during the episode. In patients with only occasional syncope related to selective triggers, suppressing the trigger can be sufficient [5,6]. In other cases, treatment of the esophageal pathology can relieve the symptoms. Pacemaker implantation is indicated in cases in which the cardioinhibitory response is not controllable by other means.

References

1 Sanchis J, García Civera R, García Sacristán J, Burguera M. Síncope deglutorio. In: García Civera R, Sanjuán R, Cosín J, López Merino V, eds. *Síncope.* MCR, Barcelona, 1989: 209–19.

2 Armstrong PW, McMillan DG, Simon JB. Swallow syncope. *Can Med Assoc J* 1985; **132**: 1281–4.

3 Carey BJ, Panerai RB. More on deglutition syncope. *N Engl J Med* 1999; **341**: 1316–7.

4 Levin B Posner JB. Swallow syncope: report of a case and review of the literature. *Neurology* 1972; **22**: 1086–93.

5 Brick JE, Lowther CM, Deglin SM. Cold water syncope. *South Med J* 1978; **71**: 1579–80.

6 Olshansky B. A Pepsi challenge. *N Engl J Med* 1999; **340**: 2006.

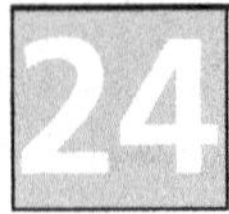

CASE 24

Transient glossopharyngeal syncope

E. Puggioni, P. Donateo, F. Croci, R. Maggi, A. Solano, M. Brignole

Case report

In July 2002, a 43-year-old woman was referred to hospital due to several episodes of loss of consciousness that occurred suddenly during painful swallowing when she was in both the supine and upright positions. They were not preceded by any prodromal signs, and were followed by jerking movements and rapid recovery of consciousness. Trauma had occurred in some cases. The patient reported having suffered pharyngodynia in the right side of the neck for a few weeks, with exacerbation during swallowing, and having taken antibiotic therapy in the previous days for fever. She was unable to drink or eat because each swallow caused asystole and symptoms.

The initial evaluation (history, physical examination, electrocardiography, and blood-pressure measurements in the supine and upright positions), conducted in the emergency department, confirmed the syncopal nature of the episode and excluded the suspicion of structural heart disease. Echocardiography confirmed the absence of structural heart disease. While the patient was lying in the supine position on the bed during continuous electrocardiography (ECG) monitoring, another spontaneous episode occurred during a painful swallow, and the ECG showed progressive bradycardia that led to sinus arrest, with prolonged asystole and syncope.

The patient was admitted to the cardiology department. During continuous ECG and blood-pressure monitoring, she was asked to swallow some food. She again had pain during swallowing, immediately followed by loss of consciousness; at this point, the ECG showed bradycardia with some pauses, the longest of which was 12.5 s, and the systolic blood pressure decreased to 50 mmHg (Fig. 24.1). The test was repeated after intravenous atropine administration (0.02 mg/kg) (Fig. 24.2); the drug was able to prevent bradycardia, hypotension, and syncope.

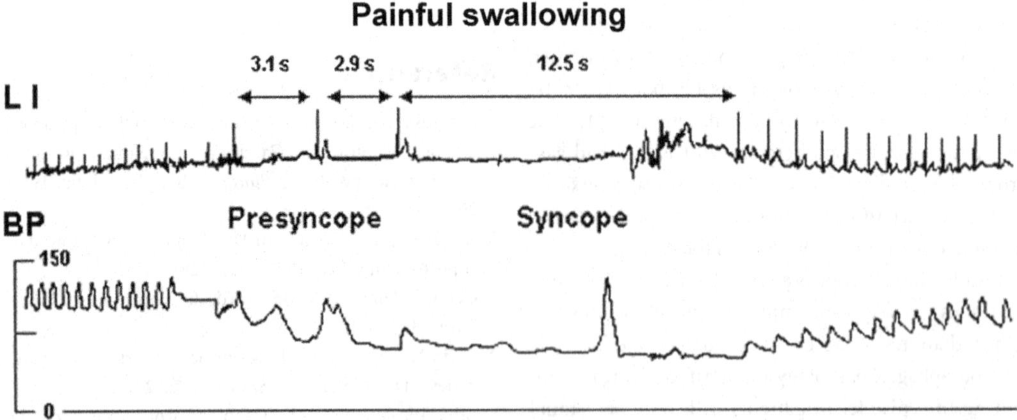

Figure 24.1 Painful swallowing associated with bradycardia and sinus arrest, with prolonged asystole and syncope. LI, Lead I; BP, blood pressure.

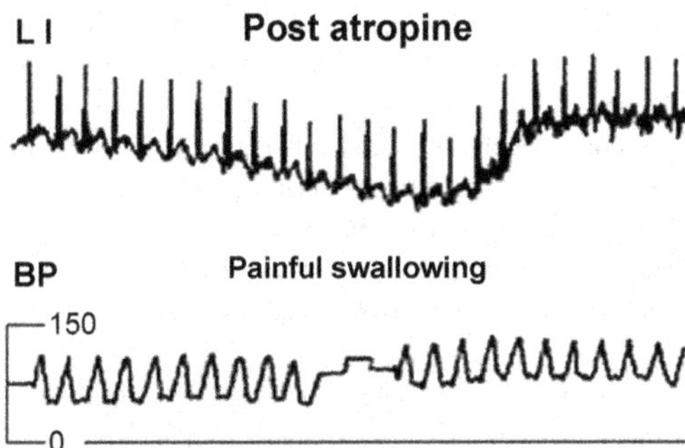

Figure 24.2 Intravenous atropine prevents bradycardia and syncope during a painful swallow. LI, Lead I; BP, blood pressure.

The patient was initially treated with atropine 1 mg i.v. every 4 h for 24 h, which prevented further episodes. An attempt was then made to prevent the symptoms with transdermic scopolamine patches, but the drug was unable to prevent the symptomatic arrhythmic episodes during swallowing or when pharyngeal pain started. A back-up temporary pacemaker was therefore positioned via the right jugular vein, which intervened properly whenever the patient had bradycardia and thus prevented symptomatic relapse.

Otorhinolaryngological and neurological evaluations were carried out, which revealed hyperesthesia in the right glossopharyngeal nerve, evoking cardioinhibitory syncope during the visit. No signs of inflammation were found during the hematological analysis, there were no significant anatomical alterations in the oropharyngeal region evident on cranial computed tomography (CT) and magnetic resonance imaging (MRI), and no gastrointestinal disease was found in the abdominal examination. A diagnosis of glossopharyngeal neuralgia was made, and treatment with gabapentin (Neurontin) 300 mg t.i.d. was started. Five days after the onset of this treatment, the pharyngodynia had completely disappeared, the patient had no further episodes of asystole or syncope, and it was possible to remove the temporary pacemaker. She was discharged on the seventh day and continued therapy for 1 month. She had no further episodes during the following 2 years.

Comment

Glossopharyngeal neuralgia is a painful syndrome characterized by paroxysms of unilateral and severe lancinating pain occurring in the area of distribution of cranial nerve IX. The pain may be spontaneous, or may be precipitated by a variety of actions that stimulate the region supplied by the nerve, such as swallowing, talking, coughing, or yawning, and it usually lasts for a few seconds or minutes [1].

Glossopharyngeal neuralgia usually occurs without any obvious cause (idiopathic glossopharyngeal neuralgia) and, in these cases, radiographic examinations, including CT, MRI, and angiography, will be normal. However, some cases of apparent "idiopathic" glossopharyngeal neuralgia may be due to vascular compression of the glossopharyngeal nerve by a vertebral or cerebellar artery at the nerve root entry zone. Surgical microvascular decompression can therefore be effective in certain cases [2]. Secondary causes of glossopharyngeal neuralgia include styloid pain (compression of the nerve against an elongated or fractured styloid process) [3], and tumors of the cerebellopontine angle or parapharyngeal space [4].

The association between glossopharyngeal neuralgia and syncope is rare. In 1981, Rushton *et al.* reported on 217 patients with glossopharyngeal neuralgia admitted to the Mayo Clinic, only four of whom had associated syncope [1]. The mechanism of the syncope in most published cases is a cardioinhibitory reflex leading to severe bradycardia or asystole [4–7]. However, in a few cases, syncope can be caused by severe hypotension without bradycardia [8].

This report describes a case of idiopathic transient glossopharyngeal neuralgia in which the occurrence of reflex symptomatic bradycardia and asystole was triggered by swallowing. The phenomenon provides clinical evidence of a close connection between the glossopharyngeal and vagus nerves.

Treatment of glossopharyngeal neuralgia depends on whether the condition involves an idiopathic or secondary type of neuralgia. Obviously, if the neuralgia is due to a compressive mass, surgical treatment must be considered. In cases of idiopathic syncope, carbamazepine treatment [9] and occasionally cardiac pacing have been suggested [10]. This report describes, perhaps for the first time, effective drug treatment with gabapentin for the transient form of glossopharyngeal syncope. Gabapentin is usually considered an optimal pharmacological treatment in patients with epileptic disease, but it is also used to control neuropathic pain [11]. Because of the possible transient and benign nature of these forms of neuralgia, pharmacological treatment should be considered the initial treatment of choice, with pacemaker implantation being reserved for cases of persistent symptomatic episodes of asystole.

References

1 Rushton JG, Stevens C, Miller RH. Glossopharyngeal (vagoglossopharyngeal) neuralgia: a study of 217 cases. *Arch Neurol* 1981; **98**: 201–5.

2 Jannetta PJ. Observations on etiology of trigeminal neuralgia, hemifacial spasm, acoustic nerve dysfunction and glossopharyngeal neuralgia: definite microsurgical treatment and results in 177 patients. *Neurochirurgia* 1977; **20**: 145–54.

3 Eagle WW. Symptomatic elongated styloid process. *Arch Otolaryngol* 1949; **49**: 490–5.

4 Cicogna R, Bonomi FG, Curnis A, *et al.* Parapharyngeal space lesions syncope syndrome: a newly proposed reflexogenic cardiovascular syndrome. *Eur Heart J* 1993; **14**: 1476–83.

5 Weinstein RE, Herec D, Friedman HJ. Hypotension due to glossopharyngeal neuralgia. *Arch Neurol* 1986; **43**: 90–2.

6 Ferrante L, Artico N, Nardacci B, Fraioli B, Cosentino F, Fortuna A. Glossopharyngeal neuralgia with cardiac syncope. *Neurosurgery* 1995; **36**: 58–63.

7 Alpert JN, Armbrust CA, Akhavi M, *et al.* Glossopharyngeal neuralgia, asystole and seizures. *Arch Neurol* 1977; **34**: 233–5.

8 Odeh M, Oliven A. Glossopharyngeal neuralgia associated with cardiac syncope and weight loss. *Arch Otolaryngol Head Neck Surg* 1994; **120**: 1283–6.

9 Saviolo R, Fiasconaro G. Treatment of glossopharyngeal neuralgia by carbamazepine. *Br Heart J* 1987; **58**: 291–2.

10 Johnston RT, Redding VJ. Glossopharyngeal neuralgia associated with cardiac syncope: long term treatment with permanent pacing and carbamazepine. *Br Heart J* 1990; **60**: 403–5.

11 Harden RN. Gabapentin: a new tool in the treatment of neuropathic pain. *Acta Neurol Scand* 1999; **173**: 43–7.

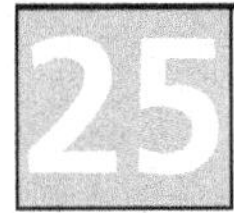

CASE 25

Tussive syncope

S. Morell Cabedo, R. Ruiz Granell, R. Sanjuán Mañez, R. García Civera

Case report

A 52-year-old man with a history of heavy smoking (40 cigarettes per day) and chronic bronchitis was referred for evaluation due to repeated syncopal episodes and an abnormal electrocardiogram (ECG). He had had four syncopal episodes over the previous year. All of the episodes were triggered by vigorous and explosive paroxysms of coughing. He denied having any palpitation paroxysms with or without syncopal spells.

The physical examination revealed thoracic hyperinflation and prolonged expiration. He had a blood pressure of 140/80 mmHg and preserved pulses. The ECG (Fig. 25.1) showed a sinus rhythm at 97 beats/min, a short PR interval (0.12 s), and a wide QRS complex with a delta wave suggestive of a left posterior accessory pathway. The response to carotid sinus massage was normal. An echocardiogram showed an absence of valvular or obstructive abnormalities and preserved left ventricular function (with a left ventricle ejection fraction of 65%).

A diagnosis of tussive syncope was made and the patient was referred to the pneumology department for treatment of chronic bronchitis. In addition, since the patient presented an asymptomatic Wolff–Parkinson–White syndrome, periodic check-ups in the outpatient cardiology clinic were scheduled.

Comment

The patient in this report had an asymptomatic Wolff–Parkinson–White syndrome, chronic bronchitis, and tussive syncope. In tussive (or cough) syncope, the loss of consciousness is associated with prolonged or explosive paroxysms of coughing. This form of

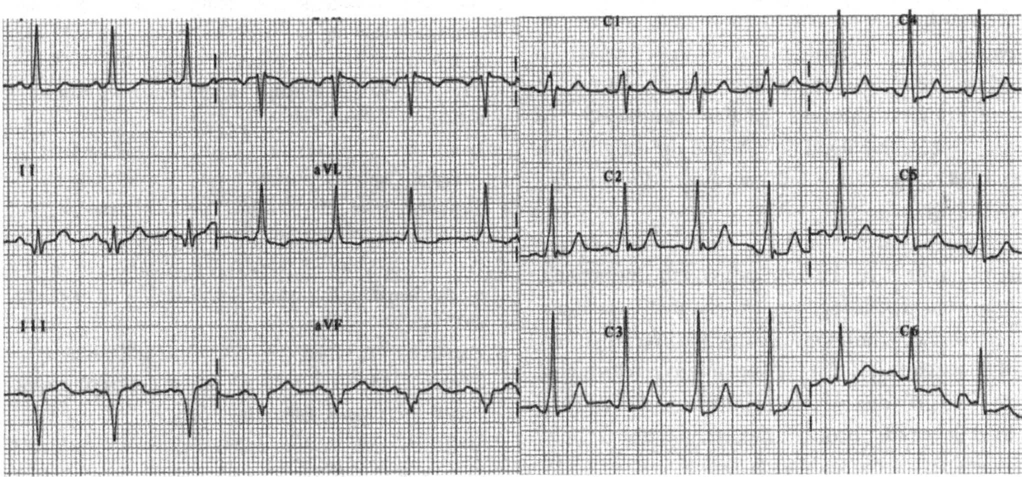

Figure 25.1 The baseline electrocardiogram.

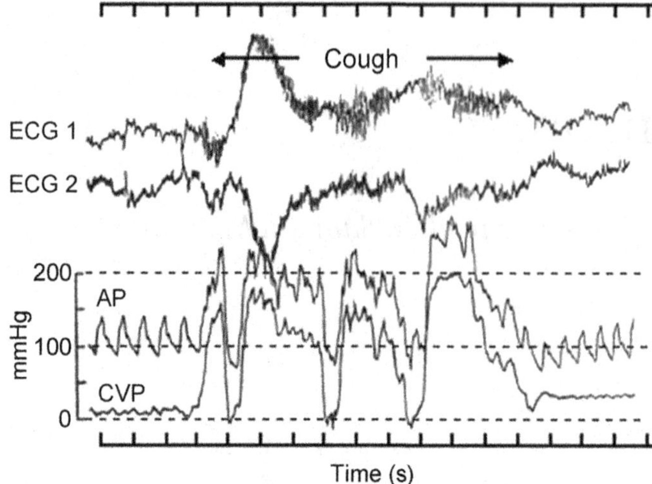

Figure 25.2 The hemodynamic response to coughing. ECG, electrocardiography; AP, arterial pressure; CVP, central venous pressure.

syncope generally occurs in obese middle-aged men with a history of smoking and chronic obstructive pulmonary disorders [1,2]. More rarely, it can be seen in adolescents with asthma or cystic fibrosis [3], or can be induced by treatment with angiotensin-converting enzyme inhibitors [4].

Cough syncope, postmicturition syncope, and defecation syncope are usually classified as "situational" faints, since they are associated with specific scenarios and the diagnosis is evident from the clinical history. However, the mechanism of the syncope is not the same in all of these cases.

Hemodynamic [5,6], cerebral [7,8], and reflex mechanisms have been postulated to explain the syncope triggered by coughing. The hemodynamic effects of a cough are depicted in Fig. 25.2. Coughing causes increases in intrathoracic, intra-arterial, and central venous pressure that produce a fall in venous return and cardiac output. In addition, the diminution of the arteriovenous pressure gradient has the effect of reducing cerebral blood flow. When the coughing fit ends, blood pressure is low and rises to the previous levels slowly.

During prolonged coughing, intrathoracic pressures are transmitted via the great veins to the intracranial compartment, causing transient elevated intracranial pressure [7,8]. The resulting reduction in cerebral perfusion pressure (arterial pressure minus cerebrospinal pressure) may cause a critical impairment of cerebral blood flow and syncope. Using transcranial Doppler sonography of the middle cerebral artery flow velocities, Mattle *et al.* [9] have demonstrated a transient cerebral circulatory arrest coinciding with loss of consciousness.

It has been suggested that neurally mediated reflexes triggered by the increased intrathoracic pressure might explain isolated cases of atrioventricular block coinciding with cough syncope. However, these are very rare cases, and tilt-table tests in patients with cough syncope are by contrast usually normal.

References

1 Kerr A, Derbes VJ. The syndrome of cough syncope. *Ann Med Intern* 1953; **39**: 1240–53.

2 Norton M, Newton JL, Gieroba Z, Kenny RA. Cough syncope: an uncommon but important cause of syncope [abstract]. *Europace* 2003; **4** (Suppl 2): B6.

3 Bonekat HW, Miles RM, Staats BA. Smoking and cough syncope: follow-up in 45 cases. *Int J Addict* 1987; **22**: 413–9.

4 Katz RM. Cough syncope in children with asthma. *J Pediatr* 1970; **77**: 48–51.

5 Jayarajan A, Prakash O. Cough syncope induced by enalapril. *Chest* 1993; **103**: 327–8.

6 Sharpey-Schafer EP. The mechanism of syncope after coughing. *Br Med J* 1953; **ii**: 860–3.

7 Pedersen A, Sandoe E, Hvidberg E, *et al.* Studies on the mechanism of tussive syncope. *Acta Med Scand* 1966; **179**: 653–61.

8 Hamilton WF, Woodbury RA, Harper HT. Atrial, cerebrospinal and venous pressures in man during cough and strain. *Am J Physiol* 1944; **141**: 42–50.

9 Mattle HP, Nirkko AC, Baumgartner RW, Sturzenegger M. Transient cerebral circulatory arrest coincides with fainting in cough syncope. *Neurology* 1995; **45**: 498–501.

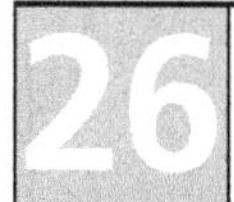

CASE 26
Laughter-induced syncope

S. Sarzi Braga, R.F.E. Pedretti

Case report

A 63-year-old patient was evaluated in our department due to a history of recurrent episodes of syncope preceded by laughter. The patient reported a total of 10 syncopal episodes during the previous 20 years. In one case, syncope occurred during forced expiration while he was undergoing pulmonary function testing. All of the other episodes typically occurred during social gatherings while the patient was laughing heartily. His wife witnessed most of the episodes and described the husband sitting, becoming unconscious while laughing, then bending forward toward the table, and spontaneously and completely recovering from the episode after a few seconds. No abnormal movements or bowel or bladder incontinence were observed on any of the occasions. After the first episodes, the patient learned to control the laughing and consciously to stop the progression of prodromal symptoms (blurred vision, light-headedness) before fainting.

The clinical evaluation, electrocardiogram, and neurological examination were normal, except for a mild and pharmacologically well controlled diabetes mellitus. The patient underwent cardiovascular autonomic evaluation, including carotid sinus massage, a head-up tilt test, and a Valsalva maneuver. Carotid sinus massage revealed a hypersensitive response, but without evoking symptoms. During the head-up tilt test, a mixed vasovagal syncope was induced (Vasovagal Syncope International Study classification type 1) (Fig. 26.1). The patient recognized the prodromal symptoms as being typical.

During the Valsalva maneuver, performed with the patient in the sitting position, an abnormal pattern was observed (Fig. 26.2). Blood pressure initially rose clearly above the expected values, and soon after rapidly declined; no reflex increase in the heart rate was observed. About 8 s after the start of the maneuver, the patient lost consciousness (blood pressure 20 mmHg, heart rate 67 beats/min), and jerking movements appeared. After a few seconds in the recumbent position, he completely recovered (blood pressure 90 mmHg, heart rate 70 beats/min) and described the prodromal symptoms as having been typical. On the basis of the available clinical and test data, as well as the occurrence of the typical symptoms during the Valsalva maneuver and head-up tilt test, a case of neurally mediated laughter-related syncope was diagnosed.

Comment

Laughing is a natural maneuver triggered by emotions. Changes in respiration during laughter have been described [1], but no definitive data on the cardiovascular dynamics have been reported. It is known that when laughter is intense and "hysterical," a normal physiological phenomenon known as the Valsalva maneuver occurs [2,3]. This is a common event in everyday life, occurring for example during coughing, vomiting, and defecation, and consists of forced expiration against a closed airway, resulting in increased pressure in the chest that affects cardiac output and blood pressure, modulating the heart rate, via baroreceptor system activity.

Several types of syncope associated with the increased intrathoracic and intra-abdominal pressure evoked by the Valsalva maneuver have been described: micturition, coughing, defecation, and trumpet blower's syncope are a few examples.

By contrast, syncope resulting from laughter has not been widely reported in the literature, most likely due to the rarity of such cases. In addition, because of the similar clinical presentation, it is possible that some laughter-related syncope has been misdiagnosed

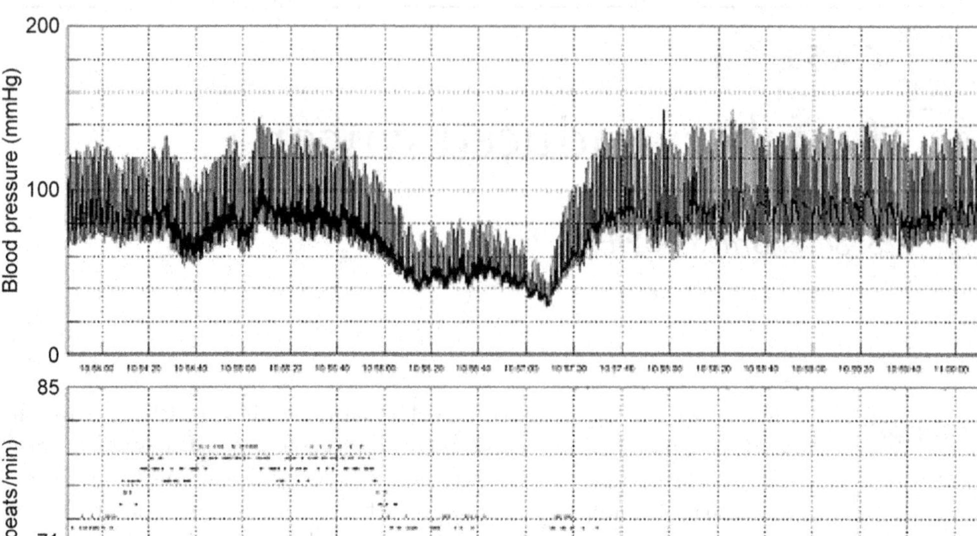

Figure 26.1 The head-up tilt test.

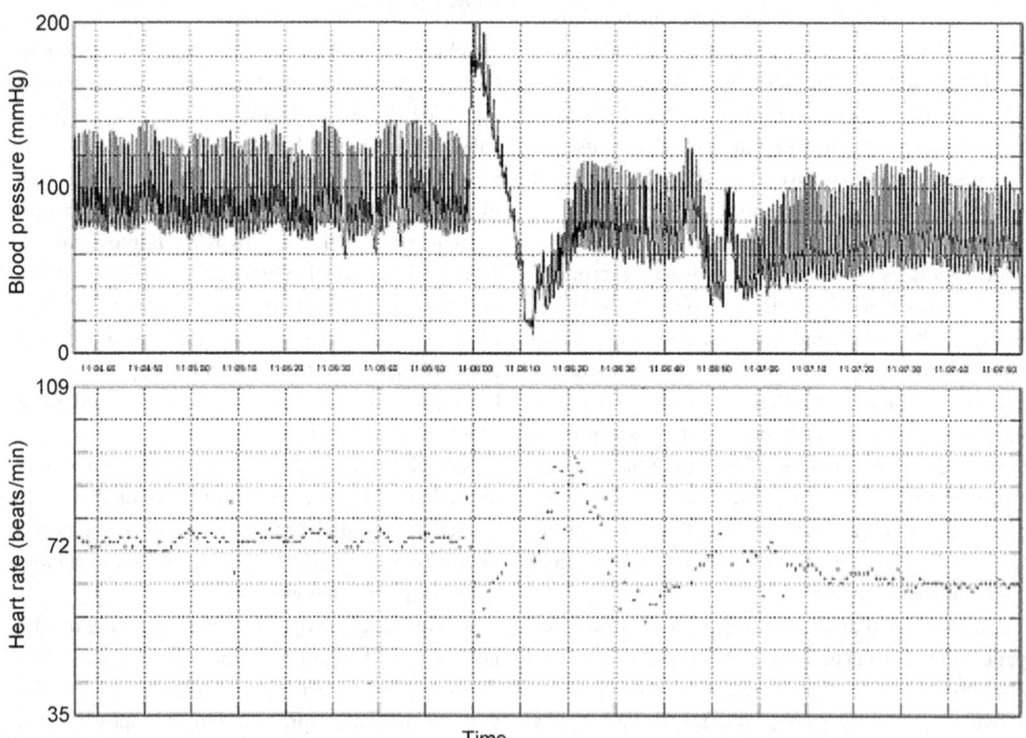

Figure 26.2 The Valsalva maneuver.

as cataplexy [4]. Cox *et al.* [5] reported a case of syncope that occurred after "hysterical" laughter in a patient affected by cerebrovascular atherosclerosis and resolved after revascularization. The present report provides data on a patient who suffered several episodes of syncope preceded by intense laughter. Age, normal neurological examination, loss of consciousness during the episodes, the relationship with the intensity of the laughter, and the voluntary capacity to stop the progression of prodromal symptoms made it possible to exclude the diagnosis of cataplexy [6]. In addition, it was possible in this patient to evoke the typical symptoms during cardiovascular autonomic evaluation, particularly during the Valsalva maneuver—the mechanism presumed to be responsible for laughter-related syncope. After a large increase in blood pressure and the expected decrease in heart rate (phase 1 of the maneuver), the autonomic system was not able during the second phase to increase the heart rate and peripheral vasoconstriction adequately in order to return the blood pressure to baseline values. As a consequence, the blood pressure rapidly dropped, and the patient experienced prodromal symptoms until syncope. Assessment of the cardiovascular autonomic system made it possible to correlate the symptoms with the pathophysiological substrate of this rare cause of syncope.

References

1 Filippelli M, Pellegrino R, Iandelli I, *et al.* Respiratory dynamics during laughter. *J Appl Physiol* 2001; **90**: 1441–6.
2 Boothe R, Ryan J, Mellett H, Swiss E, Neth E. Hemodynamic changes associated with the Valsalva maneuver in normal men and women. *J Lab Clin Med* 1962; **59**: 275–85.
3 Porth C, Bamrah VS, Tristiani FE, Smith JJ. The Valsalva maneuver: mechanisms and clinical implications. *Heart Lung* 1984; **13**: 507–18.
4 Totah A, Benbadis SR. Gelastic syncope mistaken for cataplexy. *Sleep Med* 2002; **3**: 77–8.
5 Cox SV, Eisenhauer AC, Hreib K. "Seinfeld syncope." *Cathet Cardiovasc Diagn* 1997; **42**: 242.
6 Bassetti C, Aldrich MS. Narcolepsy. *Neurol Clin North Am* 1996; **14**: 545–71.

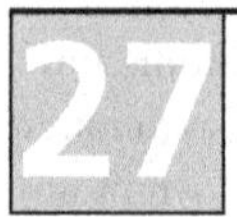

CASE 27

Syncope and the eye

W. Wieling, R.K. Khurana

Case report

A 52-year-old male physician was referred to the syncope unit for evaluation of unexplained loss of consciousness. He had no history of cardiovascular or other medical problems. He was physically active and was not taking any medication. The patient had been playing tennis when he was hit hard on the left eye by a tennis ball. Immediately after the impact, he fell to the ground and lost consciousness for a few seconds. On regaining consciousness, he felt well and continued playing at his normal capacity. He visited his general practitioner the next day. His general physical and somatic neurological examination, including trigeminal nerve function, was normal. He was referred to a cardiologist. The electrocardiogram, echocardiogram, 24-h Holter monitoring study, and exercise stress test were normal. He was referred to our unit for analysis of unexplained syncope.

The patient declined further laboratory assessment. His only interest was in having an explanation of the event in order to reassure his concerned spouse. On the basis of the typical history, syncope due to eyeball pressure was diagnosed. The underlying mechanism was explained to the patient, and he felt reassured.

Comment

An unexplained attack of syncope in an otherwise healthy individual is an alarming event for the patient. Information about the mechanism involved is required in order to explain the occurrence of transient loss of consciousness to the patient [1]. In this patient, syncope due to sudden pressure on the eyeball—the oculocardiac reflex (OCR)—was diagnosed. OCR was first described in 1908 by Aschner in Vienna and Dagnini in Bologna in almost simultaneous independent reports [2,3]. The OCR is a physiological response of the heart to physical pressure on the eyeball and orbital contents, including the extraocular muscles. It is characterized by bradycardia or cardiac arrhythmia, which may lead to cardiac asystole. This is a trigeminal–brainstem–vagal reflex. Aschner demonstrated that the reflex was eliminated by cutting the trigeminal nerve [2]. Gandevia and colleagues showed that vagotomy or atropinization almost eliminated bradycardia, and a slight residual bradycardia still evoked by eyeball pressure was eliminated after propranolol administration. This suggests that vagus (predominantly) and sympathetic nerves constitute the efferent aspects of the OCR [4].

In addition to the use of OCR as a technique for producing syncope or death in unarmed combat [5], it has also been used for several diagnostic and therapeutic purposes. Gastaut found an enhanced OCR in patients who were prone to vasovagal syncope [6]. Lambroso and Lerman demonstrated a 61% incidence of asystole exceeding 2 s induced by eyeball pressure in infants with pallid breath-holding spells, while 25% of infants in the cyanotic group and 7% of those in the control group had a similar period of asystole [7]. Stephenson used the OCR to differentiate between syncopal and epileptic seizures in infants, with the syncopal group having a hypersensitive OCR with asystole ≥ 4 s [8]. The OCR has been reported to be beneficial in averting or attenuating attacks of paroxysmal atrial tachycardia. This reflex is routinely elicited by ophthalmologists during strabismus surgery, when traction is applied to the extraocular muscles [9]. It can serve as a surgical aid for identifying a slipped or lost extraocular muscle during surgery. More often, however, the OCR can occur as an intraoperative complication of the procedure and may be potentially fatal [10].

Although stimulation of the trigeminal nerve at various sites peripheral and central to the trigeminal ganglion—including the trigeminal tract and nucleus—can produce bradycardia, the present discussion is confined to ocular stimulation. In addition to pressure on the globe or traction on the extraocular muscles, OCR can be induced by several other ocular manipulations, including blepharoplasty, laser *in-situ* keratomileusis (LASIK), subconjunctival injection, cataract extraction, contact-lens insertion, acute glaucoma, removal of a foreign body from the cornea, and insertion of Schirmer's lacrimation strips [9,11–15]. It can be assumed that stimulation of the trigeminal afferents induces the OCR in all such patients. In a patient in whom application of Schirmer's lacrimation strips in each conjunctival sac caused vasodepression and cardioinhibition, chemical deafferentation with topical administration of proparacaine hydrochloride did not influence vasodepression or cardioinhibition. This indicates a lack of contribution from the trigeminal afferents and raises the possibility that some of the reported cases of bradycardia in response to ocular stimulation belong to the vasovagal type of situational syncope [15].

References

1 Sharpey-Schafer EP. Emergencies in general practice: syncope. *Br Med J* 1956; (**4965**): 506–9.

2 Aschner B. Über einen bisher noch nicht beschriebenen Reflex vom Auge auf Kreislauf und Atmung. Verschwinden des Radialpulses bei Druck auf das Auge. *Wien Klin Wochenschr* 1908; **21**: 1529–30.

3 Dagnini G. Interno ad un riflesso provocato in alcuni emiplegici colla stimulo della corneae colo pressione sul bulbo oculate. *Boll Sci Med* 1908; **8**: 380.

4 Gandevia SC, McCloskey DI, Potter EK. Reflex bradycardia occurring in response to diving, nasopharyngeal stimulation and ocular pressure, and its modification by respiration and swallowing. *J Physiol* 1978; **276**: 383–94.

5 Mallinson FB, Coombes SK. A hazard of anaesthesia in ophthalmic surgery. *Lancet* 1960; **i**: 574–5.

6 Gastaut H. Syncopes: generalized anoxic cerebral seizures. In: Magnus O, de Haas AML, eds. *Handbook of Clinical Neurology*, vol. 15: *The Epilepsies*. North-Holland, Amsterdam, 1974: 815–36.

7 Lambroso CT, Lerman P. Breathholding spells (cyanotic and pallid infantile syncope). *Pediatrics* 1967; **39**: 563–81.

8 Stephenson JBP. Two types of febrile seizure: anoxic (syncopal) and epileptic mechanisms differentiated by oculocardiac reflex. *Br Med J* 1978; **ii**: 726–8.

9 Baykara M, Dogru M, Ozmen AT, Ozcetin H. Oculocardiac reflex in a nonsedated laser in situ keratomileusis patient. *J Cataract Refract Surg* 2002; **28**: 1698–9.

10 Van Brocklin MD, Hirons RR, Yolton RL. The oculocardiac reflex: a review. *J Am Optom Assoc* 1982; **53**: 407–14.

11 Kayikcioglu O, Kayikcioglu M, Erakgun T, Guler C. Electrocardiographic changes during subconjunctival injections. *Int Opthalmol* 1999; **23**: 37–41.

12 Gao L, Qing W, Haifeng X, Higang T, Faliang W. The oculocardiac reflex in cataract surgery in the elderly. *Br J Ophthalmol* 1997; **81**: 64.

13 Mimura T, Amano S, Funatsu H, *et al.* Oculocardiac reflex caused by contact lenses. *Ophthalmic Physiol Opt* 2003; **23**: 263–4.

14 Awan KJ. Syncope during the removal of corneal foreign body. *Va Med Month* 1975; **102**: 387–9.

15 Khurana RK. Eye examination-induced syncope: role of trigeminal afferents. *Clin Auton Res* 2002; **12**: 399–403.

Treatment

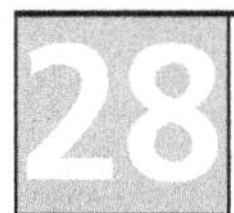

CASE 28

Long-term follow-up of vasovagal syncope with a long asystolic pause

N. Romero, G. Barón Esquivias, S. Gómez Moreno, A. Pedrote Martínez, A. Martínez Martínez, F. Errázquin Sáenz de Tejada

Case report

A 23-year-old woman presented to the emergency room in 1994 due to syncope with facial and arm injuries. She was admitted to the hospital with a history of several presyncopal and syncopal episodes, with a low vasovagal profile. The results of a physical examination were normal. The electrocardiogram, chest radiograph, and echocardiogram were also normal. After cardiac disease had been excluded, a head-up tilt (HUT) test using the Westminster protocol was carried out. The test showed a cardioinhibitory response (Vasovagal Syncope International Study type 2b) with an asystolic pause of 11.5 s (Fig. 28.1). Treatment was started with 50 mg metoprolol every 12 h, and the patient underwent a second HUT 2 weeks later when no worsening of her condition was evident. With metoprolol treatment, the patient experienced the same cardioinhibitory pattern of response during HUT, but with a longer asystole (30.5 s), and required cardiopulmonary resuscitation by chest thumping and atropine infusion (Fig. 28.2). After implantation of a temporary pacemaker, the woman underwent a further tilt test, which showed a positive result, with a predominantly vasodepressor response and no activation of the pacemaker.

At this point, it was assumed that the pacemaker was not benefiting the patient, and she was informed about ways of recognizing premonitory signs, avoiding provocative situations, and increasing her salt and fluid intake. She was discharged from hospital with drug treatment (etilefrine) alone, which she stopped taking on her own initiative after a few weeks. A review in June 2004 showed that the patient was still free of syncope after 10 years, with no further treatment other than receiving information about preventive measures.

Comment

An asystolic response during the tilting test is characteristic of the form of vasovagal syncope described as "malignant." It mainly affects young patients and is

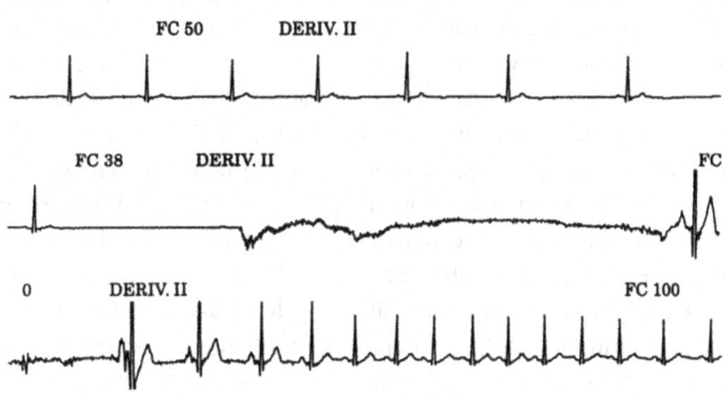

Figure 28.1 The first head-up tilt test.

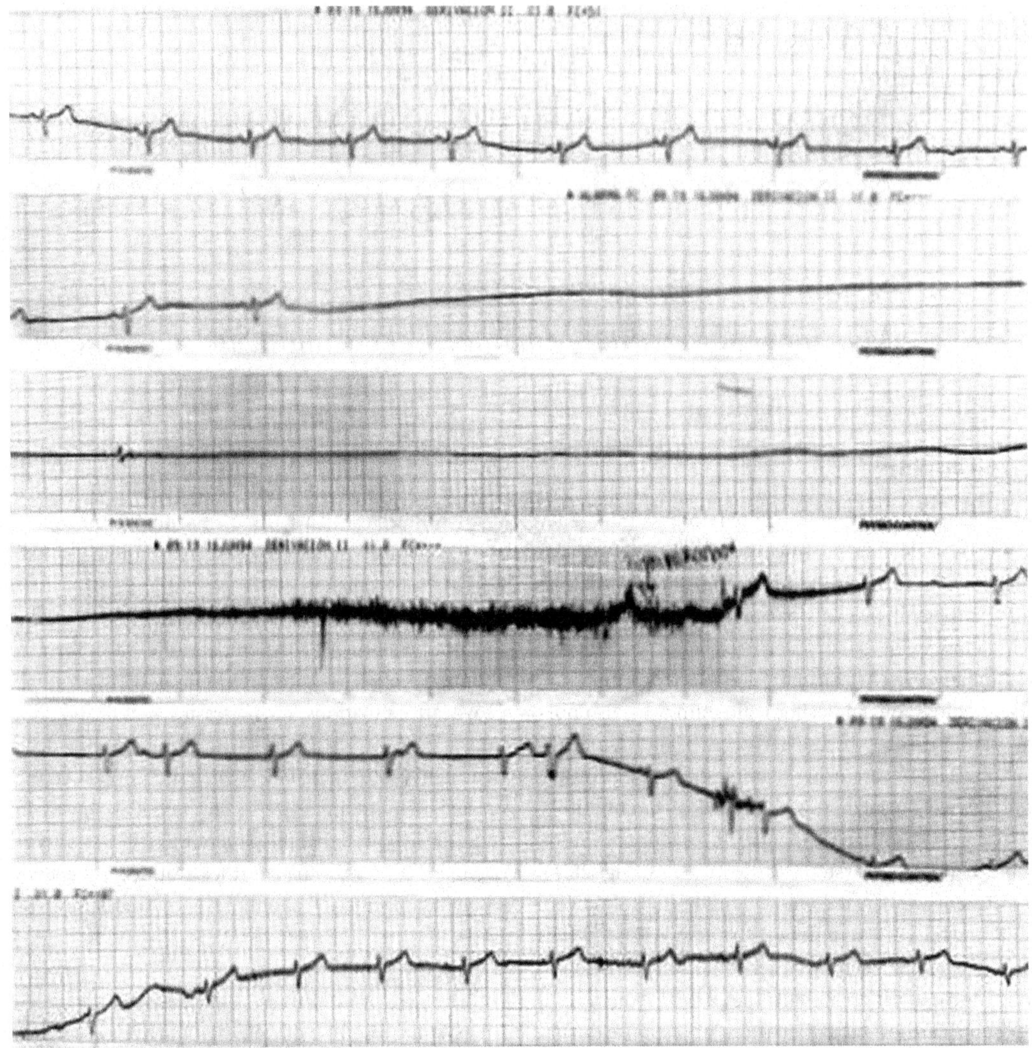

Figure 28.2 The second head-up tilt test.

associated more often with a history of trauma and several other side-effects [1]. The appropriate form of follow-up for patients with asystole in HUT was a matter of controversy for several years. However, it is now well known that the survival of patients with vasovagal syncope who have an abnormal HUT is excellent. In 2002, the present authors reported their experience with a mean follow-up period of 40.7 months in the longest series of patients with asystolic responses during HUT published to date [2]. In this series, only 12 of the 58 patients (20.6%) with asystole suffered recurrent syncope (one episode, $n = 10$; mean recurrence-free period 92.6 ± 6 months; cumulative probability of no recurrence, 70.7%). No differences in the follow-up data were observed in comparison with patients with no asystole during HUT. This recurrence rate, and in particular the absence of any cardiac deaths, suggests that the appearance of asystole during the tilt-table test does not imply a malignant outcome.

When this patient was first evaluated, some studies for the first time suggested a possible role for permanent pacing in selected patients with cardioinhibitory malignant vasovagal syndrome [3]. These theories were followed by several other studies showing that asystole during the tilt test did not appear to be a reproducible response [4], or at least did not in itself worsen the prognosis. In addition, the most recent studies on pacemaker placement, with a double-blind design, failed to show that it was superior to a placebo [5]. Although the issue is still controversial, conservative management in vasovagal syncope is now established as the initial treatment of choice, with educational measures as the first option and medical treatments being used when a further approach is needed. Only if these fail should implantation of a permanent pacemaker be considered [6].

References

1 Kouakam C, Lacroix D, Klug D, *et al.* Determinants of malignant vasovagal syncopes with asystole disclosed by the tilting test and therapeutic implications. *Ann Cardiol Angeiol (Paris)* 1997; **46**: 135–43.

2 Barón-Esquivias G, Pedrote A, Cayuela A, *et al.* Long-term outcome of patients with asystole induced by head-up tilt test. *Eur Heart J* 2002; **23**: 483–9.

3 Petersen ME, Chamberlain-Webber R, Fitzpatrick AP, Ingram A, Williams T, Sutton R. Permanent pacing for cardioinhibitory malignant vasovagal syndrome. *Br Heart J* 1994; **71**: 274–81.

4 Foglia-Manzillo G, Romano M, Corrado G, *et al.* Reproducibility of asystole during head-up tilt testing in patients with neurally mediated syncope. *Europace* 2002; **4**: 365–7.

5 Conolly SJ, Sheldon R, Thorpe KE, *et al.* Pacemaker therapy for prevention of syncope in patients with recurrent severe vasovagal syncope: Second Vasovagal Pacemaker Study (VPS II): a randomized trial. *J Am Med Assoc* 2003; **289**: 2224–9.

6 Barón-Esquivias G, Errázquin F, Pedrote A, *et al.* Long-term outcome of patients with vasovagal syncope. *Am Heart J* 2004; **147**: 883–9.

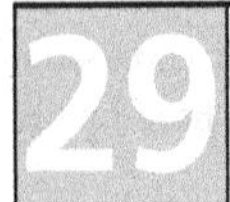

CASE 29

Averting a vasovagal faint with a combination of leg crossing and muscle tensing

C.T.P. Krediet, N. van Dijk, W. Wieling

Case report

A 28-year-old man was evaluated for recurrent episodes of transient loss of consciousness, presumably of vasovagal origin. They typically took place during prolonged standing in a hot environment. Before losing consciousness, he felt light-headed and perspired heavily. Tilt-table testing reproduced these symptoms. Figure 29.1 shows the blood pressure, heart rate, and cardiac output during this vasovagal response, measured using a Finometer/Modelflow system (FMS Finapres Medical Systems B.V., Amsterdam, Netherlands). The progressive fall in finger arterial pressure should be noted. Under the black bar in the tracing, the patient crossed his legs and tensed the leg and abdominal muscles as a physical countermaneuver to combat the vasovagal reaction (Fig. 29.1). Blood pressure recovered quickly after crossing of the legs and tensing of the leg and abdominal muscles. The rise in blood pressure was associated with a steep increase in cardiac output. Intact baroreflex function caused a short decrease in the heart rate when the blood

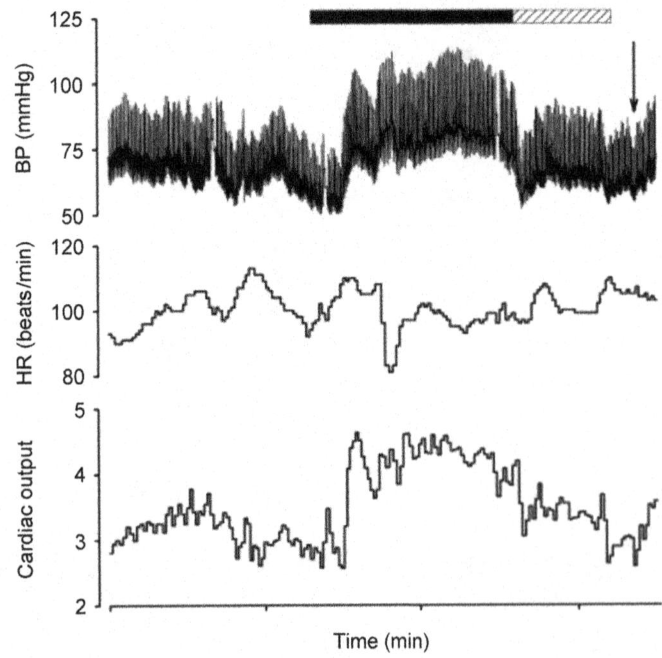

Figure 29.1 Effects of leg crossing on blood pressure and heart rate during impending vasovagal syncope. Hand gripping is not effective. The arrow indicates tilt-back. BP, blood pressure; HR, heart rate. Cardiac output is shown in arbitrary units. (Reproduced with permission from [2].)

pressure overshot the physiological set point at the start of the maneuver.

Under the striped bar in the tracing, leg crossing was replaced by single hand grip as a physical counter-maneuver. Although there was an effect, it was far less pronounced than during leg crossing, and the patient had to be tilted back due to continuing symptoms (arrow).

Comment

After observing that leg crossing and tensing of the leg muscles increased orthostatic tolerance in patients with autonomic failure (see Case 47) [1], we documented the effectiveness of leg crossing and muscle tensing for postponing or averting vasovagal syncope [2]. Brignole *et al.* reported a similar effect of arm counter-pressure maneuvers [3]. Their intervention was based on the anecdotally based advice given to patients by some general practitioners to apply muscle tension by gripping a wooden egg (of the type used for darning socks) with the hand at the start of an impending faint.

The combination of leg crossing and muscle tensing on blood pressure during a vasovagal reaction has a substantial effect (Fig. 29.1). The maneuver can induce an increase in systolic blood pressure during vasovagal syncope from an average pressure of 65 mmHg at the lowest point to 106 mmHg during the maneuver [2]. This increase is caused by mechanical and reflex effects. The acute mechanical effect of reinfusion of pooled blood due to squeezing of the veins by the skeletal muscle pressure causes a rapid increase in central venous pressure and cardiac output and consequently a rise in blood pressure and cerebral perfusion [4,5]. The reflex effects of muscle tensing are likely to be involved in the rise in systemic blood pressure as well. Tensing of skeletal muscles is associated with activation of a central nervous drive ("central command"), resulting in withdrawal of vagal outflow to the heart and an instantaneous increase in heart rate [6,7]. During maximal isometric muscle contractions, the central command also induces an increase in sympathetic outflow to the blood vessels and thus in the peripheral resistance, with stabilization of blood pressure [7].

Tensing of skeletal muscles and the consequent stimulation of mechanical receptors in these muscles elicit a reflex increase in muscle sympathetic nerve activity. Muscle chemoafferents are activated only after approximately 1 min of sustained muscle contractions. Activation of the muscle chemoreflex is therefore not likely to play an important role in the instantaneous blood pressure-increasing effect of physical counterpressure maneuvers [7]. Skeletal muscle contractions can also induce an instantaneous increase in heart rate by reducing vagal outflow to the heart (the muscle–heart reflex) [7,8]. The specific physiological effects underlying the ability to avert vasovagal syncope completely are currently under investigation.

Alternative physical counterpressure maneuvers applied to avert an impending faint are arm tensing and lower body tensing [3,9]. Arm tensing involves strong isometric contraction of both arms, achieved by gripping one hand with the other and simultaneously abducting the arms [3]. The effects of arm tensing differ in our experience from those of simple hand gripping, which is ineffective in postponing vasovagal syncope (Fig. 29.1). We would suggest that the effectiveness of arm tensing is based on the whole-body tensing that takes place during these maneuvers.

Current research experiments are focusing on the scale of the effect of the different physical countermaneuvers on blood pressure during impending fainting. When serious symptoms of an impending faint occur, squatting or sitting down with the head bent between the knees can also be used [10] (Fig. 29.2).

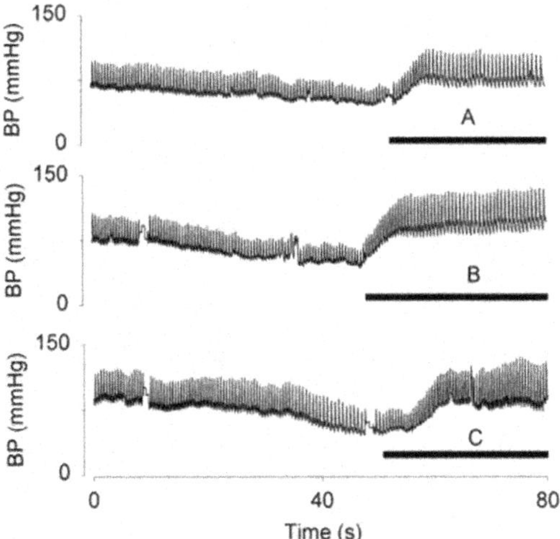

Figure 29.2 Effects of squatting (A), sitting with the head between the knees (B), and lying down (C) on blood pressure (BP) during impending vasovagal syncope. (Reproduced with permission from [10]).

The clinical effectiveness of these different maneuvers in everyday life requires further evaluation.

References

1 Wieling W, van Lieshout JJ, van Leeuwen AM. Physical manoeuvres that reduce postural hypotension in autonomic failure. *Clin Auton Res* 1993; **3**: 57–65.

2 Krediet CT, van Dijk N, Linzer M, van Lieshout JJ, Wieling W. Management of vasovagal syncope: controlling or aborting faints by leg crossing and muscle tensing. *Circulation* 2002; **106**: 1684–9.

3 Brignole M, Croci F, Menozzi C, *et al.* Isometric arm counter-pressure maneuvers to abort impending vasovagal syncope. *J Am Coll Cardiol* 2002; **40**: 2053–9.

4 Van Lieshout JJ, Pott F, Madsen PL, Goudoever J, Secher NH. Muscle tensing during standing: effects on cerebral tissue oxygenation and cerebral artery blood velocity. *Stroke* 2001; **32**: 1546–51.

5 Van Dijk N, de Bruin IG, Gisolf J, *et al.* Hemodynamic effects of leg crossing and skeletal muscle tensing during free standing in patients with vasovagal syncope. *J Appl Physiol* 2005; **98**: 584–90.

6 Thornton JM, Guz A, Murphy K, *et al.* Identification of higher brain centres that may encode the cardiorespiratory response to exercise in humans. *J Physiol* 2001; **533**: 823–36.

7 Van Dijk N, Krediet CT, de Bruin IGJM, van Lieshout JJ, Wieling W. Physical counterpressure maneuvers to prevent and abort vasovagal syncope: a novel effective treatment? In: Raviele A, ed. *Cardiac Arrhythmias 2003: Proceedings of the 8th International Workshop on Cardiac Arrhythmias.* Springer, Milan, 2003: 633–9.

8 Gladwell VF, Coote JH. Heart rate at the onset of muscle contraction and during passive muscle stretch in humans: a role for mechanoreceptors. *J Physiol* 2002; **540**: 1095–1102.

9 Sabin N. The use of applied tension and cognitive therapy to manage syncope (common faint) in an older adult. *Aging Ment Health* 2001; **5**: 92–4.

10 Krediet CT, Wieling W. Manoeuvres to combat vasovagal syncope. *Europace* 2003; **5**: 303.

11 Krediet CT, de Bruin IG, Ganzeboom KS, Linzer M, van Lieshout JJ, Wieling W. Leg crossing, muscle tensing, squatting, and the crash position are effective against vascouagal reactions solely through increases in cardiac output. *J Appl Physiol* 2005; **99**: 1697–703.

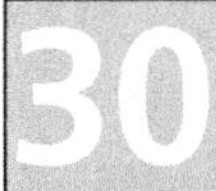

CASE 30

Vasovagal syncope averted using arm-tensing maneuvers

F. Croci, P. Donateo, D. Oddone, A. Solano, E. Puggioni, R. Maggi, M. Brignole

Case report

A 39-year-old man was referred to the syncope unit for evaluation due to a history of recurrent episodes of syncope since he was 15 years old. All of the episodes had occurred when he was in the standing position and were preceded by prodromal symptoms with gastrointestinal discomfort, nausea, sweating, and blurred vision. The duration of the prodromal signs ranged from a minimum of 1 min to a maximum of 20 min. In general, the episodes occurred without clear triggering events, but sometimes they were related to a postprandial period or a prolonged standing position. The patient had suffered minor trauma secondary to a fall in only one case. On several other occasions, he had time to sit down and avert complete loss of consciousness. He had had four episodes of syncope during the previous year. The initial evaluation excluded the presence of orthostatic hypotension and structural cardiac disease. The baseline electrocardiogram was normal. A diagnosis of vasovagal syncope was made on the basis of the typical history.

A tilt test was carried out to evaluate the mechanism of syncope and to guide therapy (Fig. 30.1A). During the passive phase, the patient had a typical vasovagal syncope, reproducing the usual symptoms, with severe hypotension and cardioinhibition and a pause of 9 s (Vasovagal Syncope International Study type 2b).

Arm counterpressure maneuvers (hand gripping and arm tensing) were prescribed in order to prevent the loss of consciousness.

A biofeedback training session was therefore scheduled to familiarize the patient with the physical maneuvers involved. A second tilt test was carried out,

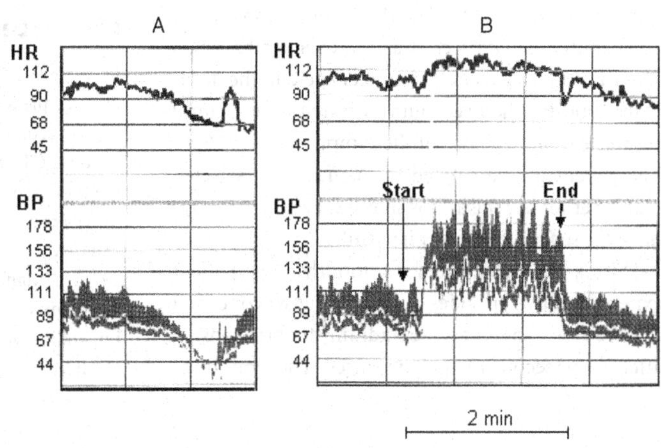

Figure 30.1 The baseline tilt-table test (A) and the effect of hand gripping during the tilt (B). HR, heart rate; BP, blood pressure.

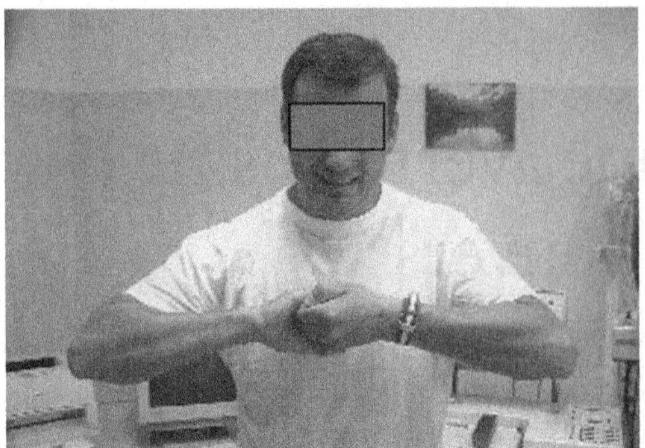

Figure 30.2 The arm-tensing (muscle-tensing) maneuver.

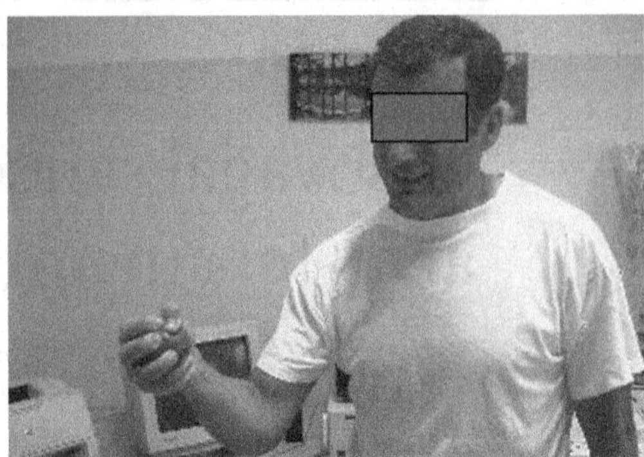

Figure 30.3 The hand-grip maneuver.

and the patient was asked to carry out a hand grip at the time of the onset of symptoms of impending syncope (Fig. 30.1B). Initially, the pattern of blood pressure and heart rate was similar to that observed in the baseline tilt. When the blood pressure decreased to 90 mmHg, symptoms occurred that were recognized by the patient as the spontaneous ones; the patient was asked to start hand gripping, which caused a rapid increase in blood pressure that persisted as long as the contraction was maintained. Initially, the heart rate increased slightly before slightly decreasing. The symptoms disappeared. During the recovery phase, systolic blood pressure fell to 90 mmHg again and the symptoms reappeared.

The patient was trained to use arm tensing and/or hand gripping when symptoms of impending syncope occurred. Arm tensing involves the maximum tolerated isometric contraction of both arms, achieved by gripping one hand with the other and simultaneously abducting (pushing away) the arms for the maximum tolerated time or until complete disappearance of the symptoms (Fig. 30.2). Hand gripping consists of a maximum voluntary contraction over a rubber ball (approximately 5–6 cm in diameter) held in the dominant hand for the maximum tolerated time or until complete disappearance of the symptoms (Fig. 30.3). The patient was instructed to maintain the selected maneuver for as long as possible and eventually move on to the second maneuver if useful.

During the subsequent 12 months, the patient experienced two episodes of impending syncope, and in both cases was able to self-administer arm tensing after a few seconds from the onset. The symptoms disappeared within a few seconds, and syncope did not occur.

Comment

Vasovagal syncope is preceded by prodromal symptoms in about two-thirds of cases. During the prodromal phase, blood pressure falls markedly, and this usually precedes the decrease in heart rate. During the phase of impending vasovagal syncope, isometric arm exercises are able to increase blood pressure through endogenous catecholamine release. Arm counterpressure maneuvers can be suggested as a new first-line treatment for patients who are able to recognize prodromal symptoms before vasovagal syncope. In some cases, the treatment will definitely avert the vasovagal reaction, while in others it can delay syncope for the duration of the maneuver, providing sufficient time to start other maneuvers for averting syncope (such as lying down) [1–3].

References

1 Brignole M, Croci F, Menozzi C, *et al.* Isometric arm counter-pressure maneuvers to abort impending vasovagal syncope. *J Am Coll Cardiol* 2002; **40:** 2054–60.

2 Krediet CT, van Dijk N, Linzer M, *et al.* Management of vasovagal syncope: controlling or aborting faints by leg crossing and muscle tensing. *Circulation* 2002; **106:** 1684–9.

3 Croci F, Brignole M, Menozzi C, *et al.* Efficacy and feasibility of isometric arm counterpressure manoeuvres to abort impending vasovagal syncope during real life. *Europace* 2004; **6:** 287–91.

CASE 31

Training patients in physical countermaneuvers using continuous on-screen blood-pressure monitoring

N. van Dijk, C.T.P. Krediet, W. Wieling

Case report

A 49-year-old man with a clinical history of vasovagal syncope underwent tilt-table testing. The vasovagal reaction provoked was averted by leg crossing and tensing of the leg, abdominal, and buttock muscles (Fig. 31.1) while the patient was still on the tilt table. He was then asked to step off the tilt table. While standing next to it, he was informed about how to apply physical countermaneuvers. Leg crossing and muscle tensing, squatting, isolated leg muscle tensing, and sitting down with the legs crossed were used to combat his continuing vasovagal hypotension. During this training session, the continuous blood-pressure tracing on the video screen was used to provide feedback to instruct the patient on how to perform the maneuvers effectively.

Comment

Patients with intermittent posture-related reflex syncope have found that leg crossing and tensing of the lower abdominal muscles, isometric arm counterpressure, and squatting are simple maneuvers that can be used to combat orthostatic hypotension [1]. They should be instructed in these physical countermaneuvers as part of the treatment program.

Patients can be advised:

- To apply leg crossing as a preventive measure to improve orthostatic tolerance during prolonged upright standing ("cocktail-party posture") [1,2].
- To combine leg crossing with tensing of the leg, abdominal, and buttock muscles to avert an impending vasovagal reaction [3,4]. An alternative is to do isometric arm counterpressure maneuvers [5,6].
- To use squatting as an emergency measure to prevent loss of consciousness when presyncopal symptoms develop rapidly. Bending over as if to tie one's shoelaces has similar results. Elderly patients may find this maneuver simpler to perform [7]. When rising again from the squatting position, patients should be advised to tense the lower abdominal muscles in order to prevent hypotension.

Patients with recurrent syncope may benefit from practicing leg crossing and lower abdominal muscle tensing while standing motionless each morning as part of their daily routine [1]. The effects of physical countermaneuvers on low blood pressure in the standing position are difficult to monitor using sphygmomanometric readings alone, but a continuous blood-pressure measuring device (e.g., Finapres, FMS Finapres Medical Systems B.V., Amsterdam, Netherlands) can be used to quantify the benefits. Patients can be shown the changes in blood pressure immediately using the continuous blood-pressure tracing on a video screen. This technique can be used to train patients to apply the maneuvers effectively [1,8].

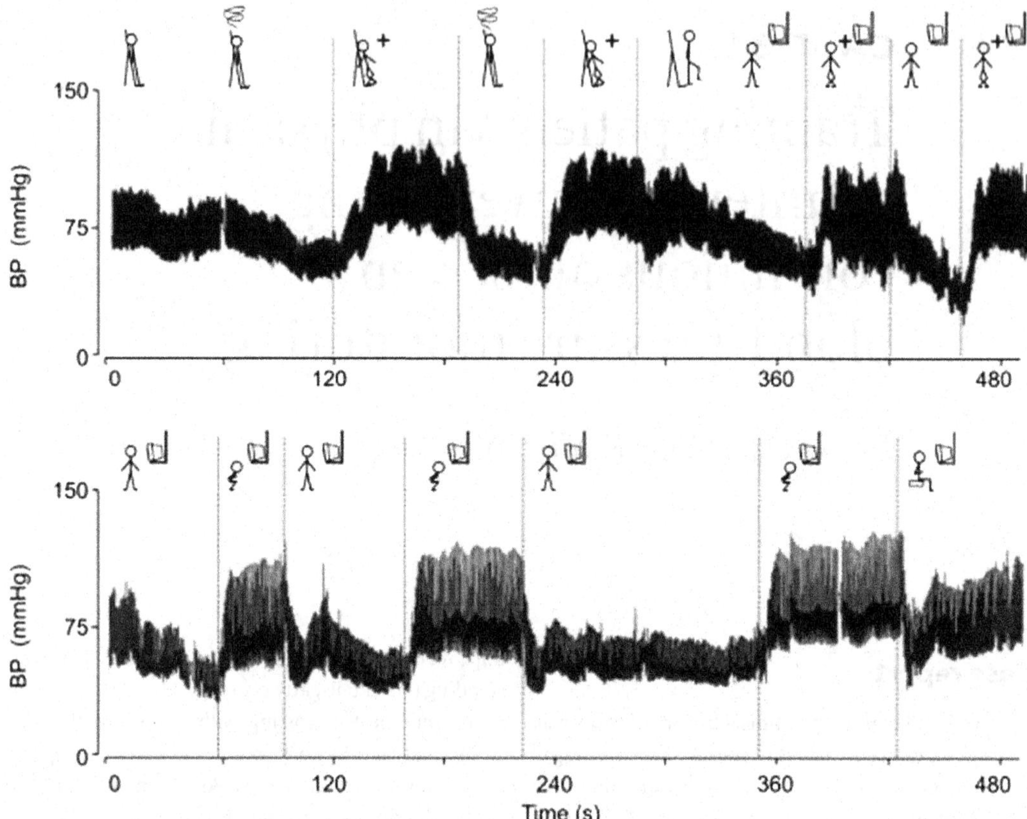

Figure 31.1 Continuous blood-pressure recordings during maneuvers; +, tensing points.

References

1 Wieling W, Colman N, Krediet CT, Freeman R. Nonpharmacological treatment of reflex syncope. *Clin Auton Res* 2004; **14** (Suppl 1): i62–i70.

2 van Dijk N, de Bruin IG, Gisolf J, *et al.* Hemodynamic effects of leg crossing and skeletal muscle tensing during free standing in patients with vasovagal syncope. *J Appl Physiol* 2005; **98**: 584–90.

3 Krediet CT, van Dijk N, Linzer M, van Lieshout JJ, Wieling W. Management of vasovagal syncope: controlling or aborting faints by leg crossing and muscle tensing. *Circulation* 2002; **106**: 1684–9.

4 van Dijk N, Krediet CT, de Bruin IGJM, van Lieshout JJ, Wieling W. Physical counterpressure maneuvers to prevent and abort vasovagal syncope: a novel effective treatment? In: Raviele A, ed. *Cardiac Arrhythmias 2003: Proceedings of the 8th International Workshop on Cardiac Arrhythmias.* Springer, Milan, 2003: 633–9.

5 Brignole M, Croci F, Menozzi C, *et al.* Isometric arm counter-pressure maneuvers to abort impending vasovagal syncope. *J Am Coll Cardiol* 2002; **40**: 2053–9.

6 Croci F, Brignole M, Menozzi C, *et al.* Efficacy and feasibility of isometric arm counter-pressure manoeuvres to abort impending vasovagal syncope during real life. *Europace* 2004; **6**: 287–91.

7 Wieling W, van Lieshout JJ, van Leeuwen AM. Physical manoeuvres that reduce postural hypotension in autonomic failure. *Clin Auton Res* 1993; **3**: 57–65.

8 Bouvette CM, McPhee BR, Opfer-Gehrking TL, Low PA. Role of physical countermaneuvers in the management of orthostatic hypotension: efficacy and biofeedback augmentation. *Mayo Clin Proc* 1996; **71**: 847–53.

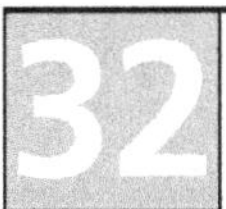

CASE 32

Vasovagal syncope treated with tilt training

G. Foglia-Manzillo, M. Santarone

Case report

A 30-year-old woman was seen at the outpatient cardiology clinic due to recurrent episodes of syncope. In her history, she described six syncopal spells over a 3-year period. All of the episodes had occurred when she was in the standing position. She had become particularly symptomatic during the previous 6 months, during which she had had five syncopal spells. All of the episodes were preceded by dizziness, sweating, and asthenia. The patient had a normal physical examination and a normal electrocardiogram.

A tilt test potentiated with 300 μg sublingual nitroglycerin (the Italian protocol) was positive for syncope after pharmacological challenge, with an asystolic response (2.7 s). The spontaneous symptoms were reproduced during tilt testing. A diagnosis of recurrent neurally mediated syncope was therefore made.

It was suggested to the patient that she should carry out a tilt training program at home by standing against a wall with the ankles together, 20 cm from the wall, once every day for a planned duration of up to 30 min, depending on her orthostatic tolerance (Fig. 32.1). After 1 month of daily tilt training at home, the patient underwent a check-up tilt test, which was negative. The patient was therefore told to continue tilt training at home.

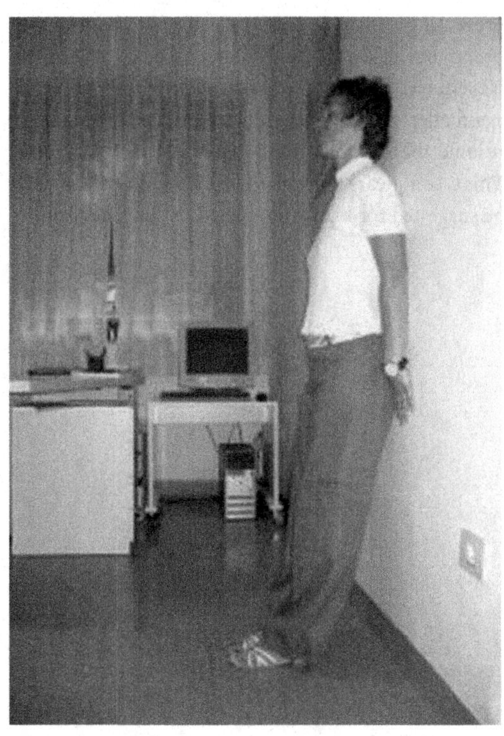

Figure 32.1 Tilt training by standing against a wall.

The patient stopped doing the tilt training after a few weeks, and a few days later had a recurrence of syncope. She spontaneously came to the outpatient cardiology clinic, requesting therapy. It was suggested that she should resume the tilt training, which had proved to be effective in preventing recurrent syncope, but she declined, saying that she did not think it was reliable. Empirical treatment with beta-blockers was then started, and after a 2-year follow-up period, she was still asymptomatic for recurrent syncope.

Comment

Ector *et al.* suggested tilt training as a new form of treatment for recurrent neurally mediated syncope [1]. After an adequate period of in-hospital training sessions (until the tilt test became negative), patients continued daily tilt training at home. In the study, patients with recurrent syncopal spells, often highly symptomatic, experienced dramatic improvement after doing tilt training. It was hypothesized that repeated orthostatic stress could be beneficial in regulating the cardiovascular mechanisms involved in neurocardiogenic syncope [2]. The efficacy of this nonpharmacological "physical" treatment was confirmed in two other nonrandomized studies [3,4]. However, a problem with this form of treatment is compliance by the patients. In a randomized study, compliance with home tilt training was found to be poor [5], affecting the efficacy of this type of treatment. In the present case, tilt training was effective in preventing recurrent syncope, with the tilt test also becoming negative after a few weeks of treatment. Nevertheless, when the patient developed syncope again after discontinuing tilt training, she refused to resume the treatment and requested drug therapy. This case appears to confirm that tilt training can only be suggested for highly motivated patients and not in the vast majority of those with recurrent vasovagal syncope.

References

1 Ector H, Reybrouck T, Heidbuchel H, *et al.* Tilt training: a new treatment for recurrent neurocardiogenic syncope or severe orthostatic intolerance. *Pacing Clin Electrophysiol* 1998; **21**: 193–6.

2 Reybrouck T, Heidbuchel H, Van de Werf F, *et al.* Tilt training: a treatment for malignant and recurrent neurocardiogenic syncope. *Pacing Clin Electrophysiol* 2000; **23**: 493–8.

3 Di Girolamo E, Di Iorio C, Leonzio L, Sabatini P, Barsotti A. Usefulness of a tilt training program for the prevention of refractory neurocardiogenic syncope in adolescents: a controlled study. *Circulation* 1999; **100**: 1798–801.

4 Abe H, Kondo S, Kohshi K, *et al.* Usefulness of orthostatic self-training for the prevention of neurocardiogenic syncope. *Pacing Clin Electrophysiol* 2002; **25**: 1454–8.

5 Foglia-Manzillo G, Giada F, Giaggioli G, *et al.* Efficacy of tilt training in the treatment of neurally mediated syncope: a randomized study. *Europace* 2004; **6**: 199–204.

CASE 33

Psychological treatment of malignant vasovagal syncope due to blood phobia

N. van Dijk, S.C.J.M. Velzeboer, A. Destrée-Vonk, M. Linzer, W. Wieling

Case report [1]

A 17-year-old boy was referred due to a long history of fainting. He had experienced his first episode at the age of 4 during venipuncture. Since then, he had fainted not only on venipuncture, but later also when thinking of blood, needles, or other hospital-associated procedures. He had no symptoms during prolonged standing. His mother had experienced the same problem when she was young.

When he was 16, he was evaluated by a pediatrician. Syncope occurred when they discussed venipuncture. The patient showed some myoclonic movements and was unconscious for less than 5 min. After regaining consciousness, he was pale, sweating, and nauseous. The physical examination, electrocardiogram (ECG), and echocardiography showed no abnormalities. On a 24-h Holter recording, a sinus rhythm with frequent bouts of sinus arrhythmia ranging from 110 to 58 beats/min was observed.

During cardiovascular reflex investigation, the patient had a blood pressure of 106/54 mmHg. Marked sinus arrhythmia was observed during deep forced breathing. Standing up elicited a normal blood-pressure and heart-rate response. The investigators discussed the normal results of the tests with the patient's mother and mentioned that a "blood-taking" provocation might be necessary on another occasion.

About 1 min later, the patient felt nauseous and started sweating. Bradycardia developed. The patient then became asystolic for almost 50 s. He was placed on the bed and cardiac massage was administered. When the ECG was reviewed afterwards, the first escape beat was almost at the same moment at which cardiopulmonary resuscitation was initiated. After 2 min, the patient regained consciousness with a normal blood pressure and bradycardia of 45 beats/min (Figs. 33.1, 33.2). Syncope due to an emotionally evoked vasovagal response with extreme bradycardia was diagnosed. In view of the clear cause of fainting, and with the patient's age in mind, it was decided not to implant a pacemaker but to refer the patient to the pediatric psychosocial department.

His blood-injury phobia was treated using systematic desensitization with muscle tensing and cognitive techniques [2,3], with surveillance by the pediatric resuscitation team. Cognitive behavioral therapy was used to teach him to apply realistic and reassuring thoughts to the physical symptoms he saw as alarming.

The experience during behavior therapy that straining his muscles immediately reduced negative bodily sensations resulted in effective control of the fear-provoking venipuncture situation. After 10 training sessions, he was able to undergo venipuncture without fainting. The patient had no further fainting episodes during a follow-up period of 18 months.

Comment

This young patient is unique in three ways. Firstly, merely thinking about venipuncture was enough to induce a vasovagal response. Secondly, he had a very

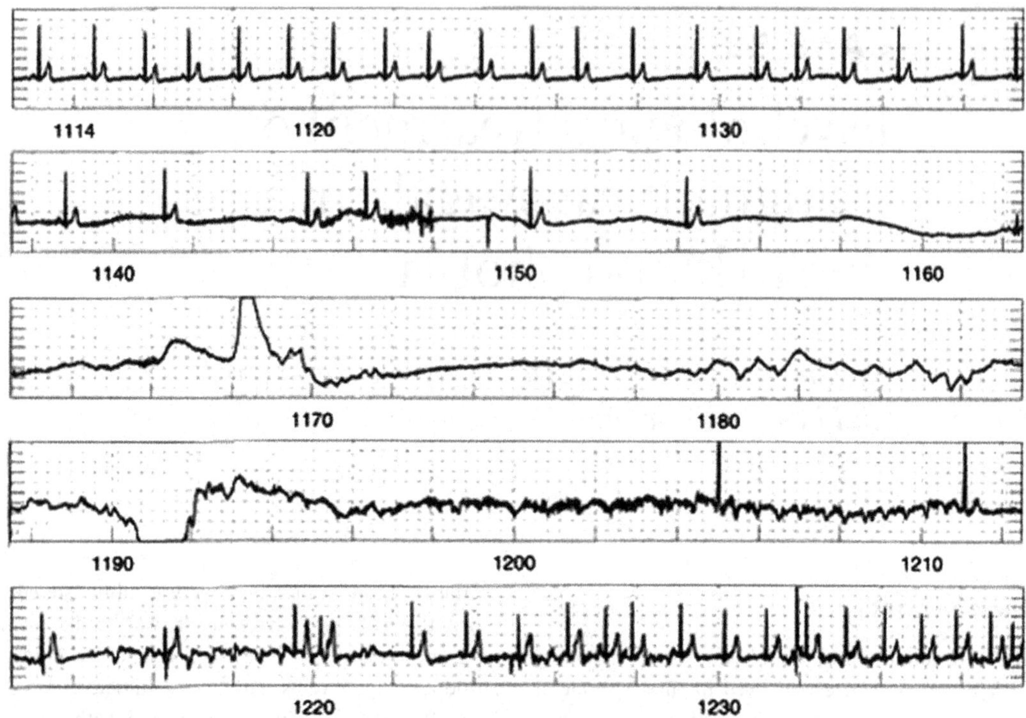

Figure 33.1 Electrocardiography. The time shown (seconds) is taken from the original recording.

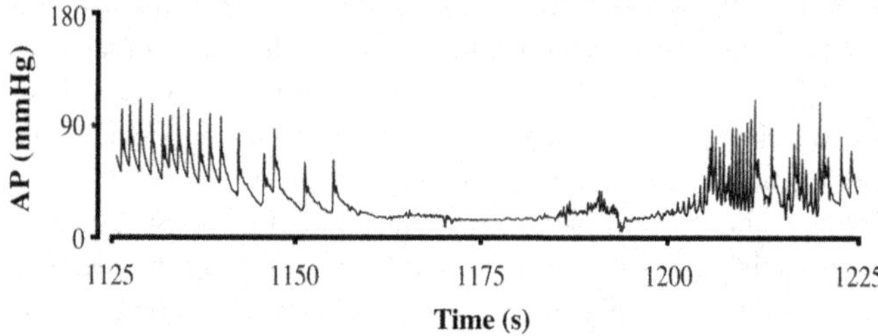

Figure 33.2 Continuous blood-pressure recordings during 50 s of asystole. AP, arterial pressure.

long period of asystole (50 s) due to the blood phobia-related vasovagal syncope. Thirdly, he was successfully treated using psychological interventions, avoiding the use of a pacemaker.

Vasovagal syncope is a frightening but usually benign condition. Vasovagal collapse can occur after certain triggers (such as emotional factors or prolonged standing), which cause a reduction in sympathetic outflow to the systemic circulation and augmentation of efferent vagal activity. In the present case, merely thinking about blood-taking induced an emotional faint. Usually, vasodilation is the most important cause of hypotension in syncope, while bradycardia is often moderate and of late onset. Treatment with a pacemaker, therefore, has no effect on hypotension in the vast majority of such patients, nor on the speed with which hypotension occurs [4–6]. The asystole was clearly instrumental in causing syncope in this patient. The pronounced sinus arrhythmia during Holter monitoring and forced breathing indicated this patient's susceptibility to vagal stimulation. Vasovagal syncope with prolonged asystole is uncommon. Deal *et al.* observed a cardioinhibitory response (asystole ≥ 5 s) in 4.5% of syncopal children during tilt-table testing [7].

Intense fear of blood is seen in 2.0–4.5% of children and adults. Blood-injury phobia usually starts in childhood, is often familial, and is a distinctive focal phobia. Exposure therapy has been described as a valuable method of treating it [8]. In serious cases such as this, great care must be taken when motivating patients to accept treatment, because of their tendency to withdraw from any confrontation with fear-provoking stimuli.

It can be concluded that vasovagal syncope due to blood phobia, even with very long periods of asystole, can be treated using psychological techniques instead of pacemaker implantation.

References

1 van Dijk N, Velzeboer SC, Destrée-Vonk A, Linzer M, Wieling W. Psychological treatment of malignant vasovagal syncope due to blood phobia. *Pacing Clin Electrophysiol* 2001; **24**: 122–4.

2 Hellstrom K, Fellenius J, Ost LG. One versus five sessions of applied tension in the treatment of blood phobia. *Behav Res Ther* 1996; **34**: 101–12.

3 Krediet CT, van Dijk N, Linzer M, van Lieshout JJ, Wieling W. Management of vasovagal syncope: controlling or aborting faints by leg crossing and muscle tensing. *Circulation* 2002; **106**: 1684–9.

4 Sra JS, Jazayeri MR, Avitall B, *et al.* Comparison of cardiac pacing with drug therapy in the treatment of neurocardiogenic (vasovagal) syncope with bradycardia or asystole. *N Engl J Med* 1993; **328**: 1085–90.

5 Hainsworth R. Syncope and fainting: classification and pathopsychological basis. In: Bannister R, Mathias CJ, eds. *Autonomic Failure: a Textbook of Clinical Disorders of the Autonomic Nervous System,* 4th ed. Oxford University Press, New York, 1999: 428–36.

6 Connolly SJ, Sheldon R, Thorpe KE, *et al.* Pacemaker therapy for prevention of syncope in patients with recurrent severe vasovagal syncope—Second Vasovagal Pacemaker Study (VPS II): a randomized trial. *J Am Med Assoc* 2003; **289**: 2224–9.

7 Deal BJ, Strieper M, Scagliotti D, *et al.* The medical therapy of cardioinhibitory syncope in pediatric patients. *Pacing Clin Electrophysiol* 1997; **20**: 1759–61.

8 Marks I. Blood-injury phobia: a review. *Am J Psychiatry* 1988; **145**: 1207–13.

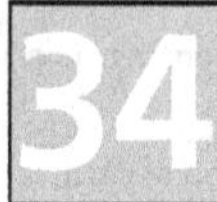

CASE 34

Syncope relapse in a patient with cardioinhibitory neuromediated syncope treated with pacing

A. Ungar, A. Landi, N. Malin, A. Maraviglia, C. Golzio, G. Masotti

Case report

A 70-year-old woman was referred to our outpatient department due to recurrent episodes of unexplained syncope (10 episodes during the previous 2 years). All of the episodes, which always occurred when she was in the upright position, were preceded by prodromal symptoms. Two events were complicated by traumatic injury (wrist and hip fractures). The patient had previously been evaluated with electrocardiography, blood chemistry, electroencephalography, and computed tomography of the brain, with negative results.

The patient's clinical history was negative for hypertension, diabetes, and heart disease. The electrocardiogram recorded at the time of the physical examination was normal. The supine blood pressure was 145/80 mmHg, and no orthostatic hypotension was present. The patient's clinical history, the number of episodes, and the absence of structural heart diseases indicated that neurally mediated syncope was likely.

Supine and upright carotid sinus massage (CSM) and a tilt test with sublingual nitroglycerin stimulation were carried out. Both supine and upright CSM were negative. The tilt test showed positive results for vasovagal syncope (Vasovagal Syncope International Study type 2b), with a 30-s asystole. As clinical data on the use of pacemakers in the treatment of vasovagal syncope are still inconclusive, it was decided not to implant a pacemaker. However, a Reveal implantable loop recorder (ILR) (Medtronic Inc., Minneapolis, Minnesota, USA) was placed. Three months later, the patient suffered a new syncope complicated by head injury. The ILR recorded an asystole of 9 s (Fig. 34.1). After this episode, a dual-chamber cardiac pacemaker was implanted. Two months later, the patient experienced another syncope. However, this time the prodromal symptoms were more pronounced and prolonged, and the patient was able to reach a chair and suffered no injury. After this, she finally decided to use the waist-height support stockings that had been prescribed during her first visit to our department. No further syncopal episodes occurred during the following 12 months.

Comment

Treatment of vasovagal syncope is difficult when recurrent episodes are very frequent. Laboratory findings with the head-up tilt test have generally reported that pacing fails to prevent syncope, although it may prolong the premonitory phase [1]. This was exactly what happened in this patient who, after receiving the pacemaker, had more prolonged prodromes that allowed her to sit down, preventing a traumatic fall. The use of cardiac pacing to treat cardioinhibitory vasovagal syncope is controversial. Positive results with pacemaker therapy were reported in three unblind trials [2–4], but two more recent blind trials (in which the patients in the control arm received a pacemaker implant that was switched off) failed to prove that pacemaker therapy was significantly better [5,6].

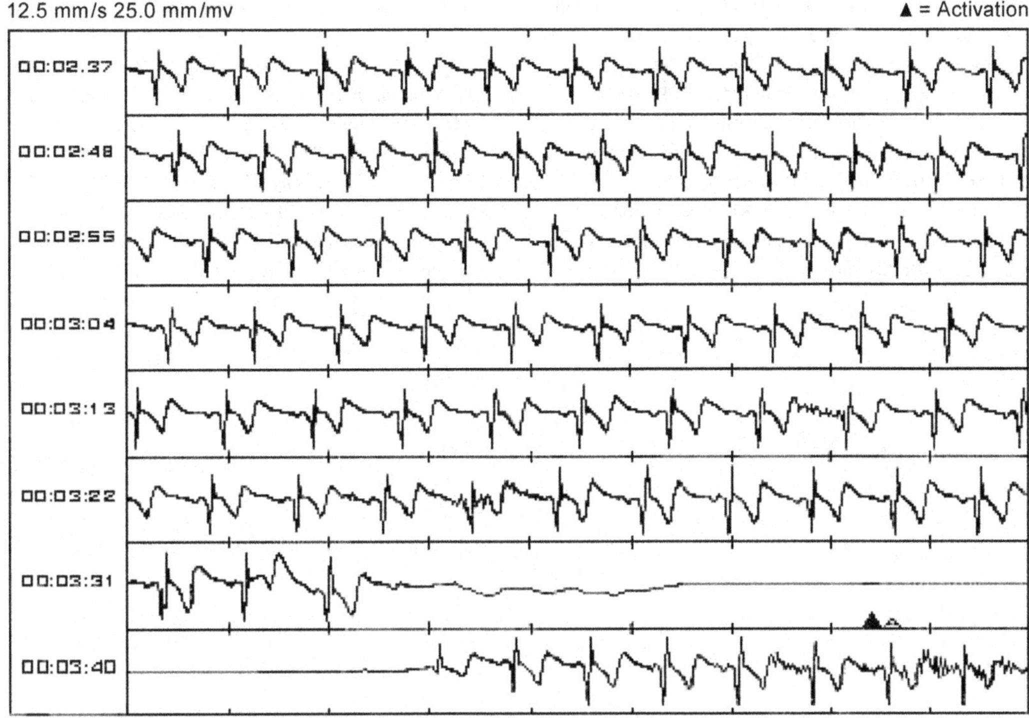

Figure 34.1 A 9-s asystole during spontaneous syncope, recorded using the Reveal implantable loop recorder.

When the results of these five trials are combined, they represent a total of 318 patients who were evaluated. Syncope recurred in 21% of the pacemaker patients (33 of 156) and in 44% of those without pacemaker treatment (72 of 162; $P < 0.001$). However, all of the studies had weaknesses, and further follow-up studies addressing many of these limitations (particularly the likely placebo effect of the pacemaker and the preimplantation criteria used to select which patients might benefit from pacemaker therapy) are needed before pacemaker treatment can be regarded as an established therapy in more than a selected group of patients with recurrent vasovagal syncope. It appears that pacemaker therapy may be effective in some patients, but not all. This is not surprising when one considers that pacemaker treatment is probably efficacious for asystolic reflex but has no role in combatting hypotension, which is frequently the dominant reflex in neurally mediated syncope. It is still uncertain how these patients should be stratified.

Usually, the selection of patients has been based on the results of the head-up tilt-table test. However, studies of patients with an ILR implant have shown a weak correlation between the type of response during the tilt test and the response observed during spontaneous syncope [7]. The role of the ILR in selecting patients who may benefit from cardiac pacing is currently being evaluated. In the present case, although a cardioinhibitory form of syncope was confirmed by the ILR recording, pacing alone was unable to control the symptoms and only the combination of cardiac pacing and the use of waist-height support stockings was effective in treating the syncope.

References

1 Sra J, Jazayeri MR, Avitall B, *et al.* Comparison of cardiac pacing with drug therapy in the treatment of neurocardiogenic (vasovagal) syncope with bradycardia or asystole. *N Engl J Med* 1993; **328**: 1085–90.

2 Sutton R, Brignole M, Menozzi C, *et al.* Dual-chamber pacing in the treatment of neurally mediated tilt-positive cardioinhibitory syncope: pacemaker versus no therapy. A multicenter randomized study. The Vasovagal Syncope International Study (VASIS) Investigators. *Circulation* 2000; **102**: 294–9.

3 Connolly SJ, Sheldon R, Roberts RS, *et al.* The North

American Vasovagal Pacemaker Study (VPS): a randomized trial of permanent cardiac pacing for the prevention of vasovagal syncope. *J Am Coll Cardiol* 1999; **33**: 16–20.

4 Ammirati F, Colivicchi F, Santini M, *et al.* Permanent cardiac pacing versus medical treatment for the prevention of recurrent vasovagal syncope: a multicenter, randomized, controlled trial. *Circulation* 2001; **104**: 52–7.

5 Connolly SJ, Sheldon R, Thorpe KE, *et al.* Pacemaker therapy for prevention of syncope in patients with recurrent severe vasovagal syncope: Second Vasovagal Pacemaker Study (VPS II). A randomized trial. *J Am Med Assoc* 2003; **289**: 2224–9.

6 Giada F, Raviele A, Menozzi C, *et al.* A randomized, double-blind, placebo-controlled study of permanent cardiac pacing for the treatment of recurrent tilt-induced vasovagal syncope. The Vasovagal Syncope and Pacing Trial (SYNPACE). *Eur Heart J* 2004; **25**: 1741–8.

7 Moya A, Brignole M, Menozzi C, *et al.* Mechanism of syncope in patients with isolated syncope and in patients with tilt-positive syncope. *Circulation* 2001; **104**: 1261–7.

Carotid sinus syndrome

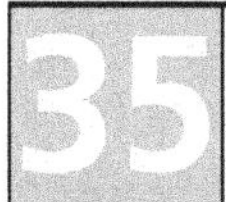

CASE 35

Carotid sinus syndrome

J.J. Blanc, P. Castellant

Case report

A 52-year-old man with an unremarkable medical history had been smoking 30 cigarettes/day for 30 years but had no other risk factors for coronary artery disease. He was referred to our department due to recurrent syncope, which on the last occasion had led to head trauma without fracture. History-taking revealed that he had had dizziness for the previous 2–3 months—always in the same situation, when descending down a spiral staircase. Two days before admission, he had in the same situation experienced a first typical syncope, with a fall but fortunately with no injury. The two syncope episodes were very abrupt, without warning symptoms, and short.

The examination was unremarkable, with normal auscultation and normal blood pressure (140/70 mmHg without orthostatic hypotension). The electrocardiography findings were also completely normal, with a normal QRS in particular. Carotid sinus massage (CSM) was carried out with the patient upright on the tilt-table for 7 s, and induced a long ventricular pause reproducing dizziness (Fig. 35.1). The blood pressure measured just after the pause was 70/40 mmHg.

In view of the recurrent syncope, the patient's need to walk downstairs regularly, and the traumatic effects of the syncope, the patient agreed to the implantation of a DDD pacemaker.

Comment

In a man older than 50 with no overt heart disease and/or electrocardiographic abnormalities, a carotid sinus syndrome should be ruled out after a normal initial evaluation. In this case, the circumstances were highly suggestive of this syndrome—walking down a spiral staircase meant that the patient had to lean his head to the side and was therefore possibly stimulating the carotid sinus.

Carotid sinus massage (CSM) is indicated, and the procedure is considered positive if there is an asystole for longer than 3 s and/or a fall in systolic blood pressure of 50 mmHg or more [1]. CSM has to be performed with the patient in the upright position in order to increase the sensitivity [2,3]. Many authors consider that the symptoms have to be reproducible for the test to be regarded as fully positive (as was the case in this patient, although massage was not continued until syncope occurred but stopped when he felt dizzy).

A positive response to CSM is considered diagnostic of carotid sinus syncope in the absence of other competing diagnoses. Implantation of a cardiac pacemaker is regarded as the treatment of choice for cardioinhibitory carotid sinus syndrome. Dual-chamber cardiac pacing is generally preferable [4].

References

1 Brignole M, Alboni P, Benditt D, *et al.* Guidelines on management (diagnosis and treatment) of syncope—update 2004. *Europace* 2004; **6**: 467–537.

2 Brignole M, Sartore B, Prato R. Role of body position during carotid sinus stimulation test in the diagnosis of cardioinhibitory carotid sinus syndrome. *G Ital Cardiol* 1983; 14: 69–72.

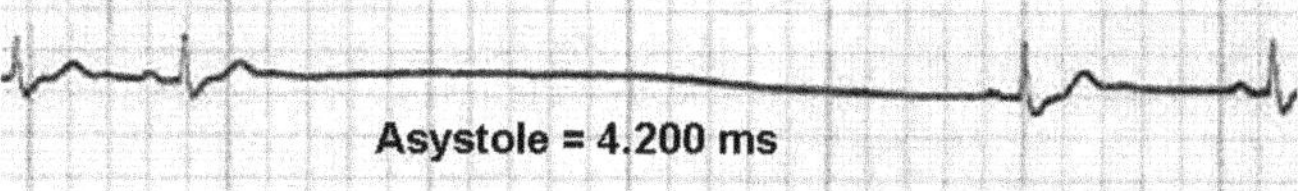

Figure 35.1 Result of the carotid sinus massage.

3 Parry SW, Richardson D, O'Shea D, *et al.* Diagnosis of carotid sinus hypersensitivity in older adults: carotid sinus massage in the upright position is essential. *Heart* 2000; **83**: 22–3.

4 Brignole M, Menozzi C. Carotid sinus syndrome: diagnosis, natural history and treatment. *Eur J Cardiac Pacing Electrophysiol* 1992; **4**: 247–54.

CASE 36

Carotid sinus hypersensitivity only during tilting

A. Bartoletti, P. Fabiani

Case report

A 76-year-old man was referred to our syncope center due to a fall that had caused severe trauma. The clinical history included a minor stroke (with complete recovery) in 1999 and recurrent, unexplained falls that had persisted since 2000. The last episode (5 days previously) was unwitnessed, and caused trauma to the head and face, with fracture of the nose and retrograde amnesia. The previous episode (1 month before) was also unwitnessed and had caused head trauma with brain concussion. Structural heart disease had been excluded in this patient during a previous hospitalization, and supine carotid sinus massage (CSM) had been carried out, with negative results.

At this presentation, the physical examination and baseline electrocardiogram were normal. The patient was not taking any cardioactive or vasoactive drugs. After orthostatic hypotension had been excluded [1], CSM was carried out in accordance with the "symptoms method" [2]. The supine CSM findings were negative (Fig. 36.1).

Repetition of CSM during 70° passive upright tilting caused a paroxysmal atrioventricular block with an asystolic pause of 5 s and clear syncope (Fig. 36.2). After bolus administration of 0.02 mg/kg atropine,

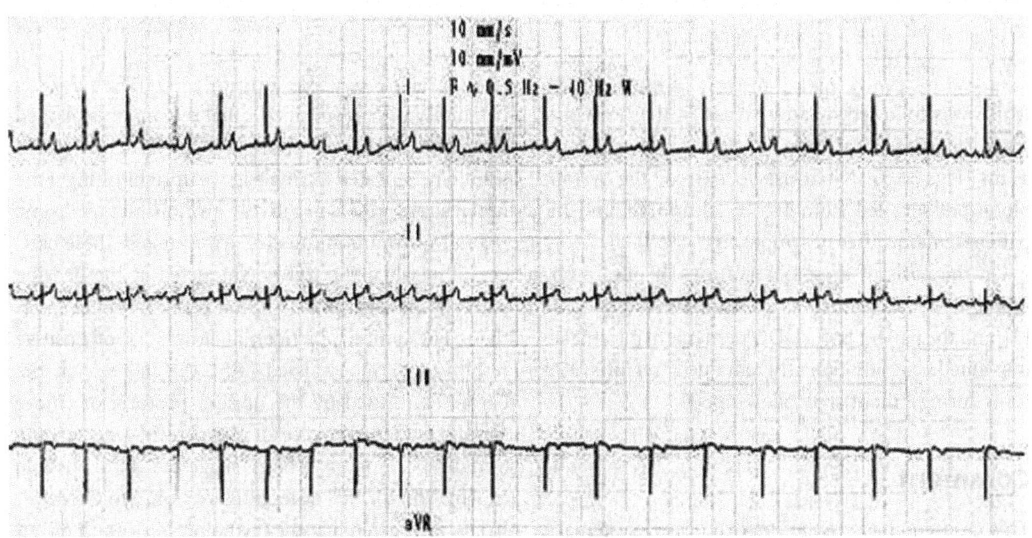

Figure 36.1 Left carotid sinus massage with the patient in the supine position.

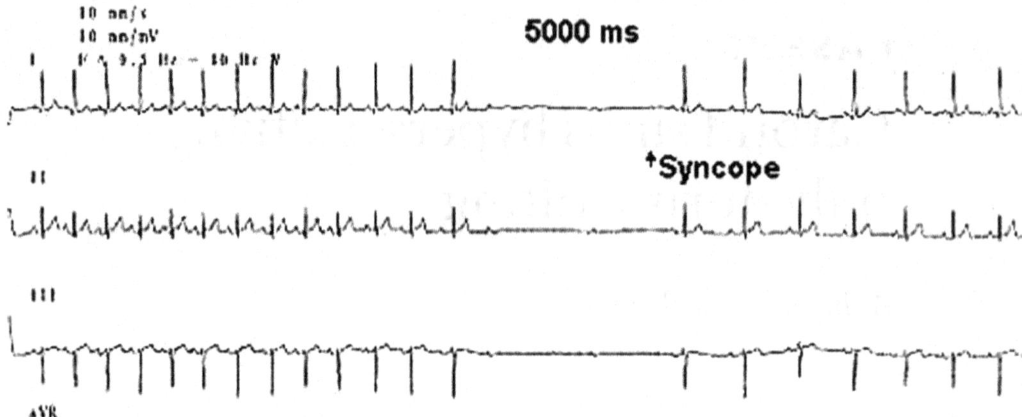

Figure 36.2 Left carotid sinus massage with the patient in the upright position.

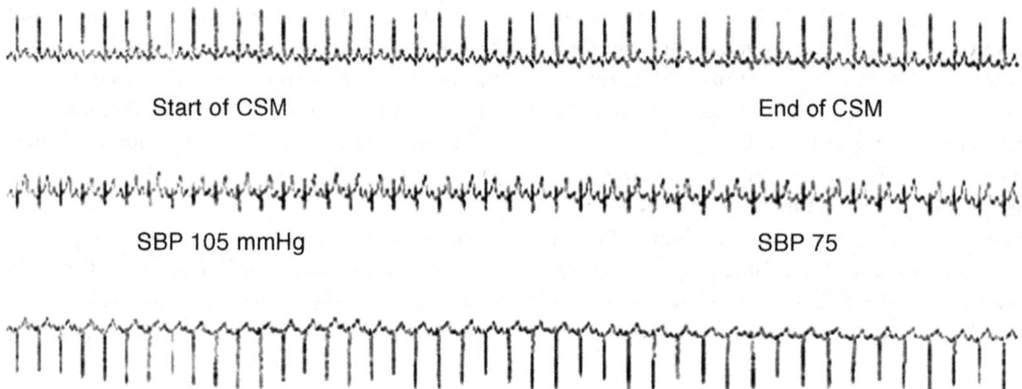

Figure 36.3 Left carotid sinus massage with the patient in the upright position after bolus administration of 0.02 mg/kg atropine. CSM, carotid sinus massage; SBP, systolic blood pressure.

which was followed by an increase in the heart rate from 76 to 108 beats/min, upright CSM was tried again (Fig. 36.3). No pauses occurred, the systolic blood pressure fell from 105 to 75 mmHg, and the patient remained free of symptoms.

On the basis of these observations, a purely cardioinhibitory carotid sinus syndrome was diagnosed [3], and the patient had a DDD permanent pacemaker implanted. He subsequently remained free of symptoms during 8 months of follow-up.

Comment

This case emphasizes the importance of systematic assessment for carotid sinus hypersensitivity in elderly patients with syncope or falls that remain unexplained after the initial evaluation [1]. In particular, CSM should be repeated during passive upright tilting if the initial supine test is negative. Carotid sinus syndrome is a not uncommon cause of symptoms in these patients, but when the test is conducted at the bedside with the patient in the supine position alone (as is the usual clinical practice), at least 30% of positive responses may be missed [4,5]. An increase in the baroreflex caused by the upright posture, or (more simply) better exposure of the carotid sinus in the upright position, has been suggested as a possible explanation for this differential response to CSM [5]. In any case, given that the cardioinhibitory and mixed subtypes of carotid sinus syndrome are amenable to effective treatment with permanent cardiac pacemaker placement [1,6], there is no doubt about the practical importance of these observations.

References

1 Brignole M, Alboni P, Benditt D, *et al.* Guidelines on management (diagnosis and treatment) of syncope. Task Force on Syncope, European Society of Cardiology. *Eur Heart J* 2001; **22:** 1256–306.

2 Brignole M, Menozzi C. Carotid sinus syndrome: diagnosis, natural history and treatment. *Eur J Cardiac Pacing Electrophysiol* 1992; **4:** 247–54.

3 McIntosh SJ, Lawson J, Kenny RA. Clinical characteristics of vasodepressor, cardioinhibitory and mixed carotid sinus syndrome in the elderly. *Am J Med* 1993; **95:** 203–8.

4 Parry SW, Richardson DA, O'Shea D, *et al.* Diagnosis of carotid sinus hypersensitivity in older adults: carotid sinus massage in the upright position is essential. *Heart* 2000; **83:** 22–3.

5 Puggioni E, Guiducci V, Brignole M, *et al.* Results and complications of the carotid sinus massage performed according to the "method of symptoms." *Am J Cardiol* 2002; **89:** 599–601.

6 Kenny RA, Richardson DA, Steen N, Bexton RS, Shaw FE, Bond J. Carotid sinus syndrome: a modifiable risk factor for nonaccidental falls in older adults. *J Am Coll Cardiol* 2001; **38:** 1491–6.

CASE 37

Complex cardioinhibitory neurally mediated syncope

P. Donateo, D. Oddone, A. Solano, F. Croci, E. Puggioni, R. Maggi, M. Brignole

Case report

A 69-year-old man presented with three syncopal episodes during the previous year. Two of the episodes occurred when he was in a standing position, without prodromal signs and with rapid recovery of consciousness. The third episode, again without prodromal signs, occurred while he was driving a car; again, consciousness returned rapidly. The patient was evaluated at the outpatient cardiology clinic. With the exception of syncope, the history and physical examination were negative. The resting electrocardiogram and echocardiogram were normal.

Assessment for neurally mediated syncope was carried out. The tilt test induced syncope during the drug-challenge phase, 6 min after nitroglycerin administration (with a 400-μg sublingual spray). The response pattern was dysautonomic, Vasovagal Syncope International Study type 2b (with progressive sinus bradycardia at 30 beats/min followed by two asystolic pauses of 6.5 and 5.0 s) (Figs. 37.1, 37.2A). Nevertheless, the patient did not recognize this as corresponding to his spontaneous clinical syncope.

Carotid sinus massage induced syncope with the patient in the supine position (14.5 s of asystolic pause, with a fall in systolic blood pressure from 135 mmHg to 40 mmHg), which was recognized by the patient as corresponding to the spontaneous syncope (Fig. 37.2B). Carotid sinus massage was repeated with the patient in the upright position and reproduced the syncope with

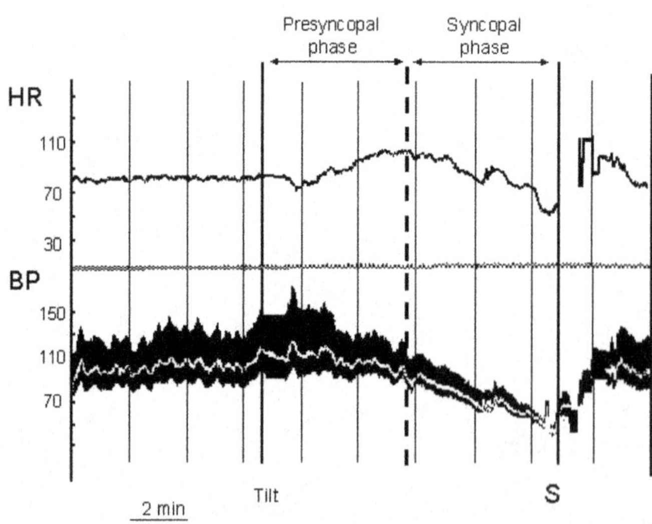

Figure 37.1 Tilt testing, showing the dysautonomic (vasovagal) syncope pattern that occurred after nitroglycerin administration. The top trace shows the heart-rate curve, while the lower trace shows the systolic, diastolic, and mean blood-pressure curves. There is an absence of adaptation of blood pressure to the upright position; during the presyncopal phase (lasting approximately 3 min), the blood pressure declines slightly; since the systolic pressure decreases more than the diastolic pressure, the pulse also declines. The heart rate rises slightly. The vertical dashed line indicates the time of onset of the vasovagal reaction, which is characterized by a decrease in heart rate until the asystolic pause (well shown in the expanded electrocardiogram in Fig. 37.2). HR, heart rate; BP, blood pressure; S, syncope.

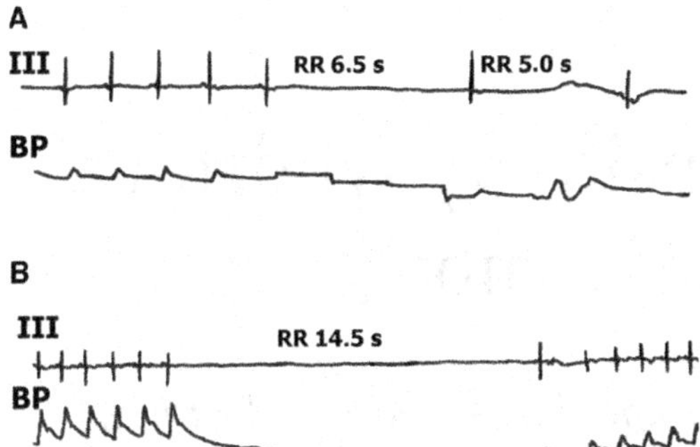

Figure 37.2 **A.** An expanded electrocardiogram tracing at the time of syncope during the tilt test shown in Fig. 37.1. **B.** Right carotid sinus massage. A long pause is recorded at the time of syncope during both the tilt test and carotid sinus massage.

an asystolic pause of 12 s and a systolic blood pressure drop from 120 mmHg to 40 mmHg (not shown). Asystole and syncope were no longer induced after atropine administration (0.02 mg/kg i.v.).

A diagnosis of complex cardioinhibitory neurally mediated syncope was therefore made. A dual-chamber pacemaker was implanted. The patient remained free of symptoms during a 14-month follow-up period.

Comment

Both carotid sinus massage and tilt testing induced syncope. Carotid sinus massage induced a dominant cardioinhibitory response, while tilt testing caused a dysautonomic hypotensive response preceded by severe bradycardia with a long asystolic pause at the time of syncope. In a recent study [1], 15% of patients affected by unexplained syncope after the initial evaluation experienced syncope during both carotid sinus massage and tilt testing. A positive response to both of these tests in patients with neurally mediated syncope has also been described in previous studies [2–4]. Syncope may therefore be precipitated by different maneuvers and by different situations (different afferent pathways); this finding suggests that neurally mediated syncope results from a central abnormality rather than from local pathology [1]. The clinical presentation of complex neurally mediated syncope is similar to that in patients with isolated carotid sinus syncope and tilt-induced syncope [1].

References

1 Alboni P, Brignole M, Menozzi C, *et al.* Clinical spectrum of neurally mediated syncopes. *Europace* 2004; **6**: 55–62.

2 Brignole M, Menozzi C, Gianfranchi L, *et al.* Carotid sinus massage, eyeball compression and head-up tilt test in patients with syncope of uncertain origin and in healthy control subjects. *Am Heart J* 1991; **122**: 1644–51.

3 Alboni P, Menozzi C, Brignole M, *et al.* An abnormal neural reflex plays a role in causing syncope in sinus bradycardia. *J Am Coll Cardiol* 1993; **22**: 30–4.

4 Brignole M, Menozzi C, Gianfrachi L, *et al.* Neurally mediated syncope detected by carotid sinus massage and head-up tilt test in sick sinus syndrome. *Am J Cardiol* 1991; **68**: 1032–6.

CASE 38

Carotid hypersensitivity syndrome secondary to neck tumor

S. Gómez Moreno, G. Barón Esquivias, A. Pedrote Martínez, F. Errázquin Sáenz de Tejada, A. Martínez Martínez

Case report

A 65-year-old man was admitted to the hospital for scheduled surgery due to a tumor of the right tonsil. While the patient was in the operating room and preparation was being carried out before the procedure, he suffered a syncopal episode, and the monitor showed a prolonged asystole. The procedure was therefore postponed and the surgeons and anesthesiologists requested a cardiologic evaluation.

There were no relevant findings in his medical history. The patient denied having had any symptoms suggesting angina pectoris, syncopal episodes, edema, or palpitations. Cardiopulmonary auscultation was normal; the blood-pressure value was 110/70 mmHg, and an electrocardiogram was also normal.

Right carotid sinus massage was carried out with the patient in the supine position and a positive response was obtained, with an asystole of 5 s without symptoms (Fig. 38.1). Left carotid sinus massage was normal. Carotid sinus hypersensitivity secondary to the tumor was therefore considered the most probable cause of the syncopal episode.

As the intervention required resection of the right lymphatic nodes and manipulation or stimulation of the carotid sinus was expected to be required, a prophylactic temporary transvenous pacing system was inserted before the intervention, and the surgical team was instructed to use vasoactive drugs if hypotension developed.

The procedure was completed without incident, and the pacemaker was removed in the postoperative period. After the intervention, the patient remained free of syncope. A repeated right carotid sinus massage before he was discharged from the hospital was normal, and no treatment for the syncope was scheduled.

Comment

It is well known that certain tumors of the head, neck, and retropharyngeal space can present with syncopal episodes that resemble vasovagal reactions due to the presence of cardioinhibition and hypotension [1–3]. Compression and irritation of the carotid sinus [1] or direct involvement of the glossopharyngeal or vagus nerves appears to be the most probable cause of these

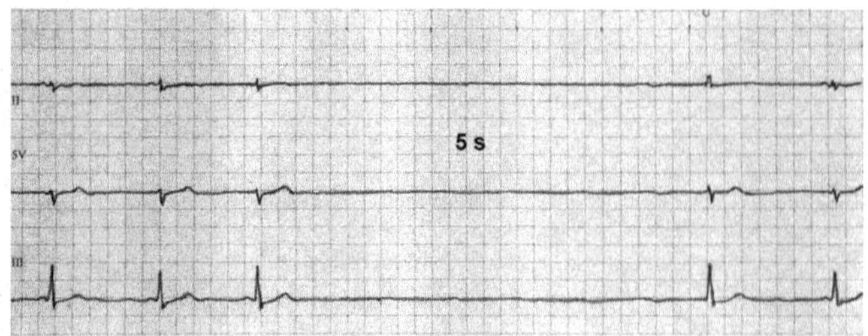

Figure 38.1 A sinus pause of 5 s was recorded during right carotid sinus massage.

types of syncope [4,5]. There are at least three clinical forms of presentation of syncope related to neck tumors:

• The syncope may be associated with carotid sinus hypersensitivity [1,2].

• The syncope may be associated with pain episodes, as a typical form of glossopharyngeal neuralgia [2,6].

• The syncope may not be associated with carotid sinus hypersensitivity or pain.

To explain the latter form, Cicogna *et al.* [4] suggested that the mechanism of the attacks could be similar to that in glossopharyngeal neuralgia, but without involving pain pathways. Syncopal episodes usually become manifest in the form of bradycardia/asystole and hypotension, but there have been reported cases of hypotension alone [2].

The management of patients with syncope secondary to neck tumors is complex. Surgical resection of the tumor should be attempted when possible. Cardiac pacemaker placement may fail, as it does not preclude the vasodepressor component. Other treatments include anticholinergic drugs, carbamazepine, and intracranial sectioning of the glossopharyngeal nerve [2].

In the present case, the patient, with a tonsillar tumor, had had no episodes of syncope until the moments just before the intervention. In the subsequent investigation, only an abnormal response to carotid sinus massage ipsilateral to the location of the tumor was demonstrated. A temporary pacemaker was inserted before the surgical procedure due to the risk of vasovagal reactions during it [7]. After surgical resection of the tumor and lymphatic nodes, no further hypersensitivity of the carotid sinus was observed.

References

1 Patel AK, Yap VU, Fields J, Thomsen JH. Carotid sinus syncope induced by malignant tumors in the neck. *Arch Intern Med* 1979; **139**: 1281–4.

2 McDonald DR, Strong E, Nielsen S, Posner JB. Syncope from head and neck cancer. *J Neurooncol* 1983; **1**: 257–67.

3 Yue AM, Thomas RD. Neurocardiogenic syncope due to recurrent tonsillar carcinoma: successful treatment by dual chamber cardiac pacing with rate hysteresis. *Pacing Clin Electrophysiol* 2002; **25**: 121–2.

4 Cicogna R, Curnis A, Dei Cas L, Visioli O. Syncope and tumours in the neck: carotid sinus or glossopharyngeal syndrome? *Eur Heart J* 1985; **6**: 979–84.

5 Prentice DA, Trotter JM, Edis RH. Syncope: a clue to malignant compression of the glossopharyngeal nerve. *Med J Aust* 1986; **144**: 547–9.

6 Rumoroso JR, Arana J, Montes PM, Gonzalez-Liebana J, Cembellin JC, Barrenetxea JL. Síncope asociado a neuralgia del glosofaringeo y tumoración parafaríngea. *Rev Esp Cardiol* 1996; **49**: 704–6.

7 Al-Ebrahim K, el-Azam M, el-Kholy A, Shafei H. Arterial and venous paragangliomas: the value of preoperative pacemaker and a multidisciplinary approach. *Br J Neurosurg* 1997; **11**: 233–7.

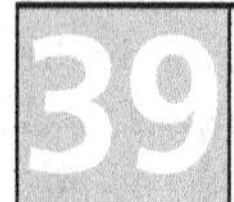

CASE 39

Syncope in a case of carotid body paraganglioma

J. García Sacristán, C. Almodóvar, M. Atienzar

Case report

A 61-year-old man was admitted to the emergency department due to recurrent episodes of syncope during the preceding 3 months. Sudden syncopal attacks developed when he was in the supine or standing position, without any apparent precipitating cause. Shortly after admission, the patient had a syncopal attack and bradycardia, and an atrioventricular block was observed on the electrocardiography (ECG) monitor. He was transferred to the intensive-care unit, where an electrical catheter was inserted via the femoral route, advanced to the right ventricular apex, and connected to an external temporary pacemaker. In the intensive-care unit, the patient experienced new syncopal episodes despite normal ventricular pacing.

The patient was a smoker (20 cigarettes/day), and had a history of mild arterial hypertension and chronic bronchitis. He denied having headaches, palpitations, or tremor. During an examination of the neck, a mobile and pulsatile mass approximately 5 cm in diameter was observed on the left side, next to the angle of the mandible. The rest of the physical examination was unremarkable, and the baseline ECG was normal.

With the patient in the supine position and the pacemaker disconnected, carotid sinus massage was carried out. Right carotid sinus massage was normal. Left carotid sinus massage (over the neck mass) induced syncope, and the ECG showed a primary sinus pause of around 15 s followed by secondary pauses and bradycardia (Fig. 39.1). The left carotid sinus massage was repeated after intravenous administration of 2 mg of atropine, and a fall in the systolic arterial pressure of more than 50 mmHg was observed (Fig. 39.2). A diagnosis of carotid sinus hypersensitivity of the mixed type (cardioinhibitory and vasodepressor) secondary to a neck tumor was therefore made.

Computed tomography (Fig. 39.3A) revealed a mass 5.3 × 3.5 × 3.8 cm in size on the bifurcation of the left common carotid artery. Arteriography (Fig. 39.3B) demonstrated widening of the carotid bifurcation, with a well-defined tumor blush (the "lyre sign"). The provisional diagnosis was paraganglioma of the carotid body. Values for urinary metanephrines and vanillylmandelic acid were within the normal limits.

Surgical excision of the tumor was uneventful. Histological examination showed well-defined nests of cuboidal cells with moderately abundant granular

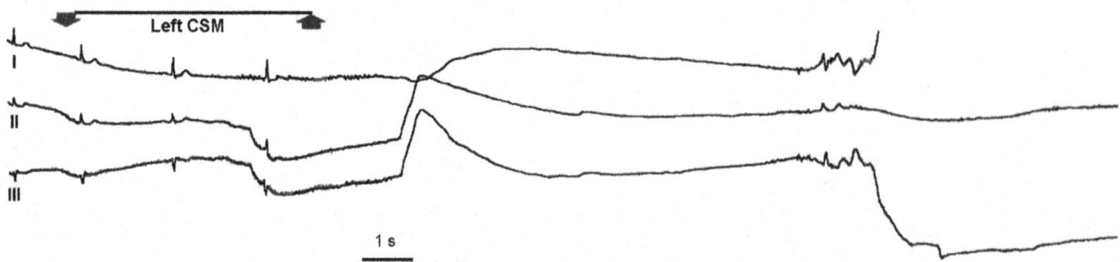

Figure 39.1 Left carotid sinus massage (CSM) induced a primary sinus pause lasting approximately 15 s, followed by secondary pauses, bradycardia, and syncope.

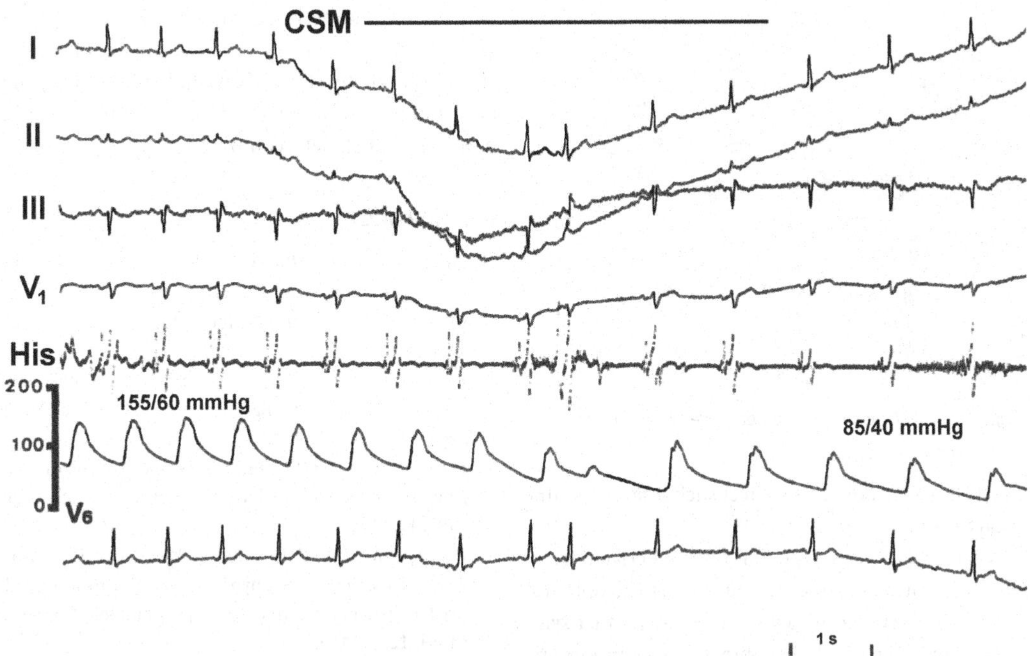

Figure 39.2 Left carotid sinus massage (CSM) after intravenous administration of 2 mg of atropine.

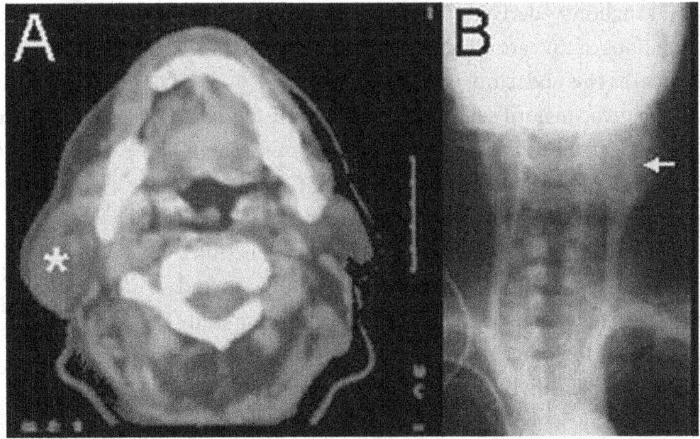

Figure 39.3 Computed tomogram (A) and angiogram (B), showing the tumor (asterisk and arrow).

cytoplasm, separated by highly vascularized fibrous septa (Fig. 39.4). Immunohistochemically, the lesion was found to be positive for neuron-specific enolase, chromogranin, serotonin, and synaptophysin. The final diagnosis was carotid body paraganglioma.

During a follow-up period of 14 years, the patient did not suffer any further syncopal episodes.

Comment

Syncope is a rare but important complication of tumors located in the neck and parapharyngeal space [1–9]. The mechanism of syncope in these cases is an intense vasovagal reaction due to carotid sinus hypersensitivity [1–5] or direct irritation/compression of the glossopharyngeal nerve [6–9]—a mechanism similar to that occurring in glossopharyngeal neuralgia syncope, except for the absence of pain. An association of syncope with glossopharyngeal neuralgia due to a parapharyngeal tumor has been described [10].

In the majority of the reported cases, neck tumors associated with syncope have been malignant [1–5], but cases of benign paragangliomas of the carotid sinus body, as in the present case, have also been described

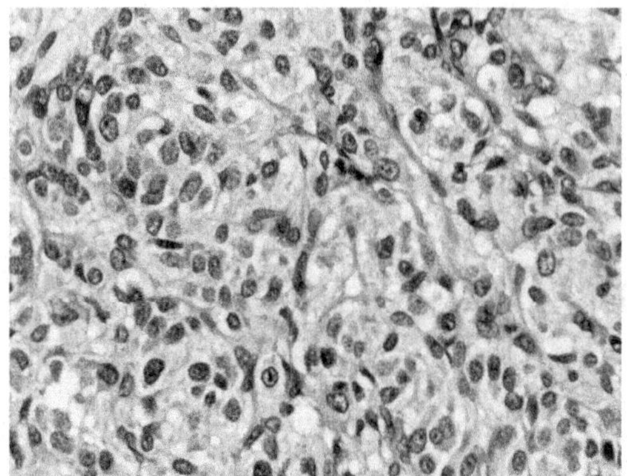

Figure 39.4 The histological appearance of the tumor.

[11,12]. It is important to detect such lesions, as surgical treatment is possible.

There are several types of tumor derived from embryonic neural crest cells. Some of these neoplasms contain endocrine cells (chromaffin tissue) that synthesize and excrete catecholamines. These tumors are termed extra-adrenal pheochromocytomas, while the nonchromaffin tumors are known as paragangliomas. Paragangliomas derived from the chemoreceptor terminations of the carotid body and glomus jugulare are known as chemodectomas.

The great majority of paragangliomas of the head and neck are nonfunctional [13] (not secreting chemical mediators), and the clinical presentation is therefore dominated by local mass effect symptoms (neck masses, tinnitus, and cranial nerve dysfunction). Alternatively, the tumors may be asymptomatic and may be diagnosed incidentally during an imaging study conducted for other reasons. Syncope due to carotid sinus hypersensitivity is a rare presentation [13].

Carotid angiography is the most useful diagnostic test for carotid body paragangliomas. This technique can establish the diagnosis, determine the size of the lesion and its relationship with the carotid arteries, and evaluate the tumor blood supply. Radiographically, a carotid body paraganglioma presents as a rounded, well-delimited, and extremely vascular soft-tissue mass located in the carotid bifurcation. The information provided by angiography is extremely important for assessing the relative risk of surgery and for planning the intervention.

Surgical resection is the treatment of choice for most paragangliomas. Although catecholamine excess is unusual in patients with paragangliomas located in the head and neck region, all patients should be screened for this in order to prevent or block the effects of an acute release of catecholamines during the induction of anesthesia and surgery, which could potentially lead to fatal complications.

References

1 Holmes FA, Glass JP, Ewer MS, Terjanian T, Tetu B. Syncope and hypotension due to carcinoma of the breast metastatic to the carotid sinus. *Am J Med* 1987; **82**: 1238–42.

2 Patel AK, Yap VU, Fields J, Thomsen JH. Carotid sinus syncope induced by malignant tumors in the neck. *Arch Intern Med* 1979; **139**: 1281–4.

3 Frank J, Ropper AH, Zuñiga G. Vasodepressor carotid sinus syncope associated with a neck mass. *Neurology* 1992; **42**: 1194–7.

4 Hawkins J, Lewis HD, Emmot W, Vacek JL. Vasodepressive carotid sinus hypersensitivity with head and neck malignancy: treatment with propranolol. *Am Heart J* 1991; **122**: 234–5.

5 Murata M, Ojima K, Morikawa M, Aizawa Y, Arai Y, Shibata A. Recurrent paroxysmal hypotension and bradycardia in a patient with pharynx tumor metastasis to cervical lymph nodes. *Jpn Circ J* 1986; **50**: 278–82.

6 Cordoba Lopez A, Torrico Roman P, Bueno Alvarez-Arenas I, Monterrubio Villar J, Corcho Sanchez G. Sincope secundario a síndrome del espacio parafaringeo. *Rev Esp Cardiol* 2001; **54**: 649–51.

7 Cicogna R, Bonomi FG, Curnis A, *et al.* Pharyngeal space lesions syncope-syndrome: a newly proposed reflexogenic cardiovascular syndrome. *Eur Heart J* 1993; **14**: 1476–83.

8 Cicogna R, Curnis A, Dei Cas L, Visioli O. Syncope and tumors of the neck: carotid sinus or glossopharyngeal syndrome? *Eur Heart J* 1985; **6**: 979–84.

9 Prentice DA, Trotter JM, Edis RH. Syncope: a clue to malignant compression of the glossopharyngeal nerve. *Med J Aust* 1986; **144**: 547–9.

10 Rumoroso JR, Arana J, Montes PM, Gonzalez-Liebana J, Cembellin JC, Barrenetxea JL. Síncope asociado a neuralgia del glosofaringeo y tumoración parafaríngea. *Rev Esp Cardiol* 1996; **49**: 704–6.

11 Rosenkranz L, Schell AR. Carotid body tumor as reversible cause of recurrent syncope. *NY State J Med* 1984; **84**: 38–9.

12 Vincelj J, Kirin M, Borkovic Z, Lajtman Z, Horzic M. Syncope caused by carotid body tumor. *Acta Med Croatica* 1996; **50**: 213–5.

13 Erickson D, Kudva YC, Ebersold MJ, *et al.* Benign paragangliomas: clinical presentation and treatment outcomes in 236 patients. *J Clin Endocrinol Metab* 2001; **86**: 5210–6.

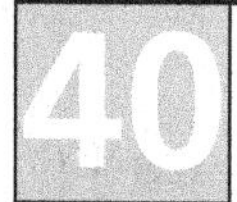

CASE 40

Recurrent syncope in a carotid sinus patient treated with a pacemaker

A. Del Rosso

Case report

A 91-year-old man had a permanent VVI pacemaker implanted due to a cardioinhibitory carotid sinus syndrome (CSS). Three years after the implantation, he experienced several presyncopal episodes and a recurrence of syncope. The syncope occurred when he was in the standing position, without prodromal signs, and the fall caused mild head trauma. The patient had a history of hypertension that had been treated with diuretics. The clinical examination was normal, and the electrocardiogram showed a normal sinus rhythm. Carotid sinus massage with the patient in the standing position induced a paced ventricular rhythm with a fall in systolic blood pressure from 130 mmHg to 70 mmHg and reproduction of the presyncope. A head-up tilt test with sublingual nitroglycerin administration was carried out. In the third minute after nitroglycerin administration, the patient experienced vasodepressor syncope (Fig. 40.1). The diuretic treatment was switched to a dihydropyridine calcium antagonist. The patient did not experience any recurrence of the symptoms during the follow-up period.

Comment

Syncope recurs in up to 10% of patients who receive pacemaker treatment for CSS, and hypotension is the main mechanism of the recurrences. Cardiac pacemaker placement appears to be beneficial in CSS when a cardioinhibitory mechanism is prevalent [1]. Dual-chamber cardiac pacing is preferable. A single-chamber ventricular pacemaker may be sufficient in cases in which there is an absence of both a vasodepressor component and what is known as the "ventricular pacing effect"—a sudden drop in blood pressure and

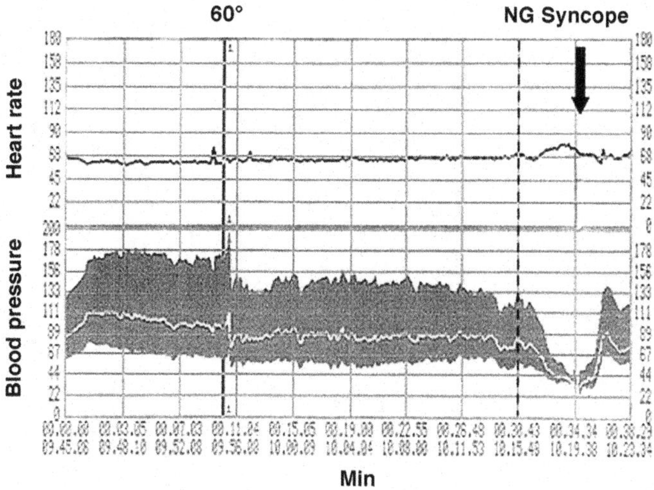

Figure 40.1 The tilt-table test. NG, nitroglycerin.

related symptoms caused by the onset of stimulation in the standing position [2].

A positive response to the head-up tilt test identifies a group of patients who have an increased risk of recurrent syncope after pacemaker implantation for cardioinhibitory CSS [3]. Non-asystolic symptoms can be expected to occur in these patients. In the present case, both a "ventricular pacing effect" and a susceptibility to an orthostatic vasodepressive response probably played a role in the genesis of the symptoms.

Treatment of the vasodepressor component of the reflex is difficult. Chronic vasodilator therapy has been shown to enhance susceptibility to CSS [4]. Discontinuation or reduction of these drugs is therefore advisable in susceptible patients.

References

1 Brignole M, Menozzi C, Lolli G, Bottoni N, Gaggioli G. Long-term outcome of paced and nonpaced patients with severe carotid sinus syndrome. *Am J Cardiol* 1992; **69**: 1039–43.

2 Brignole M, Sartore B, Barra M, Menozzi C, Lolli G. Ventricular and dual chamber pacing for treatment of carotid sinus syndrome. *Pacing Clin Electrophysiol* 1989; **12**: 582–90.

3 Gaggioli G, Brignole M, Menozzi G, *et al.* A positive response to head-up tilt testing predicts syncopal recurrence in carotid sinus syndrome patients with permanent pacemakers. *Am J Cardiol* 1995; **76**: 720–2.

4 Brignole M, Menozzi C, Gaggioli G, *et al.* Effects of chronic vasodilator therapy in patients with carotid sinus hypersensitivity. *Am Heart J* 1998; **136**: 264–8.

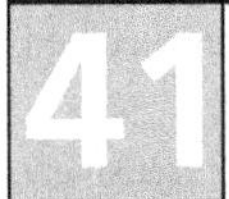

CASE 41

Unexplained falls in older patients

A. Ungar, N. Malin, T. Cellai, A. Landi, A. Maraviglia, G. Masotti

Case report

A 79-year-old woman who was suffering from hypertension, diabetes, obesity, and chronic obstructive pulmonary disease, but was totally independent in basic and instrumental activities of daily living (she worked as a hotel director), fell at home in February 2002. The fall was complicated by a humeral fracture, which was not treated surgically because of her age. The cause of the fall was not evaluated. Pain in the upper limb and an unstable gait associated with postural imbalance led to a progressive disability in instrumental and partly also basic activities of daily living and to the development of a depressive syndrome. As she was unable to live alone, she was admitted to a nursing home and, after 8 months there, was referred to us due to dyspnea on exertion and severe functional impairment.

The physical examination showed only a limitation in the movement of the right shoulder. The clinical history was positive for a syncopal episode that had occurred 2 years before the previously described fall. The syncopal episode had been evaluated at that time only with a brain computed tomography and electroencephalography, both of which were negative. To evaluate the cause of the fall, carotid sinus massage was carried out, which was negative with the patient in the supine position but positive when she was in the upright position for a mixed carotid sinus response with retrograde amnesia (asystole of 3.7 s, with a drop in systolic blood pressure of 50 mmHg) (Fig. 41.1). A tilt test was positive, with a dysautonomic pattern.

A dual-chamber pacemaker was implanted, and the existing antihypertensive treatment (diuretics and doxazosin) was replaced with angiotensin-converting enzyme inhibitors. A radiograph of the right humerus was obtained (Fig. 41.2), confirming the fracture, and the fracture was treated surgically with a prosthesis. The patient was started on a physical rehabilitation program, with progressive improvement in her

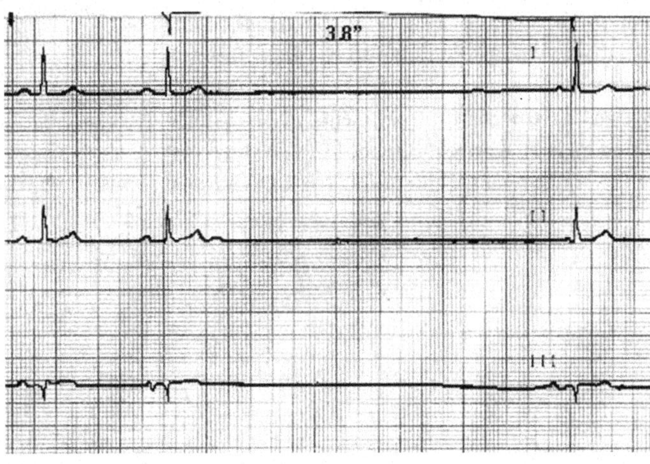

Figure 41.1 Asystole lasting 3.8 s during upright carotid sinus massage.

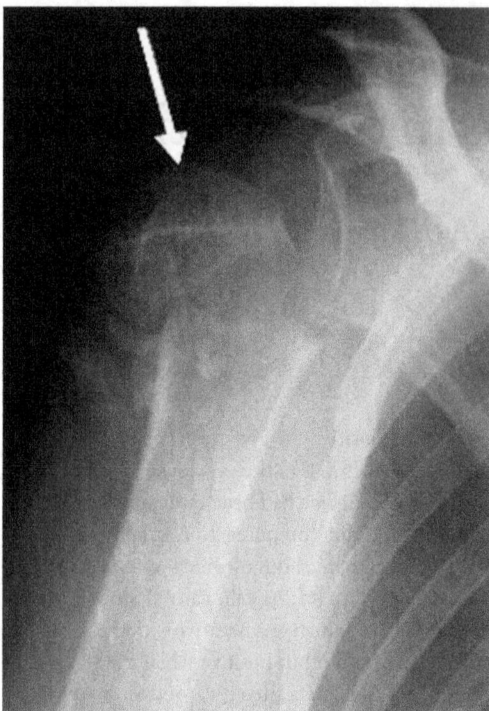

Figure 41.2 Fracture of the right humerus (arrow).

functional capacity and quality of life. At the time of discharge from the acute ward, the patient was independent in all basic activities of daily living. No more falls or episodes of syncope occurred during the following year.

Comment

Unexplained falls and unexplained syncope in older patients may overlap [1]. In particular, retrograde amnesia, an absence of witnesses, and cognitive decline may mask a syncopal episode with an unexplained fall. A recent paper showed that 30% of 647 721 falls referred to emergency departments in the United Kingdom in 1999 were unspecified [2]. The total cost of falls was substantial and mainly related to hospital admissions and social costs, particularly for unspecified falls in the oldest patients (over the age of 75).

Older patients with falls have to be extensively evaluated and promptly treated, due to the severe consequences of fall-related trauma on disability and quality of life, as illustrated by the present case [3,4]. A comprehensive geriatric assessment has to be carried out in every patient with a fall. When an unexplained fall is reported by the patient, the diagnostic protocol for unexplained syncope may be useful [5]. In addition, a neuroautonomic evaluation, particularly the tilt test potentiated with nitroglycerin, and carotid sinus massage—often regarded as potentially dangerous in older subjects—are in fact very well tolerated and useful in the geriatric population [6,7].

References

1 Rubenstein LZ, Josephson KR. The epidemiology of falls and syncope. *Clin Geriatr Med* 2002; **18**: 141–58.

2 Scuffham P, Chaplin S, Legood R. Incidence and costs of unintentional falls in older people in the United Kingdom. *J Epidemiol Community Health* 2003; **57**: 740–4.

3 Marottoli RA, Berkman LF, Cooney LM Jr. Decline in physical function following hip fracture. *J Am Geriatr Soc* 1992; **40**: 861–6.

4 Stel VS, Smit JH, Pluijm SM, Lips P. Consequences of falling in older men and women and risk factors for health service use and functional decline. *Age Ageing* 2004; **33**: 58–65.

5 Kenny RA, Richardson DA, Steen N, Bexton RS, Shaw FE, Bond J. Carotid sinus syndrome: a modifiable risk factor for nonaccidental falls in older adults (SAFE PACE). *J Am Coll Cardiol* 2001; **38**: 1491–6.

6 Del Rosso A, Ungar A, Bartoli P, *et al.* Usefulness and safety of shortened head-up tilt testing potentiated with sublingual glyceryl trinitrate in older patients with recurrent unexplained syncope. *J Am Geriatr Soc* 2002; **50**: 1324–8.

7 Puggioni E, Guiducci V, Brignole M, *et al.* Results and complications of the carotid sinus massage performed according to the "method of symptoms." *Am J Cardiol* 2002; **89**: 599–601.

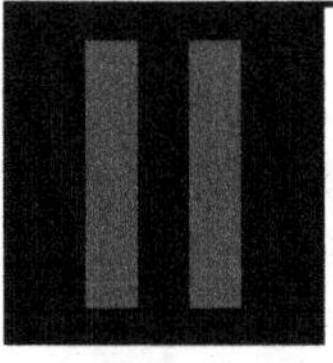

PART II
Orthostatic hypotension

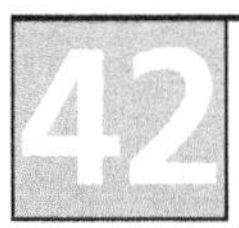

CASE 42

Initial orthostatic hypotension as a cause of syncope in an adolescent

N. van Dijk, M.P.M. Harms, W. Wieling

Case report

A 20-year-old man was referred for evaluation of complaints of light-headedness and muscle weakness shortly (5–10 s) after standing up, or when standing still after physical exercise. He had fainted on numerous occasions just after standing up. He had already had the symptoms for 8 years. He had visited five different medical specialists and had been referred for psychiatric evaluation, but no diagnosis was made [1].

The patient was tall (197 cm) and slim (73 kg). He was examined using a Finometer (FMS Finapres Medical Systems B.V., Amsterdam, Netherlands), which measures rapid changes in blood pressure continuously, accurately, and noninvasively [2]. In the supine position, finger arterial pressure was 105/60 mmHg with a heart rate of 70 beats/min. The initial drop in blood pressure (Fig. 42.1A) was abnormally large (–65 mmHg systolic and –30 mmHg diastolic). During the drop in blood pressure, the patient had recognizable symptoms. His complaints disappeared within 20 s after he had stood up. After 1 and 5 min, his blood pressure was 80/55 mmHg and 100/65 mmHg, respectively, and his heart rate was 120 beats/min. During head-up tilting, there was no drop in blood pressure and the patient did not report any symptoms (Fig. 42.1B).

The patient was diagnosed with initial orthostatic hypotension. He was relieved when we explained the origin of his symptoms. The patient was advised to increase his water and salt intake and was prescribed a mineralocorticoid (fludrocortisone 0.1 mg/day). He was also advised to use lower body muscle tensing as a preventive measure in case of symptoms. Over the years, his symptoms have significantly declined.

Comment

Syncope, and in particular presyncope on standing, is observed much more commonly in younger individuals than in adults. Almost all teenagers and adolescents are familiar with a brief feeling of light-headedness and some visual blurring within a few seconds of standing up quickly. The symptoms typically resolve spontaneously within 20 s. Such complaints are most common after prolonged supine resting or after rising from a squatting position [1–3] (see Cases 43 and 44). The complaints are caused by a transient fall in arterial pressure that occurs when actively standing up. This transient fall in blood pressure during active standing is a physiological response [4]. However, blood pressure does not normally drop by more than –40 mmHg systolic and –20 mmHg diastolic [2]. This initial drop in blood pressure is less dramatic, or is not seen at all, during passive head-up tilting. In some instances, the symptoms are severe and true syncope may develop after standing up in otherwise healthy individuals. A recent study including 394 medical students showed that standing up triggered syncope in 8% [5].

The initial transient fall in pressure in normal young individuals is caused by vasodilation in active muscles during standing [4]. Patients with the most severe symptoms tend to be tall, with an asthenic habitus and poorly developed musculature [6]. The patients often also have postural tachycardia and a tendency to faint during prolonged standing [7,8]. In this condition, history-taking is the most important diagnostic tool. The onset of symptoms between 5 and 10 s and disappearance of the symptoms within 20 s are typical of this clinical condition. The diagnosis can only be confirmed by an active standing test with

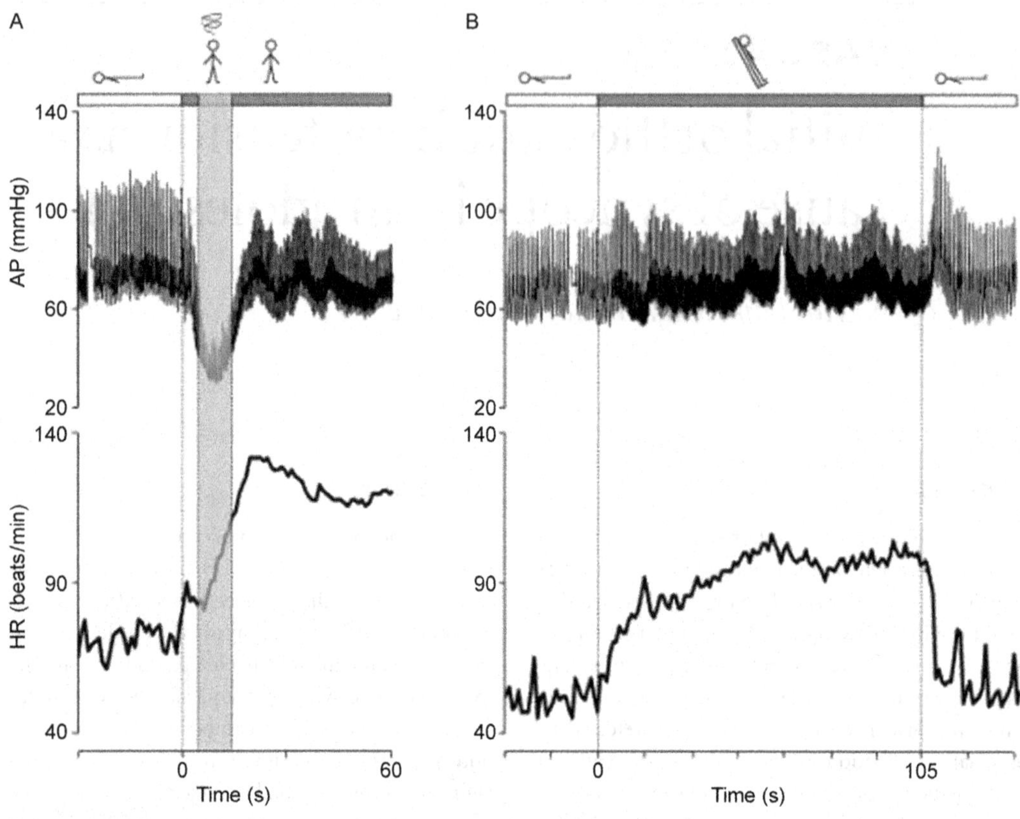

Figure 42.1 Continuous blood-pressure monitoring during active standing (A) and head-up tilting (B). AP, arterial pressure; HR, heart rate.

continuous blood-pressure monitoring using a Finometer [2]. Treatment is symptomatic, the aim being to reduce the drop in blood pressure during standing. Giving the patient a clear explanation of the underlying mechanism and about ways of avoiding the main trigger (rapid rising) is the principal treatment option. A second step is to provide training in maneuvers that increase blood pressure. We have found that muscle tensing in the lower body immediately after standing up is very effective in reducing the fall in pressure [9] (see also Case 44). In the most severe cases, volume expansion can be achieved by raising the patient's intake of water and salt [10]. If necessary, pharmacological treatment with mineralocorticoids (fludrocortisone) can be started (see Case 48).

Acknowledgment

Parts of this case were previously published in van Dijk *et al.* [1]. We are grateful to the *Nederlands Tijdschrift voor Geneeskunde* for granting permission to reprint.

References

1 van Dijk N, Harms MPM, Wieling W. Three patients with unrecognized orthostatic intolerance. *Ned Tijdschr Geneeskd* 2000; **144**: 249–54.

2 Wieling W, Karemaker JM. Non-invasive continuous recording of heart rate and blood pressure in the evaluation of neurovascular control. In: Mathias CJ, Bannister R, eds. *Autonomic Failure: a Textbook of Clinical Disorders of the Autonomic Nervous System*, 4th ed. Oxford University Press, Oxford, 1999: 197–210.

3 Wieling W, Ganzeboom KS, Saul JP. Reflex syncope in children and adolescents. *Heart* 2004; **90**: 1094–1100.

4 Sprangers RL, Wesseling KH, Imholz AL, Imholz BP, Wieling W. Initial blood pressure fall on stand up and exercise explained by changes in total peripheral resistance. *J Appl Physiol* 1991; **70**: 523–30.

5 Ganzeboom KS, Colman N, Reitsma JB, Shen WK,

Wieling W. Prevalence and triggers of syncope in medical students. *Am J Cardiol* 2003; **91**: 1006–8.

6 van Dijk N, Immink RV, Mulder BJ, van Lieshout JJ, Wieling W. Orthostatic blood pressure control in Marfan's syndrome. *Europace* 2005; **7**: 25–7.

7 Dambrink JH, Imholz BP, Karemaker JM, Wieling W. Postural dizziness and transient hypotension in two healthy teenagers. *Clin Auton Res* 1991; **1**: 281–7.

8 Tanaka H, Yamaguchi H, Matushima R, Tamai H. Instantaneous orthostatic hypotension in children and adolescents: a new entity of orthostatic intolerance. *Pediatr Res* 1999; **46**: 691–6.

9 Krediet CT, Wieling W. Physical counter maneuvers are effective in diminishing initial orthostatic hypotension. *Clin Auton Res* 2004; **14**: 311–2.

10 Shichiri M, Tanaka H, Takaya R, Tamai H. Efficacy of high sodium intake in a boy with instantaneous orthostatic hypotension. *Clin Auton Res* 2002; **12**: 47–50.

CASE 43

Initial orthostatic hypotension and syncope due to medications in a 60-year-old man

W. Wieling, M.P.M. Harms, R.A.M. Kortz, M. Linzer

Case report

A 60-year-old man presented with a 6-month history of recurrent unexplained syncope. The spells occurred suddenly, usually after he stood up. The patient was taking pipamperone (a neuroleptic), fluvoxamine (an antidepressant), and clobazam (a benzodiazepine) for depression, and sotalol and acenocoumarol for paroxysmal atrial fibrillation [1]. The patient had recently been hospitalized after an episode of transient loss of consciousness, which occurred after he stood up from a squatting position while doing a painting job. The spell was accompanied by myoclonic jerks, and the fall caused a large hematoma in the lumbar region. During his 2-week hospital stay, he had an entirely negative evaluation, including physical examination, electrocardiography, echocardiography, and blood analysis. On 24-h electrocardiographic monitoring, a sinus rhythm was observed during episodes of near-syncope. His blood pressure at one time decreased from supine values around 100/70 mmHg to values around 80 mmHg systolic after 2–3 min standing, but there were no accompanying symptoms of near-collapse and this finding could not be reproduced. He was referred to the syncope unit for tilt-table testing.

The patient reported severe symptoms of light-headedness and near-syncope, which occurred reproducibly on rising from a lying or sitting position several times a day. The symptoms usually disappeared within 1 min. An active standing-up maneuver was therefore performed to test the initial orthostatic adjustment [2]. His supine brachial blood pressure was 109/59 mmHg, and simultaneous noninvasive finger blood pressure using a Finapres model 5 (FMS Finapres Medical Systems B.V., Amsterdam, Netherlands) was 85/43 mmHg. His heart rate was 55 beats/min (Fig. 43.1). After he stood up, the finger systolic blood pressure almost immediately decreased to below 40 mmHg, with a reflex increase in heart rate. The patient reported light-headedness, which lasted for only 20 s and then gradually disappeared as his blood pressure rose.

During a second standing-up maneuver, an almost identical drop in blood pressure was observed. When he stood up from a squatting position, an even larger fall in the finger arterial pressure (from 120/75 mmHg to 40/30 mmHg) and near-fainting were observed. The patient recognized the symptoms as being the same as those that preceded his syncopal spells.

It was explained to the patient that the cause of his syncope was initial orthostatic intolerance related to the use of antidepressants, and he was advised to rise slowly from supine positions. Changing his medication was problematic due to the severity of his psychiatric disorder, and orthostatic symptoms, including syncope, therefore continued to be a significant problem.

Comment

Most people experience a brief feeling of light-headedness 5–10 s after standing up, especially after prolonged supine rest. Such common spells of light-headedness are caused by a transient fall in systemic blood pressure that occurs after active standing, but *not* after passive head-up tilting [3]. This initial transient fall in blood pressure is attributed to vasodilation

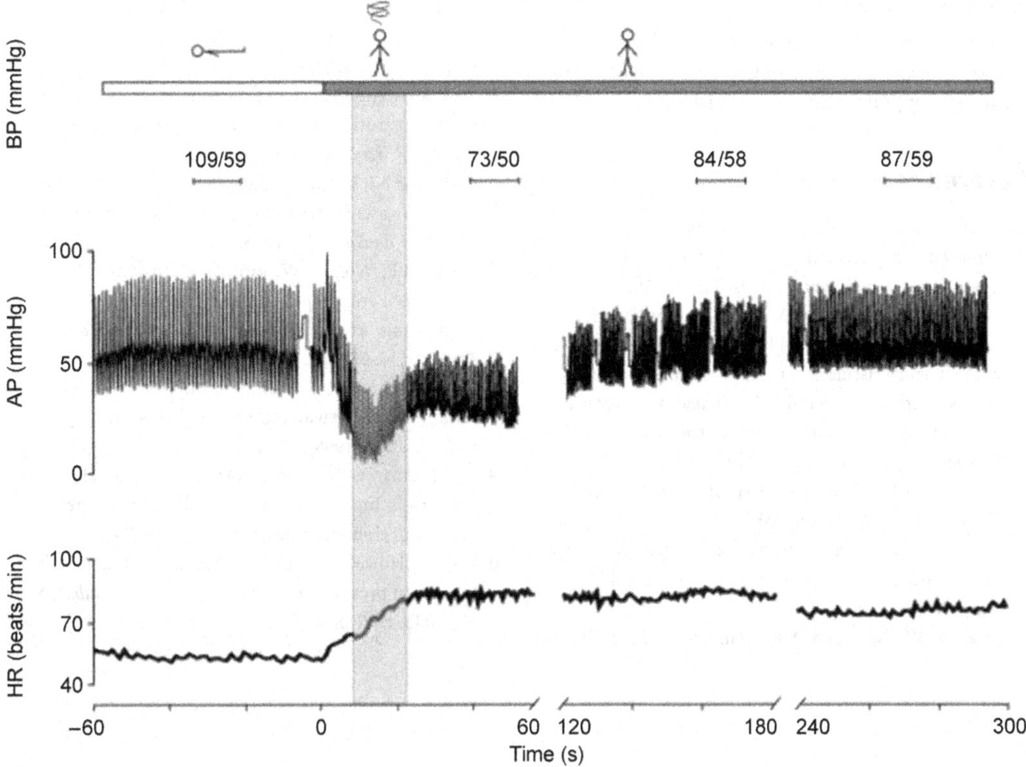

Figure 43.1 Continuous blood-pressure and heart-rate recordings during active standing. AP, arterial pressure; BP, blood pressure; HR, heart rate.

in the active muscles during standing, and it is characterized by its time of onset and short duration. The transient fall in systemic blood pressure does not increase with age and a fall of up to 40 mmHg systolic and 20 mmHg diastolic is considered normal (the 95% confidence limits obtained in 74 healthy individuals aged 10–86 years) [4]. Larger falls in blood pressure are considered abnormal [2].

Since initial orthostatic hypotension is only associated with active standing, tilt testing (i.e., passive head-up tilting) is not a helpful diagnostic provocation test. The tilt test, for which the patient was referred, was therefore not indicated.

Recent studies have reported that an abnormally large initial fall in blood pressure occurs in a variety of conditions that affect arterial baroreflex control of the sympathetic activation of resistance vessels. Examples are patients with deafferented carotid sinus baroreceptors after neck surgery (impairment of the afferent pathways [5]; see Case 50) and those receiving clonidine (with blockade of central pathways) [6].

The patient's description of his episodes of fainting indicated that initial orthostatic hypotension was the cause of the syncope. The cardiovascular examination documented the postulated abnormally large initial fall in pressure (Fig. 43.1). The combination of medications the patient was taking was almost certainly involved in the initial orthostatic hypotension. Pipamperone, fluvoxamine, clobazam, and sotalol have all been reported to impair orthostatic blood-pressure control [1].

This case shows the importance of continuous noninvasive blood-pressure measurement on standing, as the rapid blood-pressure changes cannot be assessed using the cuff and stethoscope [7,8]. Studies in patients taking drugs that are known to interfere with sympathetic function are needed, in order to assess how often abnormal initial falls in blood pressure after standing—which may predispose them to falls and injury—are overlooked [8]. Examples of such medications are antidepressants and drugs used to treat benign prostatic hyperplasia [9,10].

Acknowledgment

This case was previously published in Wieling *et al.* [1]. We are grateful to Springer Verlag (Darmstadt, Germany) for granting permission to reprint.

References

1 Wieling W, Harms MPM, Kortz RAM, Linzer M. Initial orthostatic hypotension as a cause of recurrent syncope: a case report. *Clin Auton Res* 2001; **11**: 269–70.

2 Wieling W, Karemaker JM. Non-invasive continuous recording of heart rate and blood pressure in the evaluation of neurovascular control. In: Mathias CJ, Bannister R, eds. *Autonomic Failure: a Textbook of Clinical Disorders of the Autonomic Nervous System*, 4th ed. Oxford University Press, Oxford, 1999: 197–210.

3 Sprangers RLH, Wesseling KH, Imholz ALT, Imholz BPM, Wieling W. The initial blood pressure fall upon stand up and onset to exercise explained by changes in total peripheral resistance. *J Appl Physiol* 1991; **70**: 523–30.

4 Wieling W, Veerman DP, Dambrink JHA, Imholz BPM. Disparities in circulatory adjustment to standing between young and elderly subjects explained by pulse contour analysis. *Clin Sci* 1992; **83**: 149–55.

5 Smit AAJ, Timmers HJLM, Wieling W, *et al.* Long-term effects of carotid sinus denervation on arterial pressure in humans. *Circulation* 2002; **105**: 1329–35.

6 Coupland NJ, Wilson SJ, Nutt D. The effects of clonidine on cardiovascular responses to standing in healthy volunteers. *Clin Auton Res* 1995; **5**: 171–7.

7 Imholz BP, Wieling W, van Montfrans GA, Wesseling KH. Fifteen years experience with finger arterial pressure monitoring: assessment of the technology. *Cardiovasc Res* 1998; **38**: 605–16.

8 Caine SE, Alsop K, MacMahon M. Overlooking orthostatic hypotension with routine blood-pressure equipment [letter]. *Lancet* 1998; **352**: 458.

9 Schlingemann RO, Smit AAJ, Lunel HF, Hydra A. Amaurosis fugax on standing and angle-closure glaucoma with clomipramine [letter]. *Lancet* 1996; **347**: 465.

10 Wilt TJ, Howe RW, Rutks IR, MacDonald R. Terazosin for benign prostatic hyperplasia. *Cochrane Database Syst Rev* 2002; **4**: CD003851.

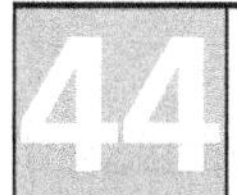

CASE 44

Initial orthostatic hypotension induced by standing up from squatting

C.T.P. Krediet, W. Wieling

Case report

A 37-year-old woman who was an enthusiastic horse rider underwent cardiovascular reflex assessment after losing consciousness. The episode occurred after she had squatted to bandage her horse's legs and then stood up. The patient reported that before the loss of consciousness, she saw black spots and felt light-headed. She was unconscious for less than 1 min and was well oriented when she regained consciousness [1].

During her medical examination, the patient was asked to mimic the procedure of bandaging the four legs of her horse. Figure 44.1 shows her continuous noninvasively measured finger blood pressure at heart level (Finapres model 5; FMS Finapres Medical Systems B.V., Amsterdam, Netherlands) and derived heart rate. The patient was asked to squat (Fig. 44.1, white bar) for about 30 s and to stand up quickly (black bar). This was repeated three times. After the fourth time, the patient remained standing. Each

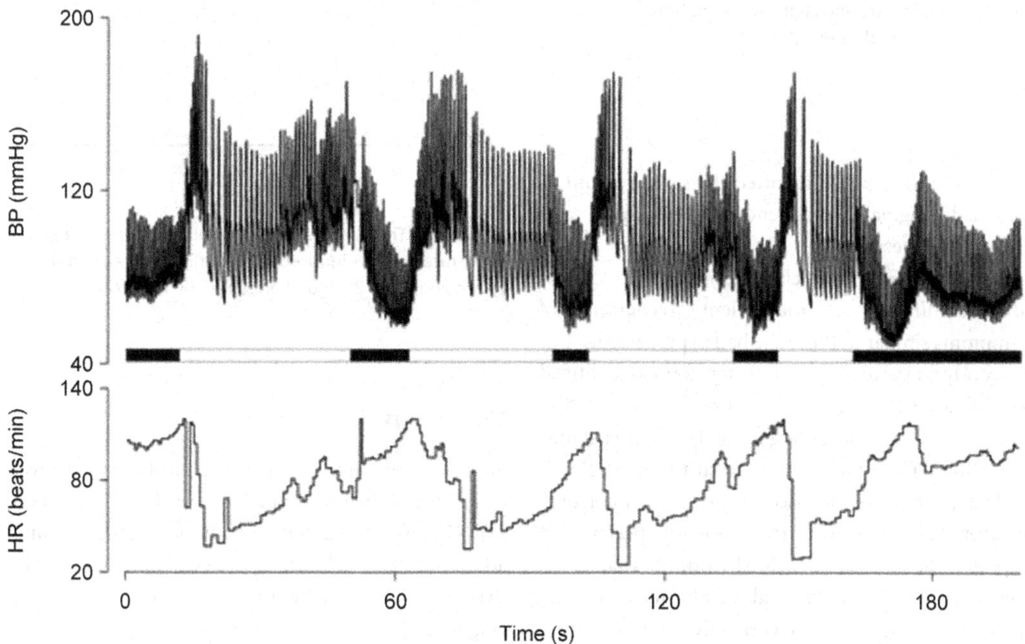

Figure 44.1 Continuous monitoring of blood pressure and instantaneous heart rate during the squat–stand test. BP, blood pressure; HR, heart rate.

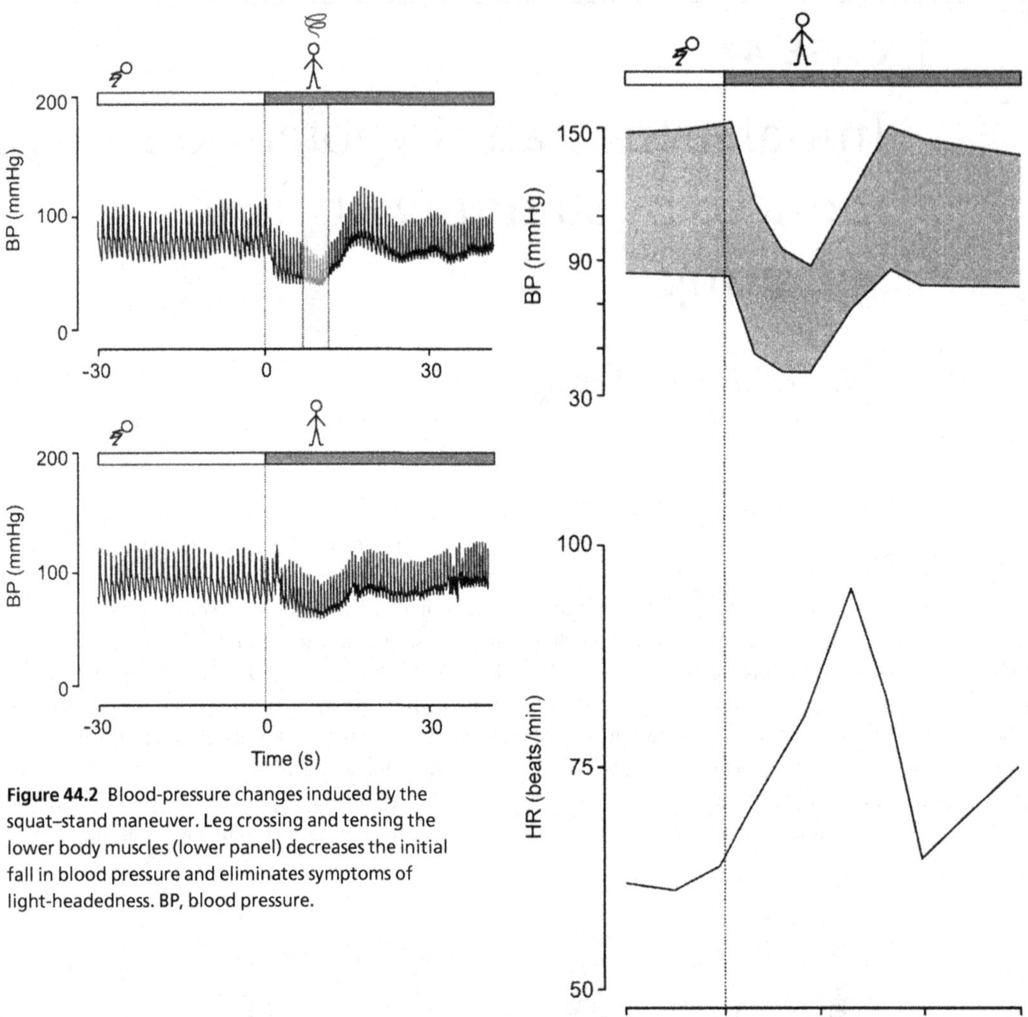

Figure 44.2 Blood-pressure changes induced by the squat–stand maneuver. Leg crossing and tensing the lower body muscles (lower panel) decreases the initial fall in blood pressure and eliminates symptoms of light-headedness. BP, blood pressure.

Figure 44.3 The average intra-arterial blood-pressure and heart-rate changes induced by squatting in three healthy young adults [3]. BP, blood pressure; HR, heart rate.

time she stood up, she reported the same symptoms she had originally experienced (black spots and light-headedness).

Based on this reproducible blood-pressure change after standing up and the patient's recognition of symptoms similar to those she had experienced spontaneously, initial orthostatic hypotension was identified as the cause for her loss of consciousness [1]. Leg crossing with muscle tensing immediately after standing reduced the drop in blood pressure (Fig. 44.2).

The patient was advised to use this maneuver in everyday life. During the follow-up period, she reported that she had benefited from the maneuver. Tensing of the leg, abdominal, and buttocks muscles alone was found to be just as effective and more convenient. She had not lost consciousness since the cardiovascular reflex test.

Comment

Standing up from the squatting position involves a considerable hemodynamic–i.e., orthostatic–stress [2]. On average, blood pressure in healthy young adults falls by –60 mmHg systolic and –40 mmHg diastolic, with a nadir about 7 s after standing up (Fig. 44.3) [3].

Two factors are likely to be involved in the rapid fall in pressure. Firstly, a sudden decrease in total peripheral resistance in the legs due to the ischemic effect of squatting, allowing a very rapid inflow of arterial blood into the legs. Secondly, marked pooling of blood in the veins in the legs and abdomen, which are squeezed in the squatting position, resulting in a decrease in venous return and thereby in cardiac output. The combination of these two factors results in a rapid translocation of a large amount of arterial blood from the chest to the distensible venous capacitance system below the diaphragm. The accelerative force during rapid standing up may play an additional role in the fall in pressure [4].

Rising to an erect posture from squatting is a recognized trigger for fainting in everyday life. Squatting in combination with hyperventilation and straining can induce fainting in almost everybody (the fainting lark; see Case 45). In the older literature in German, standing up from squatting was widely reported as a test for assessing initial orthostatic adjustments [5,6]. The squat–stand test was also recently described as an orthostatic stress test in the English-language literature [7,8].

Little is known regarding the best form of treatment for symptomatic initial orthostatic hypotension. Increasing salt intake has been advised (see Case 42). The present case and additional recent observations [9] strongly suggest that muscle tensing in the lower body immediately after standing up is an effective way of preventing the abnormally large initial fall in pressure after standing.

Acknowledgment

Parts of this case were previously published in *Clinical Autonomic Research* [1]. We are grateful to Springer Verlag (Darmstadt, Germany) for permission to reprint.

References

1 Krediet CT. A woman with transient loss of consciousness. *Clin Auton Res* 2004; **14**: 49–51.
2 Sharpey-Schafer EP. Effects of squatting on the normal and failing circulation. *Br Med J* 1956; **i**: 1072–4.
3 Rossberg R, Penaz J. Initial cardiovascular response on change of posture from squatting to standing. *Eur J Appl Physiol* 1988; **57**: 93–7.
4 Brown GE, Wood EH, Lambert EH. Effects of tetra-ethyl-ammonium chloride on the cardiovascular reactions in man to changes in posture and exposure to centrifugal force. *J Appl Physiol* 1949; **2**: 117–32.
5 de Marees H. Zur orthostatischen Sofortregulation. *Cardiology* 1976; **61** (Suppl 1): 78–90.
6 Barbey K, Barbey K, Kutscha W. Über die orthostatische Sofortregulation. *Med Welt* 1966; **32**: 1648–53.
7 Convertino VA, Tripp LD, Ludwig DA, Duff J, Chelette TL. Female exposure to high G: chronic adaptations of cardiovascular function. *Aviat Space Environ Med* 1998; **69**: 875–82.
8 Rickards CA, Newman DG. A comparative assessment of two techniques for investigating initial cardiovascular reflexes under acute orthostatic stress. *Eur J Appl Physiol* 2003; **90**: 449–57.
9 Krediet CT, Wieling W. Physical counter maneuvers are effective in diminishing initial orthostatic hypotension. *Clin Auton Res* 2004; **14**: 311–2.

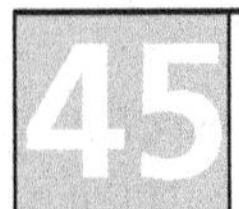

CASE 45

Self-induced syncope: the fainting lark

W. Wieling, J.J. van Lieshout

Case report

The fainting lark is a self-applied maneuver that induces fainting [1]. Self-induced fainting has been used by children, high-school students, and military recruits as entertainment for their friends [2–4]. The fainting lark has also been applied as a research tool to document the sequence of events that take place during abrupt-onset syncope in young individuals [4].

The classical procedure consists of squatting in a full knee-bend and overbreathing by taking about 20 deep breaths. The subject then stands up suddenly and performs a forced expiration against a closed glottis.

Figure 45.1 documents the resulting precipitous and deep fall in arterial pressure and cerebral blood flow in one of the authors (W.W.) [1], who briefly (2–3 s) lost consciousness, preceded by an extremely short period of light-headedness and black-out. The blood pressure overshoots after lying down.

Comment

The fainting lark combines the effects of systemic arterial hypotension, induced by acute vasodilation of the lower limbs (the ischemic effect of squatting) and decreased cardiac output (the effects of standing up and increased intrathoracic pressure), and cerebral vasoconstriction, induced by hypocapnia (due to hyperventilation) [2]. The fainting lark can trigger syncope in almost anyone, and myoclonic jerks directly after falling down are observed in the majority of cases [2,5]. The high cerebral venous pressure induced by straining can be expected to play an important adjunctive role in the effectiveness of the fainting lark in inducing fainting [6].

Another maneuver used to induce syncope is known as the "mess trick" [2], recently also described as "suffocation roulette" [7]. During this trick, the individual is instructed to take a deep breath; a companion grasps him or her unexpectedly from behind around the chest and squeezes as hard as possible. The subject automatically closes the glottis, intrathoracic pressure is increased, and the subject faints. This is liable to be done as entertainment, usually with the effects of alcohol being added to the mechanical effects.

Self-induced fainting is reported to be safe, but injuries may occur due to falling. Moreover, severe complications and even death have been reported [8–10].

References

1 Wieling W, van Lieshout JJ. The fainting lark. *Clin Auton Res* 2002; **12**: 207.

2 Howard P, Leathart GL, Dornhorst AC, Sharpey-Schafer EP. The "mess trick" and the "fainting lark." *Br Med J* 1951; **ii**: 382–4.

3 Johnson RH, Lambie DG, Spalding JMK. Syncope without heart disease. In: Johnson RH, Lambie DG, Spalding JMK, eds. *Neurocardiology: the Interrelationships between Dysfunction in the Nervous and Cardiovascular Systems.* Saunders, London, 1984: 159–63.

4 Lamb LE, Green HC, Combs JJ, Cheeseman SA, Hammond J. Incidence of loss of consciousness in 1980 air force personnel. *Aerosp Med* 1960; **31**: 973–88.

5 Lempert T, Bauer M, Schmidt D. Syncope: a videometric analysis of 56 episodes of transient cerebral hypoxia. *Ann Neurol* 1994; **36**: 233–7.

6 Gastaut H. Syncopes: generalized anoxic cerebral seizures. In: Magnus O, de Haas AML, eds. *Handbook of Clinical*

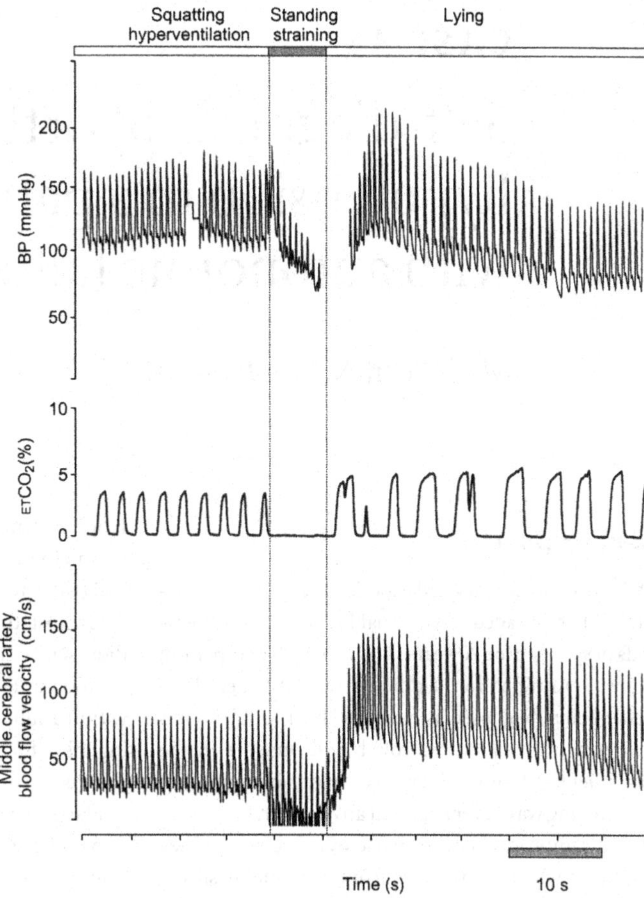

Figure 45.1 Continuous monitoring of changes in finger blood pressure, end-tidal CO_2, and cerebral blood flow velocity induced by the fainting lark. BP, blood pressure.

Neurology, vol. 15: *The Epilepsies*. North-Holland, Amsterdam, 1974: 815–36.

7 Shlamovitz GZ, Assia A, Ben-Sira L, Rachmel A. "Suffocation roulette": a case of recurrent syncope in an adolescent boy. *Ann Emerg Med* 2003; **41**; 223–6.

8 Murphy JV, Wilkinson IA, Pollack NH. Death following breath holding in an adolescent. *Am J Disease Children* 1981; **135**: 180–1.

9 Rumball A. Pulmonary oedema with neurological symptoms after the fainting lark and mess trick. *Br Med J* 1963; **5349**: 80–3.

10 Chow KM. Deadly game among children and adolescents. *Ann Emerg Med* 2003; **42**: 310.

CASE 46

Self-diagnosis of orthostatic hypotension in a patient with autonomic failure

M.C. Boer, N. van Dijk, W. Wieling

Case report

A 56-year-old teacher had experienced spells of "dizziness" (light-headedness), visual black-outs, and periods of syncope for 20 years [1]. Over a 12-year period, he was examined by 11 different medical specialists. After being diagnosed as having a "burn-out," he was declared unfit for work. Low blood pressure in the standing position was identified on one occasion, but this finding was never explored any further.

His symptoms became worse over the years. They occurred when he switched from a supine or sitting position to a standing position, after transitions from moderate to strenuous physical exercise, and after straining. During these provocations, he experienced blurring of vision and sometimes visual black-outs, aching pain in his neck muscles and shoulder muscles, and sometimes loss of consciousness. He had had symptoms of erectile dysfunction and loss of perspiration for 3–4 years. The symptoms were more severe on warm days and resolved when he sat down, squatted, or bent over. He discovered that the symptoms were also decreased if he placed one leg on a chair during prolonged standing (see Case 48). Despite these impediments, he led an active life; he played badminton, although he needed to squat (see Case 48) every three hits to prevent syncope from occurring.

These symptoms were hard to understand for the patient and his relatives, especially since the patient was perfectly healthy in every other respect. He thought the complaints might be related to a low upright blood pressure and therefore carried out an Internet search for "hypotension" and found the John Hopkins University web site (www.jhu.edu). On this site he found, among others, the name of our group, and contacted us by e-mail.

Orthostatic hypotension was obvious during cardiovascular reflex testing. Finger blood pressure was 125/60 mmHg in the supine position and dropped within 1 min to 45/30 mmHg after he stood up, forcing him to sit down. On standing, his heart rate increased from 58 to 80 beats/min.

Plasma levels of norepinephrine, epinephrine, and dopamine were low and did not increase on standing. The patient's medical history, cardiovascular reflex tests, and laboratory results were characteristic for "pure autonomic failure," a condition of unknown origin with postganglionic deficits in the autonomic nervous system [2].

The patient received extensive information and explanation of his condition; he was advised to use the maneuvers he had discovered to improve orthostatic tolerance (see Case 48), to increase his daily fluid intake (above 2 L/day), to use ample dietary salt (10 g/day), and to sleep in a head-up position [3]. In addition, the patient received a prescription for fludrocortisone 0.1 mg/day. As a result of these measures, the patient's orthostatic symptoms diminished considerably. During repeated cardiovascular testing, his finger blood pressure dropped from 120/55 mmHg to "only" 60/40 mmHg after standing up (Fig. 46.1A).

Comment

Orthostatic faints are most readily identified by taking a careful medical history in which the association with

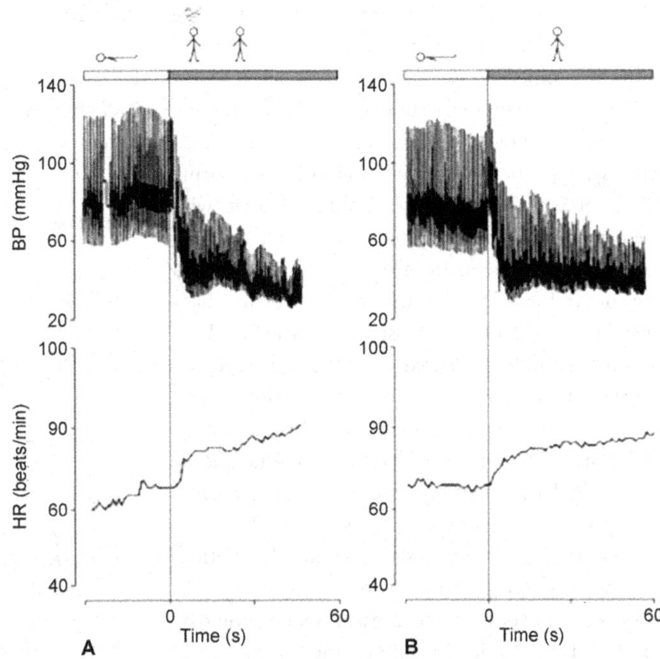

Figure 46.1 Finger arterial pressure and heart-rate changes before (A) and after (B) extracellular fluid volume expansion. BP, blood pressure; HR, heart rate.

posture is documented (i.e., syncope occurring shortly after changing from lying or sitting to a standing position or prolonged orthostatic stress). The underlying diagnosis is of particular importance for patients with orthostatic hypotension. It is important to identify reversible causes of orthostatic hypotension, such as volume depletion and the effect of medication [2,3]. The drugs most frequently associated with orthostatic syncope are vasodilators and diuretics [4]. Alcohol can also be associated with orthostatic syncope, by causing orthostatic intolerance (vasodilation and volume depletion), as well as by inducing autonomic and somatic neuropathy. Elimination of the responsible drug or offending agent is usually sufficient to improve symptoms.

A mismatch between intravascular volume and the required cardiac output on standing up is the most common cause of orthostatic hypotension. In a small minority of cases, however, orthostatic hypotension is not caused by volume depletion, but by impairment of the autonomic reflexes required to maintain blood pressure in the upright position. This disorder is known as autonomic failure [2]. Autonomic failure can be due to a primary disease (pure autonomic failure, multiple-system atrophy), secondary to other diseases that affect the autonomic nervous system (such as diabetes or amyloidosis), or due to drugs [2]. In patients with autonomic failure, orthostatic hypotension is caused by an impaired capacity of sympathetic nerves to increase vascular resistance. Downward pooling of venous blood and a consequent reduction in stroke volume and cardiac output lead to the orthostatic fall in arterial pressure [5]. With a significant and persistent decrease in arterial pressure, characteristic features occur. The symptoms include light-headedness and blurring of vision. A neck ache radiating to the occipital region of the skull and to the shoulders (with a coat-hanger distribution) often precedes actual loss of consciousness. The postulated mechanism of this virtually unique symptom of postural hypotension is ischemia in continuously contracting postural muscles. Other symptoms suggesting impaired perfusion of muscle tissue are lower back and buttock ache or angina pectoris. Typically, symptoms develop within minutes on standing up or walking and resolve on lying down [2,6]. Patients with autonomic failure quickly learn to use these symptoms as a warning signal that they need to lie down to restore an adequate perfusion pressure. If the patient remains upright, a gradual fading of consciousness occurs and the patient slowly falls to his or her knees. Sudden postural attacks and true syncope may, however, also occur. Symptoms and signs of autonomic activation, such as sweating or vagally induced bradycardia, are absent in patients with autonomic failure.

Orthostatic syncope can be diagnosed when there is documentation of orthostatic hypotension associated with syncope or presyncope. Carefully measuring blood pressure using a sphygmomanometer with the patient in the supine position and after standing suffices for routine assessment of orthostatic blood pressure in the office or at the bedside. For the diagnosis of orthostatic hypotension, the arterial blood pressure has to be measured when the patient adopts the standing position after 5 min in the supine position. Orthostatic hypotension is defined as a decline in blood pressure of at least 20 mmHg systolic and/or 10 mmHg diastolic within 3 min of standing, regardless of whether or not symptoms occur [2]. If the patient does not tolerate standing for this period, the lowest systolic blood pressure during the upright position should be recorded. Measurements should be continued after 3 min of standing if the blood pressure is still falling at 3 min. In some patients with syncope who have a history suggestive of impaired orthostatic blood-pressure control, blood-pressure measurements in the upright position may be normal. In these patients, additional tests using provocative stimuli, such as food ingestion and exercise, may be needed to unmask orthostatic hypotension. A useful alternative is ambulatory blood-pressure recording for 24 h or longer in everyday circumstances similar to those associated with symptoms in the individual patient.

Acknowledgment

Parts of this case were previously published in van Dijk *et al.* [1]. We are grateful to the *Nederlands Tijdschrift voor Geneeskunde* for granting permission to reprint.

References

1 van Dijk N, Harms MPM, Wieling W. Three patients with unrecognized orthostatic intolerance. *Ned Tijdschr Geneeskd* 2000; **144**: 249–54.

2 Bannister R, Mathias CJ. Management of postural hypotension. In: Mathias CJ, Bannister R, eds. *Autonomic Failure: a Textbook of Clinical Disorders of the Autonomic Nervous System*, 4th ed. Oxford University Press, Oxford, 1999: 342–56.

3 Wieling W, Cortelli P, Mathias CJ. Treating neurogenic orthostatic hypotension. In: Appenzeller O, ed. *The Autonomic Nervous System, Part 2. Dysfunctions. Handbook of Clinical Neurology*, vol. 75 (rev. ser. 31). Elsevier, Amsterdam, 2000: 713–29.

4 Hanlon JT, Linzer M, McMillan JP, Lewis IK, Felder AA. Syncope and presyncope associated with probable adverse drug reactions. *Arch Intern Med* 1990; **150**: 2309–2312.

5 Smit AAJ, Halliwill JR, Low PA, Wieling W. Pathophysiological basis of orthostatic hypotension in autonomic failure. *J Physiol* 1999; **519**: 1–10.

6 Bleasdale-Barr K, Mathias CJ. Neck and other muscle pains in autonomic failure: their association with autonomic failure. *J R Soc Med* 1998; **91**: 355–9.

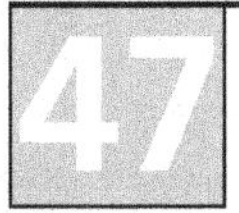

CASE 47

Unexplained transient loss of consciousness in a 58-year-old man after *Legionella* pneumonia

N. van Dijk, C.T.P. Krediet, W. Wieling

Case report

A 58-year-old man was referred to our syncope unit by a cardiologist for evaluation of an unexplained episode of transient loss of consciousness. Four years before this visit, he had been admitted to an intensive-care unit due to *Legionella* pneumonia. After his recovery, urinary bladder dysfunction and erectile dysfunction became evident. A urologist diagnosed prostate hypertrophy, and a transurethral resection of the prostate was carried out. However, the problems did not improve. Autonomic dysfunction of the bladder was considered and self-catheterization was started. Before the *Legionella* pneumonia, the patient's general health and sexual and urinary bladder functions had been normal.

In the years following this episode, the patient experienced progressive problems with fatigue and dyspnea during stair climbing. The symptoms were attributed to diminished pulmonary function after the *Legionella* pneumonia. He also complained of light-headedness during prolonged standing and near-syncope during toilet visits at night. A few months before the visit to our unit, he had lost consciousness on a very hot day shortly after standing up from a chair. He had also fallen into a swimming pool and almost drowned.

Cardiological assessment was carried out after this episode. An electrocardiogram (ECG) and echocardiogram were normal. During a tilt-table test, a large drop in blood pressure was observed after administration of nitroglycerin (to 60 mmHg systolic), but the patient did not faint and the test result was interpreted as negative. During bicycle exercise testing, the patient had to stop at a load of only 120 W due to fatigue and light-headedness. His blood pressure dropped from 150/60 mmHg as he was sitting on the bicycle to 60/40 mmHg directly post-exercise. No ECG changes were noted. Because the fall in blood pressure during exercise was unexplained, cardiac catheterization, including ventricular and coronary angiography, was carried out to exclude cardiac disease. No abnormalities were found.

On examination in our syncope unit, the patient was found to be in good general health. His finger arterial pressure was 190/93 mmHg supine, with an asymptomatic fall to 175/93 after 3 min standing. During an exercise test (the step test), his blood pressure decreased in 1 min from values around 175/95 mmHg to levels of 114/64 (Fig. 47.1).

During a Valsalva test there was a large fall, with hardly any recovery in pressure during straining and no overshoot of blood pressure after release of the strain (Fig. 47.2). The heart rate followed the changes in blood pressure, suggesting intact afferent, central, and efferent cardiac arterial baroreflex pathways. The lesion therefore appeared to be located in the efferent sympathetic vasoconstrictor pathways.

On the basis of the symptoms of orthostatic hypotension and abnormalities in urinary bladder and sexual function, autonomic neuropathy was diagnosed clinically and confirmed by autonomic testing. Autonomic neuropathy has previously been reported as a complication of a *Legionella* infection [1]. The patient received an explanation of his condition and instructions (see Case 46).

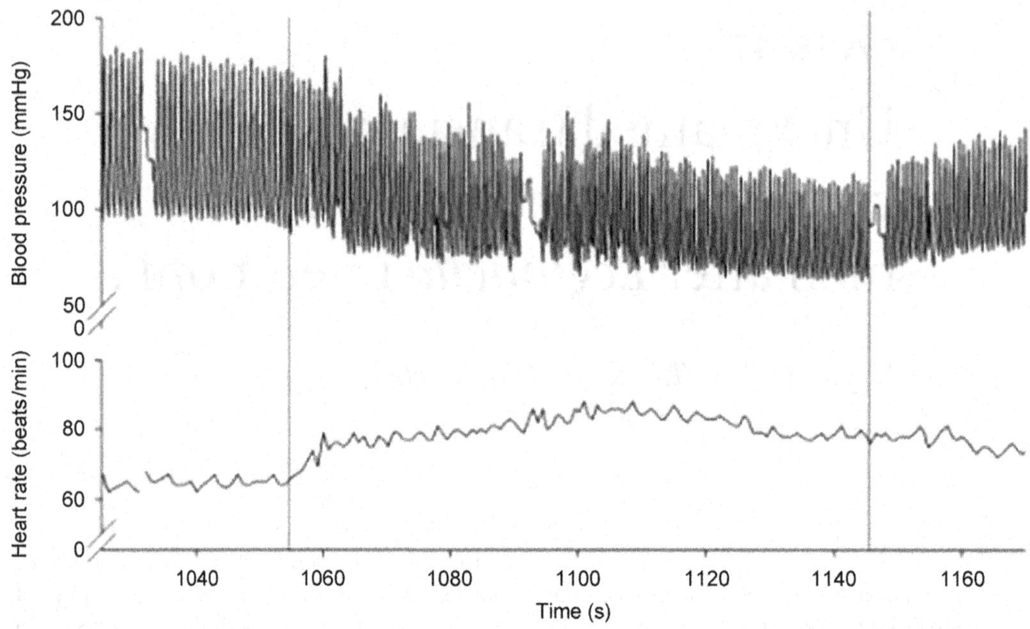

Figure 47.1 The patient's blood-pressure and heart-rate response to exercise. Note the progressive fall in blood pressure.

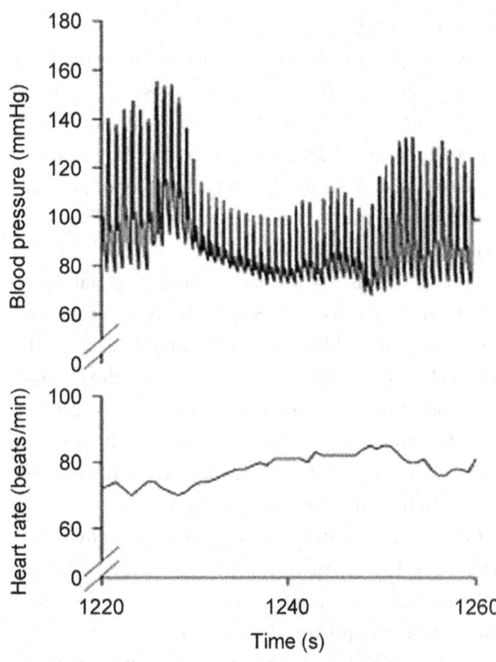

Figure 47.2 The blood-pressure and heart-rate response during the Valsalva maneuver. Note the fall in pressure during straining and the lack of blood pressure overshoot after release of the strain.

Comment

Light-headedness induced by exercise is a recognized presenting feature of ischemic heart disease [2]. The referring cardiologist was therefore puzzled when he was unable to demonstrate a cardiac abnormality. However, an adequate rise in blood pressure during exercise is dependent not only on normal cardiac function, but in particular also on an intact efferent sympathetic innervation of the blood vessels. Vasoconstriction in nonexercising skeletal muscle and in the splanchnic and renal vascular beds is a prerequisite for obtaining an adequate physiological increase in blood pressure in response to exercise. However, vasoconstriction is blunted in patients with autonomic neuropathy [3].

Autonomic neuropathy is a rare disorder, but the presentation in this patient was classical [4]. Exercise-induced hypotension during common daily activities in patients with autonomic failure was recognized by earlier investigators. Climbing stairs in particular was noted to elicit symptomatic hypotension [5,6]. The symptoms during stair climbing in the present patient were at first attributed to his diminished pulmonary function, but laboratory testing disclosed that stair climbing induced symptomatic hypotension (Fig. 47.1).

The absence of sympathetic vasoconstrictor activity in nonactive and active muscles, with excessive peripheral vasodilation during muscular work, is not compensated for by the increase in cardiac output that occurs during dynamic exercise [7]. As a consequence, blood pressure falls even if the exercise is carried out in the supine position and, as the patient develops muscle fatigue and stops exercising, a further drop in blood pressure occurs [8,9].

Another frequently reported finding in these patients is syncopal or presyncopal symptoms during toilet visits at night and in the early morning [2,3], as in this case.

In conclusion, in patients with syncope or presyncope during exercise combined with urination, defecation, sweating, or erectile problems in the absence of cardiac disorders, autonomic dysfunction is likely to be present, and autonomic evaluation, including exercise testing and a Valsalva maneuver, should be carried out. The diagnosis may be overlooked if blood pressure is only tested with the patient in the supine and standing positions.

References

1 Bernardi DL, Lerrick KS, Hoffman K, Lange M. Neurogenic bladder: new clinical finding in Legionnaires' disease. *Am J Med* 1985; **78**: 1045–6.

2 Weiner DA, Macabe CH, Cutler SS, Ryan TJ. Decrease in systolic blood pressure during exercise testing: reproducibility, response to coronary by-pass grafting, and prognostic significance. *Am J Cardiol* 1982; **49**: 1627–32.

3 Rowell LB. *Human Cardiovascular Control.* Oxford University Press, Oxford, 1993.

4 Bannister R, Mathias CJ. Management of postural hypotension. In: Mathias CJ, Bannister R, eds. *Autonomic Failure: a Textbook of Clinical Disorders of the Autonomic Nervous System*, 4th ed. Oxford University Press, Oxford, 1999: 342–56.

5 Bradbury S, Eggleston C. Postural hypotension: a report of three cases. *Am Heart J* 1925; **1**: 73–86.

6 Wieling W, van Lieshout JJ, van Leeuwen AM. Physical manoeuvres that reduce postural hypotension in autonomic failure. *Clin Auton Res* 1993; **3**: 57–65.

7 Rowell LB. Neural control of muscle blood flow: importance during dynamic exercise. *Clin Exp Pharmacol Physiol* 1997; **24**: 117–25.

8 Marshall RJ, Schirger A, Shepherd JT. Blood pressure during supine exercise in idiopathic orthostatic hypotension. *Circulation* 1961; **24**: 76–81.

9 Smith GD, Bannister R, Mathias CJ. Post-exertion dizziness as the sole presenting symptoms of autonomic failure. *Br Heart J* 1993; **69**: 359–61.

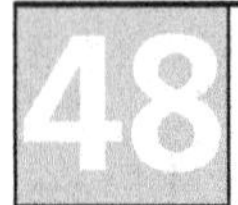

CASE 48

Physical maneuvers that reduce postural hypotension in autonomic failure

W. Wieling, J.J. van Lieshout, A.M. van Leeuwen

Case report

A young woman was healthy until she presented with severe disabling orthostatic hypotension, shortly after Hodgkin's disease was diagnosed at the age of 23 [1]. She even fainted when attempting to sit upright, and was only able to move around sitting in her wheelchair with her knees drawn up. She also had a dry mouth, anhidrosis, constipation, and urinary retention. Acute pandysautonomia was diagnosed. On formal testing, she had the features of a hypoadrenergic orthostatic hypotension syndrome. In the cardiovascular system, she had an isolated sympathetic postganglionic lesion, but despite other features of parasympathetic impairment, had parasympathetic control of heart rate [2,3].

Treatment with chemotherapy and radiation resulted in complete remission of the Hodgkin's disease. Her saliva production, bowel movements, and urinary bladder function returned to normal. Severe orthostatic hypotension persisted, however, despite treatment with fludrocortisone 200 μg/day. During this period, she discovered a series of maneuvers that helped reduce the symptoms of orthostatic hypotension. The light-headedness that developed soon after she rose from the supine position was relieved by squatting (Fig. 48.1).

Orthostatic tolerance improved distinctly when she stood with the head bent and with contracted abdominal muscles. By applying these techniques, she was able to walk short distances at home. When shopping or needing an item that was out of reach, she rose from her wheelchair, lifted her arms quickly to pick up the item from the shelves, and squatted immediately afterward, thereby preventing syncope. Climbing stairs was impossible, and she reached her first-floor apartment by hopping backwards up the stairs.

A year after the onset of symptoms of orthostatic hypotension, she was admitted for further improvements in therapy. The hypoadrenergic orthostatic hypotension syndrome was still present. She was able to stand still in the upright position for only about 1 min. However, her orthostatic tolerance improved

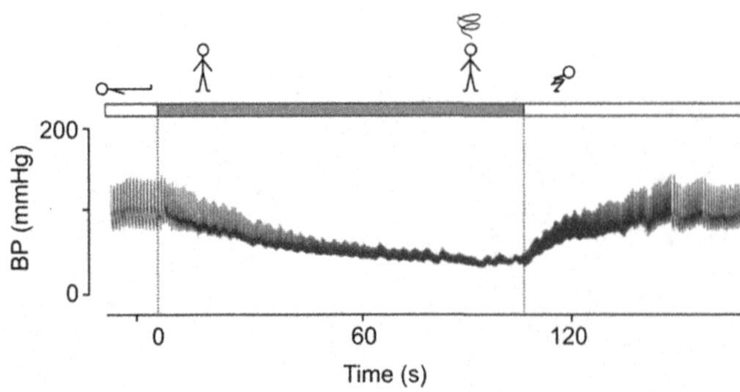

Figure 48.1 Immediate reduction of orthostatic hypotension and relief of accompanying symptoms by squatting. On the verge of syncope (after about 115 s in the upright position), the patient squatted. BP, blood pressure.

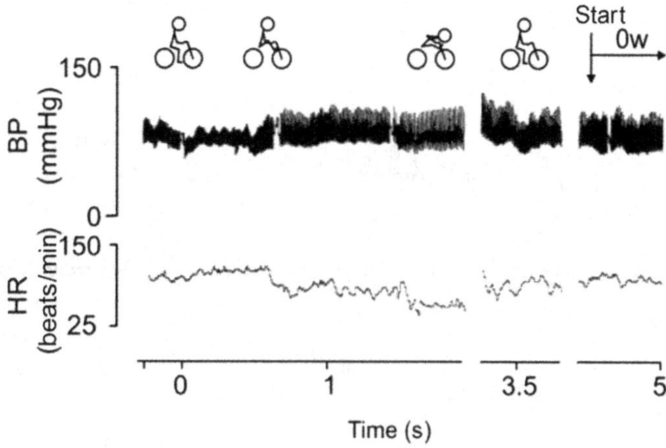

Figure 48.2 Blood-pressure and heart-rate tracings during "bicycle maneuvers" before the start of cycling. When the patient was sitting quietly with her feet on the pedals, the blood pressure was low. When she pulled up her legs and put them on the bicycle frame, it induced an increase in blood pressure, with an additional increase in pulse pressure when she bent over the handle-bars. A rapid fall in blood pressure was observed when she lowered her feet. BP, blood pressure; HR, heart rate.

distinctly after chronic expansion of plasma volume. She was discharged, walking upright, with a regimen of fludrocortisone (300 μg), sodium chloride (around 12 g), and sleeping at night in a 12° head-up tilted position. This has been described in detail elsewhere [4].

After discharge, she reported that she felt reasonably well and was not seriously restricted in her everyday activities. At this point, she started a laborious part-time job as a social worker in an institution for battered women. She regularly went for bicycle rides, initially with her friend on a tricycle or as the rear rider on a tandem, covering distances of up to 60 km a day, but in due course on her own as well. This faced her with a new problem: light-headedness during and immediately after cycling. She prevented fainting by short intermittent resting periods with her knees pulled up on the frame. A further difficulty was stopping at red traffic lights, as stopping cycling almost instantaneously caused dizziness. She discovered that bending over the bicycle's handle-bars prevented fainting. During investigation of her "bicycle maneuvers" in the laboratory (Fig. 48.2), her blood pressure fell progressively while she was sitting motionless on the bicycle. When she pulled up her legs, her blood pressure increased; bending over the handle-bars resulted in an additional increase in pulse pressure. When she returned her feet from the frame to the pedals, her blood pressure dropped again.

During later visits to the laboratory, she was instructed to use other maneuvers to improve orthostatic tolerance, such as leg crossing and putting a foot on a chair. We have taught these two maneuvers to other patients [5]; leg crossing has been particularly helpful. At present, this patient uses a combination of these maneuvers almost automatically in everyday life (Fig. 48.3).

Comment

Patients with autonomic failure soon experience the dangers of standing still. They learn to shift weight from one leg to another and discover specific maneuvers useful for combatting orthostatic light-headedness during standing [1].

Leg crossing. The beneficial effect of leg crossing has been attributed to mechanical compression of the venous beds in the legs, buttocks, and abdomen, into which blood pools during standing, causing an increase in the thoracic blood volume [6]. This results in an increase in cardiac filling pressure, stroke volume, and output, and thereby leads to a rise in systemic arterial pressure.

Leg crossing can also be used to prevent hypotensive light-headedness in the sitting position in patients with autonomic failure [7]. Leg crossing has the advantage that it can be done casually without much effort and without drawing attention to the patient's problem. It is our experience that, after proper instruction and training, patients automatically apply leg crossing in everyday life. When it is practiced routinely, standing systolic/diastolic blood pressure can be increased by about 20/10 mmHg [5,6,8]. Larger increases of about 30/15 mmHg can be seen with the additional contraction of the leg musculature, thighs, and buttocks [9].

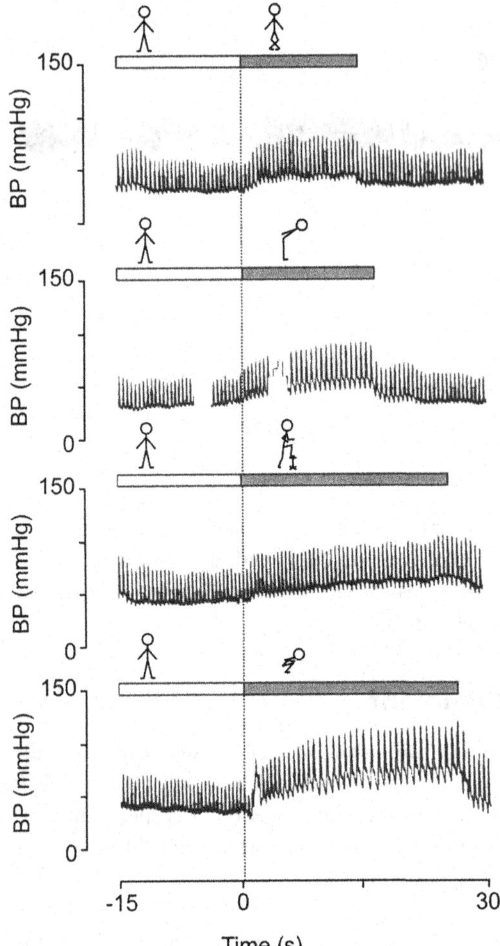

Figure 48.3 The effects of crossing the legs, bending forward, placing a foot on a chair, and squatting on orthostatic blood pressure. The patient was standing quietly before the maneuvers. The bars indicate the duration of the maneuvers. BP, blood pressure.

Squatting. When healthy individuals squat, the mean arterial pressure and pulse pressure increase, because the maneuver forces blood out of the vessels in the leg and splanchnic veins, thereby restoring cardiac filling pressure and cardiac output [1]. It is a highly effective physical maneuver for increasing venous return rapidly. It can produce an increase in systolic/diastolic blood pressure of about 60/35 mmHg [8,9]. This can be used as an emergency measure to prevent loss of consciousness when presyncopal symptoms develop rapidly (Fig. 48.1). Bending over as if to tie one's shoes has similar effects and is simpler for elderly patients to perform. The beneficial effects of sitting in the knee–chest position or placing one foot on a chair while standing are comparable to those of squatting [1].

Acknowledgment

This case was previously published in Wieling *et al.* [1]. We are grateful to Springer Verlag (Darmstadt, Germany) for granting permission to reprint.

References

1 Wieling W, van Lieshout JJ, van Leeuwen AM. Physical manoeuvres that reduce postural hypotension in autonomic failure. *Clin Auton Res* 1993; **3**: 57–65.

2 Van Lieshout JJ, Wieling W, van Montfrans GA, *et al.* Acute dysautonomia associated with Hodgkin's disease. *J Neurol Neurosurg Psychiatry* 1986; **49**: 830–2.

3 Van Lieshout JJ, Wieling W, Wesseling KH, Karemaker JM. Pitfalls in the assessment of cardiovascular reflexes in patients with sympathetic failure but intact vagal control. *Clin Sci* 1989; **76**: 523–8.

4 Van Lieshout JJ, ten Harkel AD, van Leeuwen AM, Wieling W. Contrasting effects of acute and chronic volume expansion on orthostatic blood pressure control in a patient with autonomic circulatory failure. *Neth J Med* 1991; **39**: 72–83.

5 van Lieshout JJ, Ten Harkel ADJ, Wieling W. Combatting orthostatic dizziness in autonomic failure by physical manoeuvres. *Lancet* 1992; **339**: 897–8.

6 Ten Harkel AD, van Lieshout JJ, Wieling W. Effects of leg muscle pumping and tensing on orthostatic arterial pressure: a study in normal subjects and patients with autonomic failure. *Clin Sci (Lond)* 1994; **87**: 553–8.

7 Takishita S, Touma T, Kawazoe N, Muratani H, Fukiyama K. Usefulness of leg-crossing for maintaining blood pressure in a sitting position in patients with orthostatic hypotension: case reports. *Angiology* 1991; **42**: 421–5.

8 Bouvette CM, McPhee BR, Opfer-Gehrking TL, Low PA. Role of physical countermaneuvers in the management of orthostatic hypotension: efficacy and biofeedback augmentation. *Mayo Clin Proc* 1996; **71**: 847–53.

9 Smit AAJ, Halliwill JR, Low PA, Wieling W. Pathophysiological basis of orthostatic hypotension in autonomic failure. *J Physiol* 1999; **519**: 1–10.

CASE 49

Disabling orthostatic hypotension caused by sympathectomies for hyperhidrosis

J.J. van Lieshout, W. Wieling

Case report

An otherwise healthy 38-year-old woman had suffered from severe hyperhidrosis of the hands and the feet since childhood, as a result of which she felt socially withdrawn. Since medical treatment of the hyperhidrosis proved ineffective, she was referred to a clinic for neurovisceral surgery. Extensive sympathectomies were carried out over a period of 2 years (Fig. 49.1). After thoracoscopic sympathetic ganglionotomies bilaterally at the upper thoracic levels (T2–T6), the excessive sweating on her hands disappeared. In the following year, the procedure was extended to lumbar levels L2–L4 on the left and interganglionic sympathicotomies at L2–L4 on the right were carried out, with a salutary effect on plantar hyperhidrosis. After these procedures, abnormal sweating developed, located on both the dorsal and ventral parts of the trunk. A further right-sided extension of the sympathectomies was carried out at T7–T12, including a repeat ganglionotomy at T6 and an interganglionic sympathicotomy at T10–T12. This resulted in relief of the hyperhidrosis over the right hemithorax. Abnormal sweating persisted on the left side of the trunk, while palmar hyperhidrosis returned on the left, for which the following procedure was performed on the left side: repeat ganglionotomy at T2–T5, ganglionotomy at T7–T9, and interganglionic sympathicotomy at T3, T4, T11, and T12. Two days before the last procedure she had played a field hockey game in the highest veteran league, indicating excellent exercise tolerance. Directly after the last operation, she complained of dizziness on standing, which caused

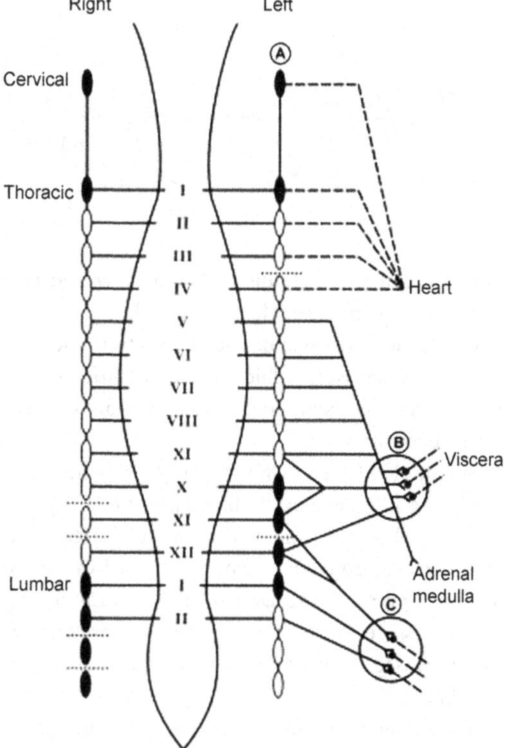

Figure 49.1 The adrenergic part of the autonomic nervous system. The sites of the lesions in the sympathetic thoracolumbar chain are indicated. For clarity, the adrenergic innervation of the heart, splanchnic vascular bed, and adrenal medulla is shown on the left side only. ....., Interganglionic sympathicotomy; ___, preganglionic fiber; ---, postganglionic fiber; 0, intact sympathetic ganglion; ▮, ganglionotomy; A, cervical ganglia; B, celiac and superior mesenteric ganglia; C, lower abdominal sympathetic ganglia.

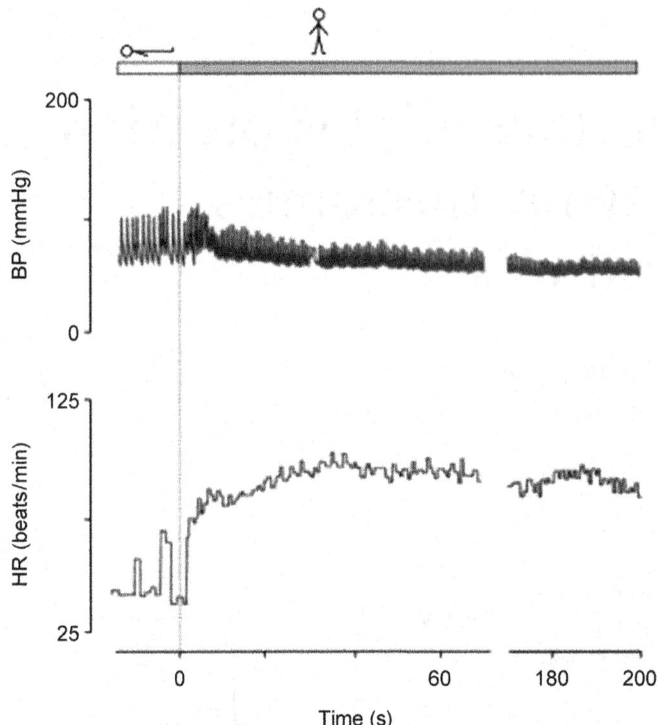

Figure 49.2 Blood-pressure and heart-rate responses after standing. A progressive fall in the blood pressure is accompanied by an instantaneous heart-rate increment, indicating sympathetic vasomotor lesions and intact vagal heart-rate control. BP, blood pressure; HR, heart rate.

her to become severely disabled and prevented her acutely from carrying out housework [1].

On physical examination, small scars from the surgical procedures were visible in the dorsal thoracic and lumbar regions. Neurological examination showed no abnormalities.

Supine blood pressure was normal. When she stood up, the systolic and diastolic blood pressures dropped markedly (Fig. 49.2) and dizziness ensued. Her heart rate increased from 50 to 85 beats/min in 15 s and to 100 beats/min after 35 s. Despite the progressive fall in blood pressure, the heart rate did not increase further but decreased slightly to 95 beats/min after 2 min of standing.

The supine values for plasma norepinephrine and epinephrine were abnormally low, and there was virtually no increase after she stood up.

Comment

Hyperhidrosis is a pathological condition of excessive sweating of unknown origin. Various forms of non-surgical treatment have been considered in patients with hyperhidrosis. Although anticholinergic drugs appear to be effective, their use has been limited due to side-effects [2]. In selected cases of hyperhidrosis, destruction of the sympathetic ganglia by thoracoscopic sympathectomy is therefore regarded as the reference treatment for severe palmar hyperhidrosis [3].

Despite the patient's thoracolumbar sympathectomies, cardiovascular control remained sufficient even to meet the needs of the prolonged and intermittently vigorous exercise involved in competitive field hockey. However, after the final surgical procedure, which resulted in an almost complete sympathetic denervation of the splanchnic area (Fig. 49.1), symptoms of postural hypotension developed. The critical importance of the splanchnic area for the control of blood pressure is well known [4–10]; sympathectomies have little influence on postural blood pressure control until the major part of the sympathetic outflow to the splanchnic area is destroyed [5–7].

The sympathetic nerve supply to the heart is derived from segments T1–T4 (T5), synapsing in all of the cervical and the upper four (five) thoracic ganglia [2]. In view of the pattern of sympathectomies carried out, therefore, sympathetic innervation of the heart was expected to be at least partially intact (Fig. 49.1), and

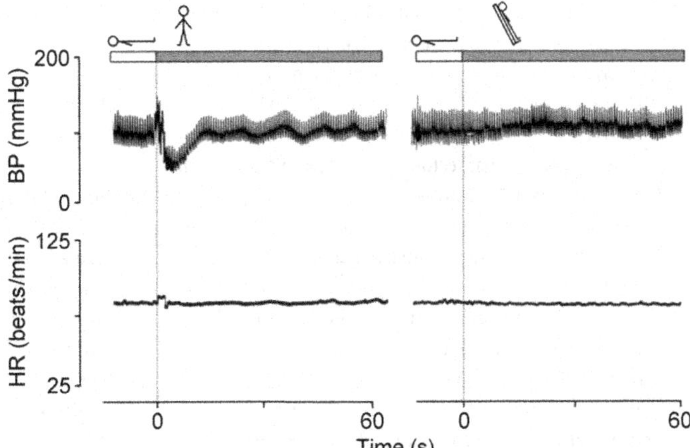

Figure 49.3 The finger blood-pressure and heart-rate responses after active standing and passive head-up tilting in a 38-year-old man with a cardiac transplant. Note the marked difference in blood-pressure adjustment in the first 15 s. BP, blood-pressure; HR, heart rate.

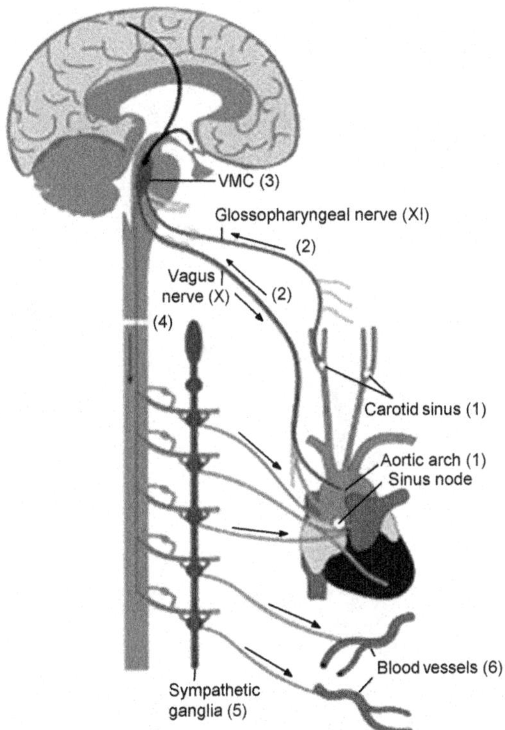

Figure 49.4 The arterial baroreceptor afferents and efferent autonomic pathways. Mechanisms that can cause failure in the baroreflex arc are indicated: 1, lesion in the carotid sinus/aortic baroreceptors; 2, lesion in the carotid sinus/aortic afferents; 3, lesion in the medulla; 4, spinal cord lesion; 5, preganglionic/ganglionic lesion; 6, postganglionic lesion. VMC, vasomotor centers.

testing showed that functional integrity was present. An abnormally large increase in the heart rate (45 beats/min) was observed. This case is therefore a rare example of a hypoadrenergic orthostatic response in a patient with intact heart-rate control (Fig. 49.2). The opposite pattern—i.e., intact vasomotor control and complete cardiac denervation—is observed in patients with a cardiac transplant. In these patients, orthostatic blood-pressure control is normal despite the lack of an increase in heart rate. Figure 49.3 shows an example of the heart-rate and blood-pressure response after active standing and passive head-up tilting in a 38-year-old fit patient with a cardiac transplant.

Patients with circumscribed anatomical lesions on the arterial baroreflex arc provide a unique opportunity to study cardiovascular control in otherwise healthy humans. Figure 49.4 provides a schematic drawing of the baroreceptor afferent and autonomic efferent pathways of the baroreflex arc, with possible mechanisms for failure of cardiovascular function, resulting in a tendency to develop orthostatic hypotension and syncope.

Acknowledgment

This case history was previously published in van Lieshout *et al.* [1]. We are grateful to Van Zuiden Communications for granting permission to reprint.

References

1 van Lieshout JJ, Wieling W, Wesseling KH, Endert E, Karemaker JM. Orthostatic hypotension caused by sympathectomies performed for hyperhidrosis. *Neth J Med* 1990; **36**: 53–7.

2 Johnson RH, Lambie DG, Spalding JMK, eds. *Neurocardiology: the Interrelationships between Dysfunction in the Nervous and Cardiovascular Systems.* Saunders, London, 1984.

3 Dumont P, Denoyer A, Robin P. Long-term results of thoracoscopic sympathectomy for hyperhidrosis. *Ann Thorac Surg* 2004; **78**: 1801–7.

4 Allen EV, Adson AW. The physiological effects of extensive sympathectomy for essential hypertension. *Am Heart J* 1937; **14**: 415–27.

5 Roth GM. The postural effects of blood pressure following interruption of the vasomotor nerves of man. *Am Heart J* 1937; **14**: 87–103.

6 Gambill EE, Hines EA, Adson AW. The circulation in man in certain postures before and after extensive sympathectomy for essential hypertension. *Am Heart J* 1944; **275**: 360–80.

7 Wilkins RW, Culbertson JW. The effect of surgical sympathectomy upon certain vasopressor responses in hypertensive patients. *Trans Assoc Am Phys* 1947; **60**: 195–207.

8 Rowell LB, Detry JM, Blackmon JR, Wyss C. Importance of the splanchnic vascular bed in human blood pressure regulation. *J Appl Physiol* 1972; **32**: 213–20.

9 Low PA, Thomas JE, Dyck PJ. The splanchnic autonomic outflow in Shy–Drager syndrome and idiopathic orthostatic hypotension. *Ann Neurol* 1978; **4**: 511–4.

10 Shepherd JT, Vanhoutte PM. *The Human Cardiovascular System: Facts and Concepts.* Raven Press, New York, 1979.

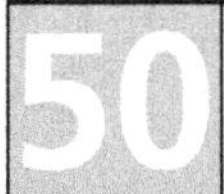

CASE 50

Orthostatic hypotension due to arterial baroreflex failure

H.J.L.M. Timmers, W. Wieling, J.M. Karemaker, J.W.M. Lenders

Case report

A 63-year-old woman had undergone radical excision of a right-sided carotid body tumor at the age of 23. Forty years later, a contralateral carotid body tumor was resected. The operation was radical, and no malignancy was found. The second operation was followed by severe, disabling postural light-headedness and near-syncope. In addition, she was suffering from attacks of severe headache, evoked by mental stress and physical exercise such as cycling. She had also developed dysphagia and voice changes. Impairment of rima glottidis closure, identified on laryngoscopy, indicated damage to the superior laryngeal nerve.

Since bilateral carotid body tumor surgery can be complicated by arterial baroreflex failure due to damage to the carotid sinus baroreceptors [1], preoperative and postoperative baroreflex control of blood pressure were documented. The mean office blood pressure was 177/98 mmHg before the second operation, in comparison with 194/116 mmHg 1 year after surgery. Ambulant blood-pressure variability during scheduled standardized activities was assessed using a 24-h beat-to-beat recording of finger arterial pressure using the Portapres device (model 1; FMS Finapres Medical Systems B.V., Amsterdam, Netherlands) [2]. A year after surgery, blood-pressure variability had increased in comparison with the preoperative findings. After the operation, 75% of the mean arterial blood-pressure values were between 66 and 110 mmHg, in comparison with 75% of blood-pressure values between 69 to 97 mmHg before the operation. Marked blood-pressure increments were observed during activities such as walking (from 111/66 to 160/79 mmHg) and cycling (from 139/68 to 160/80 mmHg). During mental activities such as watching television or speaking on the phone, her blood pressure rose to values between 192/96 and 232/123 mmHg.

In addition, orthostatic control of blood pressure was evaluated due to severe orthostatic symptoms. Before surgery, active standing resulted in a decrease from 150/80 mmHg (supine) to 135/65 mmHg (1 min standing). One month after surgery, there was an initial decrease in blood pressure of 170/110 to 90/75 mmHg, with a sluggish, inadequate recovery (Fig. 50.1). The maximal initial increase in the heart rate was abnormally low (+5 beats/min; normally > 13 beats/min). In addition, the Valsalva maneuver showed a progressive decrease in blood pressure during straining, without a blood pressure overshoot after release of the strain. The heart rate did not change during this procedure. After 1 year of follow-up, the initial blood pressure decrease during active standing was still marked (55/35 mmHg; normally < 40/25), but overt orthostatic hypotension had resolved (Fig. 50.1).

Comment

The acute form of baroreflex failure is encountered after loss of glossopharyngeal or carotid sinus nerve function due to surgical intervention or accidental injury [1,3,4]. It is characterized by severe, unremitting hypertension, tachycardia, and headache. The systolic blood pressure can exceed 250 mmHg, which may lead to hypertensive encephalopathy and (fatal) cerebral hemorrhage [5]. Hypertensive crisis may develop over days and weeks into the more chronic volatile hypertensive phase [1,6]. In addition, volatile hypertension may result from a gradual decline in baroreflex function due to neck irradiation [7]. Volatile hypertension

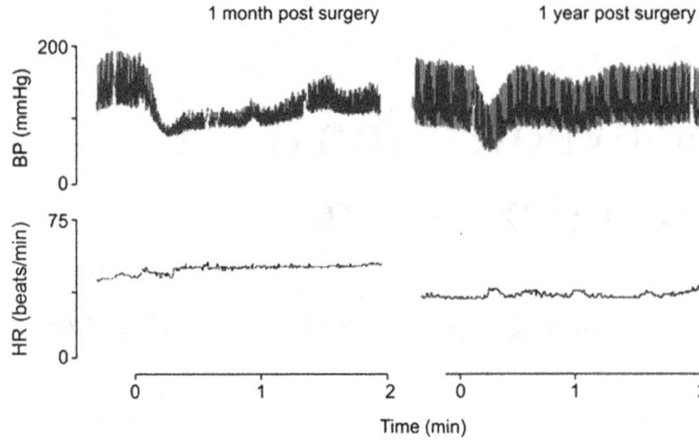

Figure 50.1 Blood-pressure and heart-rate responses to standing up, 1 month and 1 year after the second (contralateral) carotid body tumor resection. BP, blood pressure; HR, heart rate. (Adapted from [6], with permission.)

due to baroreflex failure is characterized by paroxysms of abrupt sympathetic activation, including excessive increments in plasma catecholamine levels. Surges in blood pressure and tachycardia may occur spontaneously, or can be elicited by mental stress or physical stimuli such as exercise, cold, or sexual arousal. These bouts of sympathetic activation may be accompanied by severe headaches, palpitations, diaphoresis, light-headedness, and anxiety. In addition, emotional instability appears to be a prominent feature in this phase of baroreflex failure.

Apart from hypertensive surges, hypotensive episodes may occur during sleep. In rare cases, inadequate baroreflex buffering of cardiovagal efferents is the most prominent feature, resulting in malignant vagotonia with hypotension, bradycardia, and asystole [8]. Accompanying symptoms of this so-called "selective baroreflex failure" include fatigue and dizziness, with possible progression to frank syncope. In the patient reported here, orthostatic light-headedness due to initial orthostatic dizziness and orthostatic hypotension was a prominent feature of baroreflex failure. It was originally claimed that orthostatic hypotension was not part of the baroreflex failure syndrome [1]. However, compensatory mechanisms were later shown to fail after squatting [7]. In other cases, orthostatic hypotension may not become apparent until years after baroreceptor denervation [9]. In addition, persistent orthostatic hypotension has been found in patients after bilateral carotid body tumor surgery [10]. Afferent baroreceptor denervation in these patients was shown to result in abnormal control of cardiovagal efferents and also of efferent muscle sympathetic nerve activity [11]. Abnormal orthostatic control of blood pressure and heart rate after injury to the afferent baroreceptors may occur through abnormal baroreflex-mediated adjustments of both efferent pathways during active standing. In the patient described here, orthostatic hypotension resolved within 1 year after the onset of baroreflex failure, but initial orthostatic dizziness and hypotension persisted. The remaining aortic baroreceptors and cardiopulmonary baroreceptors may in time (partially) compensate for the loss of carotid sinus baroreceptors.

References

1 Robertson D, Hollister AS, Biaggioni I, Netterville JL, Mosqueda Garcia R, Robertson RM. The diagnosis and treatment of baroreflex failure. *N Engl J Med* 1993; **329:** 1449–55.

2 Voogel AJ, van Montfrans GA. Reproducibility of twenty-four-hour finger arterial blood pressure, variability and systemic hemodynamics. *J Hypertens* 1997; **15:** 1761–5.

3 Ille O, Woimant F, Pruna A, Corabianu O, Idatte JM, Haguenau M. Hypertensive encephalopathy after bilateral carotid endarterectomy. *Stroke* 1995; **26:** 488–91.

4 Ketch T, Biaggioni I, Robertson R, Robertson D. Four faces of baroreflex failure: hypertensive crisis, volatile hypertension, orthostatic tachycardia, and malignant vagotonia. *Circulation* 2002; **105:** 2518–23.

5 Ford FR. Fatal hypertensive crisis following denervation of the carotid sinus for the relief of repeated attacks of syncope. *Johns Hopkins Med J* 1956; **100:** 14–6.

6 Smit AAJ, Timmers HJLM, Wieling W, *et al.* Long-term effects of carotid sinus denervation on arterial blood pressure in humans. *Circulation* 2002; **105:** 1329–35.

7 Timmers HJLM, Karemaker JM, Lenders JWM, Wieling W. Baroreflex failure following radiation therapy for nasopharyngeal carcinoma. *Clin Auton Res* 1999; **9**: 317–24.

8 Jordan J, Shannon JR, Black BK, *et al.* Malignant vagotonia due to selective baroreflex failure. *Hypertension* 1997; **30**: 1072–7.

9 Robertson RM. Baroreflex failure. In: Robertson D, Low PA, Polinsky J, eds. *Primer on the Autonomic Nervous System*. Academic Press, London, 1996: 197–208.

10 Timmers HJ, Karemaker JM, Wieling W, Marres HA, Folgering HT, Lenders JW. Baroreflex and chemoreflex function after bilateral carotid body tumor resection. *J Hypertens* 2003; **21**: 591–9.

11 Timmers HJ, Karemaker JM, Wieling W, Marres HA, Lenders JW. Baroreflex control of muscle sympathetic nerve activity after carotid body tumor resection. *Hypertension* 2003; **42**: 143–9.

CASE 51

Hypotension due to straining in a patient with a high spinal-cord lesion

J.J. van Lieshout, W. Wieling

Case report

A 44-year-old woman was admitted due to symptoms of dizziness (light-headedness) related to singing, debating, and car parking [1]. As the symptoms were not related to orthostatic stress, they were initially judged to be psychoneurotic. She had had an incomplete spinal-cord lesion (C5–C6) since the age of 17 due to a motorcycle accident, with partial residual function of the hands. Despite her physical disability, she had given birth to twins and had a job as a doctor's assistant. She was a singer in a steel band. In association with the spinal-cord lesion, she had related symptoms such as autonomic (reflex) bladder, spasms, recurrent urinary tract infections with stone formation, constipation, and occasional orthostatic dizziness.

During the physical examination, a dissociated sensory loss from level C5–T1 was found, with paralysis from T1 and paresis of the forearm flexors, loss of triceps tendon reflexes bilaterally, an extensor plantar reflex, and variable muscle tone with leg spasms. Magnetic resonance imaging showed narrowing of the cervical spinal canal at C2–C5 (C6), with a medullary lesion at C6–C7, which was confirmed by somatosensory evoked potentials.

Supine blood pressure was low (80/40 mmHg), with normal plasma catecholamines (norepinephrine 170–295 ng/L, epinephrine 25–40 ng/L), and elevated plasma renin activity (PRA; 4.0 ng/mL). When she sat in a wheelchair for 20 min, her blood pressure fell slightly (–8/–2 mmHg), with no changes in the catecholamine level (norepinephrine 155–235 ng/L, epinephrine 25–35 ng/L), and with a small rise in PRA to 4.8 ng/mL. Provocation of symptoms by singing showed that both systolic and diastolic blood pressure dropped markedly within a few seconds till near-fainting (Fig. 51.1). On graded 45° head-up tilting, her heart rate increased from 72 beats/min to 100 beats/min, with a slight systolic blood pressure drop (80/40 to 70/45 mmHg); on additional tilting up to 70°, her blood pressure and heart rate did not change (Fig. 51.1).

A drop in blood pressure comparable in magnitude and time course was reproduced by a low-strain Valsalva maneuver (10 mmHg). Small increments in the Valsalva straining pressure induced a rapid progressive fall in pulse pressure during the strain, to a state of disappearance of the pulsatile blood pressure signal (Fig. 51.2), indicating an absence of arterial blood flow. On echocardiography during a 30-mmHg Valsalva strain, the left heart chamber emptied almost completely.

During head-up tilting, her blood pressure gradually declined, with an inversely related increase in the heart rate. These differential effects of orthostasis and strain were reproducible [1].

Comment

Arterial pressure is usually low in patients with a high spinal-cord lesion, depending on the amount of residual spinal-cord reflex activity. Although sympathetic outflow has been isolated from control by the brain, orthostatic tolerance is usually reasonably maintained; as in the present patient, tetraplegics tend to be able to manage an upright posture in a wheelchair with minimal symptoms for much of the day [2–4].

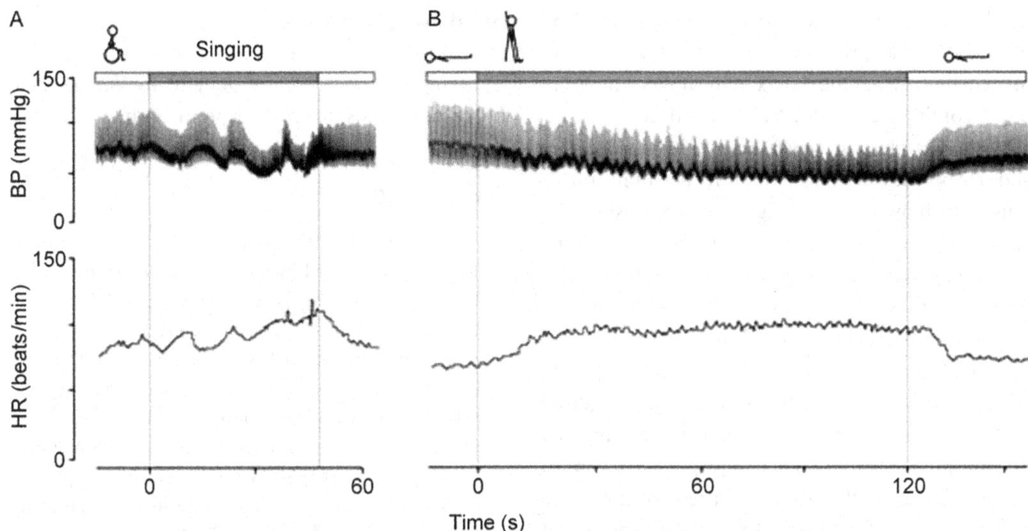

Figure 51.1 Cardiovascular responses to singing (A) and head-up tilting (B). When the patient sings a scale, her blood pressure drops sharply at high-pitched notes; this is comparable to the circulatory effects of about 10 mmHg of Valsalva straining (see Fig. 51.2). BP, blood pressure; HR, heart rate.

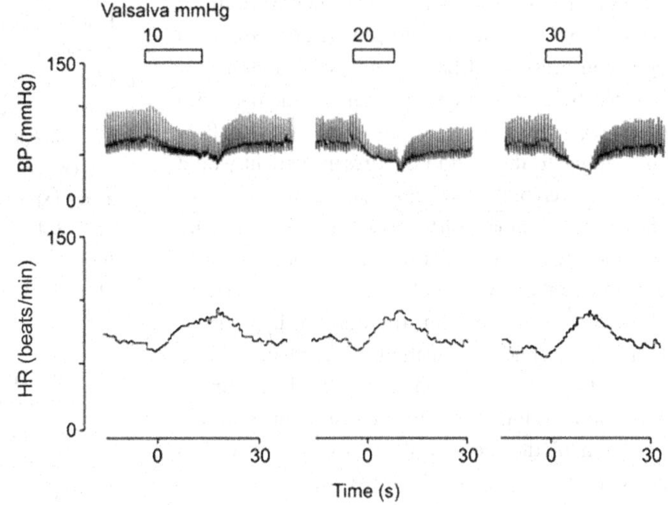

Figure 51.2 Blood-pressure responses to graded straining. Pulse pressure during Valsalva phase II drops progressively without recovery; the size of the drop is proportional to the Valsalva strain. BP, blood pressure; HR, heart rate.

Circulatory adaptation to orthostatic stress in these patients is attributed to activation of spinal sympathetic reflexes acting through the isolated spinal cord [2], to local venoarteriolar axon reflexes [4,5], and to activation of the renin–angiotensin system [2,3]. The small renin release in the sitting position in this patient is in accordance with the minimal postural fall in blood pressure [3].

A peculiar contrast was observed between the patient's relatively normal orthostatic tolerance and severe complaints of dizziness induced by singing, debating, and car parking. It was documented that the dramatic effects of a moderate strain on blood pressure, as involved in everyday physical activities, accounted for this contrast. During provocative maneuvers such as singing, a drop in blood pressure was observed that was comparable in magnitude and time course to the response to a low-strain (10 mmHg) Valsalva maneuver.

In healthy individuals, the Valsalva maneuver

involves a voluntary elevation of intrathoracic and intra-abdominal pressures, resulting in a displacement of blood from the thorax to the limbs, but not to the abdominal cavity [6]. Patients with high spinal-cord lesions lack control over their abdominal muscles and rely on the clavicular part of the pectoralis major muscle to blow against a high counterpressure [7]. Their ability to strain is less, but the effects on the circulation appear to be larger; this can be attributed to pooling in the abdominal cavity due to failure of compression by the abdominal wall muscles and loss of control of splanchnic venoconstriction. The expected fall in cardiac filling volume was indeed visualized in this patient on echocardiography. The finding of a relationship between the small stepwise increments in strain pressure and the fall in pulse pressure during the Valsalva maneuver supports our view that mechanical circulatory effects are responsible for the observed paradox of relatively normal orthostasis and debilitating hypotension on straining.

Hyperventilation and straining are important predisposing factors in syncope [8]. During hypocapnia, cerebral blood flow is markedly decreased at all perfusion pressures. Changes in cerebral blood flow induced by $P\text{CO}_2$ changes are normal in men with spinal-cord transection [9], and a decrease in $P\text{CO}_2$ comparable to the level in the present patient would halve the cerebral blood flow [10]. The effects of chronic hypocapnia on arterial cerebral blood flow are not known; however, this may have contributed to deterioration of the already compromised cerebral blood flow in this patient. In addition, hypocapnia induces systemic vasodilation. Treatment with a high-salt diet and bicarbonate improved her clinical situation and, together with the provision of an explanation of the mechanism, this was sufficient to prevent further syncope or near-syncope.

This case shows that ill-defined symptoms in such patients deserve a full physiological examination.

Acknowledgment

This case was previously published earlier in van Lieshout *et al.* [1]. We are grateful to Van Zuiden Communications for granting permission to reprint.

References

1 van Lieshout JJ, Wieling W, Wesseling KH, Karemaker JM. Singing-induced hypotension: a complication of a high spinal cord lesion. *Neth J Med* 1991; **38**: 75–9.

2 Mathias CJ, Frankel HL. Autonomic failure in tetraplegia. In: Bannister R, ed. *Autonomic Failure: a Textbook of Clinical Disorders of the Autonomic Nervous System.* Oxford University Press, Oxford, 1983: 453–88.

3 Mathias CJ, Christensen NJ, Corbett JL, Frankel HL, Goodwin TJ, Peart WS. Plasma catecholamines, plasma renin activity and plasma aldosterone in tetraplegic man, horizontal and tilted. *Clin Sci* 1975; **49**: 291–9.

4 Skagen K, Jensen K, Hendriksen O, Knudsen L. Sympathetic reflex control of subcutaneous blood flow in tetraplegic man during postural changes. *Clin Sci* 1982; **62**: 605–9.

5 Andersen EB, Boesen F, Hendriksen O, Sonne M. Blood flow in skeletal muscle of tetraplegic man during postural changes. *Clin Sci* 1986; **70**: 321–5.

6 Eckberg DL. Parasympathetic cardiovascular control in human disease: a critical review of methods and results. *Am J Physiol* 1980; **239**: H581–93.

7 De Troyer A, Estenne M, Heilporn A. Mechanism of active expiration in tetraplegic subjects. *N Engl J Med* 1986; **314**: 740–4.

8 Klein LJ, Saltzman HA, Heyman A, Sieker HO. Syncope induced by the Valsalva maneuver. *Am J Med* 1964; **37**: 263–8.

9 Nanda RA, Wyper DJ, Johnson RH, Harper AM. The effect of hypocapnia and change of blood pressure on cerebral blood flow in men with spinal cord transection. *J Neurol Sci* 1976; **30**: 129–35.

10 Hainsworth R. Fainting. In: Bannister R, ed. *Autonomic Failure: a Textbook of Clinical Disorders of the Autonomic Nervous System.* Oxford University Press, Oxford, 1983: 142–58.

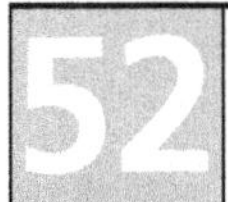

CASE 52

Orthostatic hypotension and syncope in a patient with pheochromocytoma

B. Daga Calejero, E. Gutierrez Ibáñez, A. Carmona Ainat, A. Sánchez Val, J. Pelegrín Díaz, G. Rodrigo Trallero

Case report

A 73-year-old man with a history of hypertension, treated with irbesartan and hydrochlorothiazide, was admitted to hospital due to multiple orthostatic syncopal episodes in the previous 3 months. Other symptoms included frequent and severe headache, diaphoresis, and marked variations in blood pressure.

The clinical examination showed no significant abnormalities, except for significant variations in blood pressure and heart rate related to postural changes. In the supine position, his blood pressure was 200/110 mmHg with a heart rate of 80 beats/min. In the standing position, his blood pressure was 130/70 mmHg with a heart rate of 130 beats/min. A 12-lead electrocardiogram (ECG) showed a sinus rhythm at 80 beats/min, with diffuse negative T waves, whereas a previous ECG obtained several months before had been normal. Echocardiography, chest radiography, electroencephalography, and computed tomography (CT) of the brain showed no significant abnormalities. A cardiac electrophysiological study was carried out, which showed normal sinus function and atrioventricular conduction and no inducible arrhythmia. On the basis of these data, a tilt test was carried out, which showed a slow and progressive decline in blood pressure starting immediately after he moved to the upright position, associated with a continuous increase in heart rate. On sublingual nitroglycerin administration, there was a fall in blood pressure to 69/37 mmHg, and syncope supervened.

Due to the marked oscillations in blood pressure, with a poor response to treatment, a complete hormonal screening was conducted. Serum levels of adrenocorticotropic hormone, luteinizing hormone, follicle-stimulating hormone, prolactin, thyroid-stimulating hormone, basal cortisol, and testosterone were within normal ranges, but there was a significant elevation of urinary normetanephrine (7536 mg/24 h; normal range 30–440 mg/24 h) and vanillylmandelic acid (14.2 mg/24 h; normal range 0.5–6.7 mg/24 h). On the basis of these findings, ^{123}iodinated metaiodobenzylguanidine (^{123}I-MIBG) scintigraphy was carried out, which revealed a left adrenal tumor located at the adrenal medulla (Fig. 52.1). An abdominal CT confirmed the existence of a large mass in the left adrenal gland (Fig. 52.2).

A diagnosis of orthostatic syncope due to a pheochromocytoma in the left adrenal gland was made. After adequate alpha-adrenergic block had been achieved with prazosin, the patient underwent a left subcostal laparotomy, and a left adrenal mass 70 × 45 mm in size was removed. The histopathological analysis showed that it was a capsulated tumor with a large central necrosis and a peripheral halo of chromaffin cells.

The patient has remained asymptomatic during a 4-year follow-up period, with normal blood pressure and without treatment.

Comment

Pheochromocytoma is a rare tumor arising from chromaffin tissue located in the adrenal medulla,

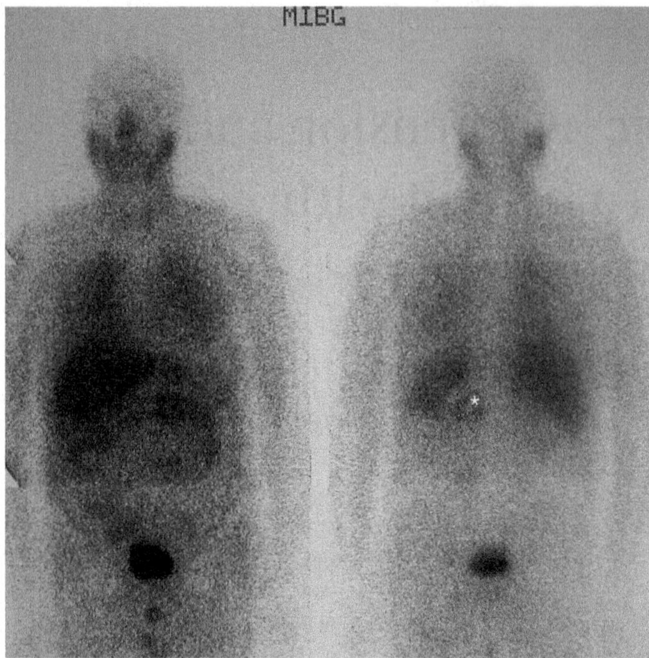

Figure 52.1 ^{123}Iodinated metaiodobanzylguanidine (^{123}I-MIBG) scintigraphy, showing a left adrenal tumor (asterisk).

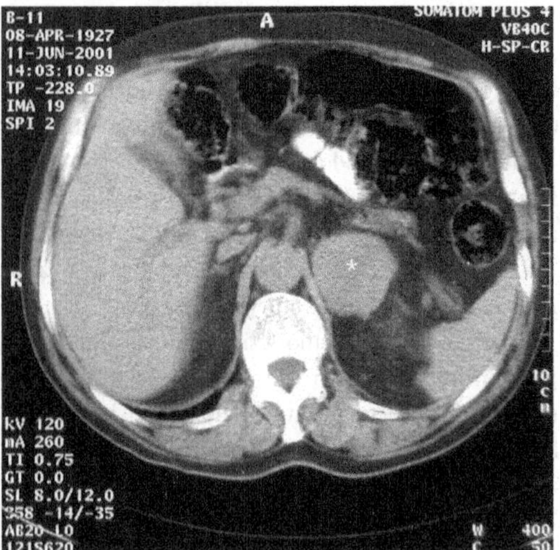

Figure 52.2 Abdominal computed tomography, showing a large mass (asterisk) in the left adrenal gland.

sympathetic ganglia, the para-aortic bodies (Zuckerkandl bodies), or urinary bladder. The epidemiological aspects of pheochromocytoma have been described with the "rule of 10": 10% are extra-adrenal and, of those, 10% are extra-abdominal; 10% are malignant; 10% are found in patients who do not have hypertension; and finally, 10% of patients have a familial presentation [1].

Pheochromocytomas secrete epinephrine and norepinephrine, and variations in the amounts, types of hormone secreted, and the pattern of release of these catecholamines may account for the variation in the clinical manifestations [2]. Patients with pheochromocytoma may present with sustained hypertension that is resistant to conventional treatment, or with paroxysmal attacks of hypertension, headache, sweating, palpitation, and tremor. However, the clinical presentation of pheochromocytoma is highly variable, making these tumors very difficult to diagnose.

Patients with pheochromocytoma can present with orthostatic hypotension and syncope. In the Italian pheochromocytoma registry [3], 5% of 258 patients had syncope and 14% had orthostatic hypotension. In another study, syncope was observed in five (20%) of 25 consecutive patients diagnosed with pheochromocytoma in a single hospital [4].

Orthostatic hypotension in pheochromocytoma has been attributed to two main causes: firstly, inadequate arteriolar and venous reflexes with orthostasis [5], probably due to down-regulation of the alpha-receptors after prolonged exposure to high plasma catecholamine levels [6] or to central inhibition of norepinephrine secretion [7]; and secondly, blood volume reduction [8].

In the present case, hypertension and orthostatic syncope were the more striking symptoms. Orthostatic hypotension was clearly demonstrated by both active orthostatic testing and passive tilt testing. A wide hormonal screen was carried out, and the pheochromocytoma was suspected due to the high urinary output of normetanephrine and vanillylmandelic acid. Finally, ^{123}I-MIBG scintigraphy and abdominal CT scanning were able to locate the tumor in the left adrenal gland. Surgical extirpation of the tumor led to control of the hypertension and syncopal attacks.

References

1 Bravo E, Gifford RW Jr. Pheochromocytoma: diagnosis, localization and management. *N Engl J Med* 1984; **311**: 1298–303.

2 Bravo E, Tagle R. Pheochromocytoma: state-of-the-art and future prospects. *Endocr Rev* 2003; **24**: 539–53.

3 Mannelli M, Ianni L, Cilotti A, Conti A. Pheochromocytoma in Italy: a multicentric retrospective study. *Eur J Endocrinol* 1999; **141**: 619–24.

4 Liao WB, Liu CF, Chiang CW, Kung CT, Lee CW. Cardiovascular manifestations of pheochromocytoma. *Am J Emerg Med* 2000; **18**: 622–5.

5 Levenson JA, Safar ME, London GM, Simon AC. Haemodynamics in patients with pheochromocytoma. *Clin Sci (Lond)* 1980; **58**: 349–56.

6 Streeten DPH, Anderson GH Jr. Mechanisms of orthostatic hypotension and tachycardia in patients with pheochromocytoma. *Am J Hypertens* 1996; **9**: 760–9.

7 Grassi G, Seravalle G, Turri C, Mancia G. Sympathetic nerve traffic responses to surgical removal of pheochromocytoma. *Hypertension* 1999; **34**: 461–5.

8 Brunjes S, Johns VJ Jr, Crane MG. Pheochromocytoma: postoperative shock and blood volume. *N Engl J Med* 1960; **262**: 393–6.

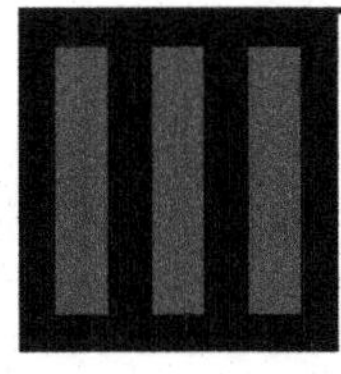

PART III
Arrhythmic syncope

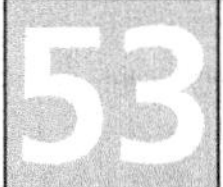

CASE 53

Syncope and the Brugada syndrome

R. García Civera, R. Ruiz Granell, S. Morell Cabedo, R. Sanjuán Mañez

Case report

A 28-year-old man was referred for cardiologic evaluation due to a syncopal attack, with no trigger, and an abnormal electrocardiogram (ECG). He had no personal history of heart disease or family history of syncope or sudden death. The physical examination was normal.

The 12-lead ECG (Fig. 53.1) shows a sinus rhythm at 60 beats/min, a 0.16-s PR interval, a QRS duration of 0.10 s, and a QT interval of 0.40 s. The QRS shows an rSR′ pattern in leads V_1 and V_2 and ST-segment elevation with a "saddleback" configuration in leads V_2 and V_3. Laboratory tests, echocardiography, and cardiac magnetic resonance imaging did not disclose any abnormalities.

An electrophysiological study (EPS) was carried out due to a suspicion of Brugada syndrome. Figure 53.2 shows the results of programmed ventricular stimulation. Two ventricular extrastimuli (with coupling intervals of 200 and 190 ms), delivered from the right ventricular apex during a basic drive cycle length of 400 ms, resulted in the induction of polymorphic ventricular tachycardia with rapid transition to

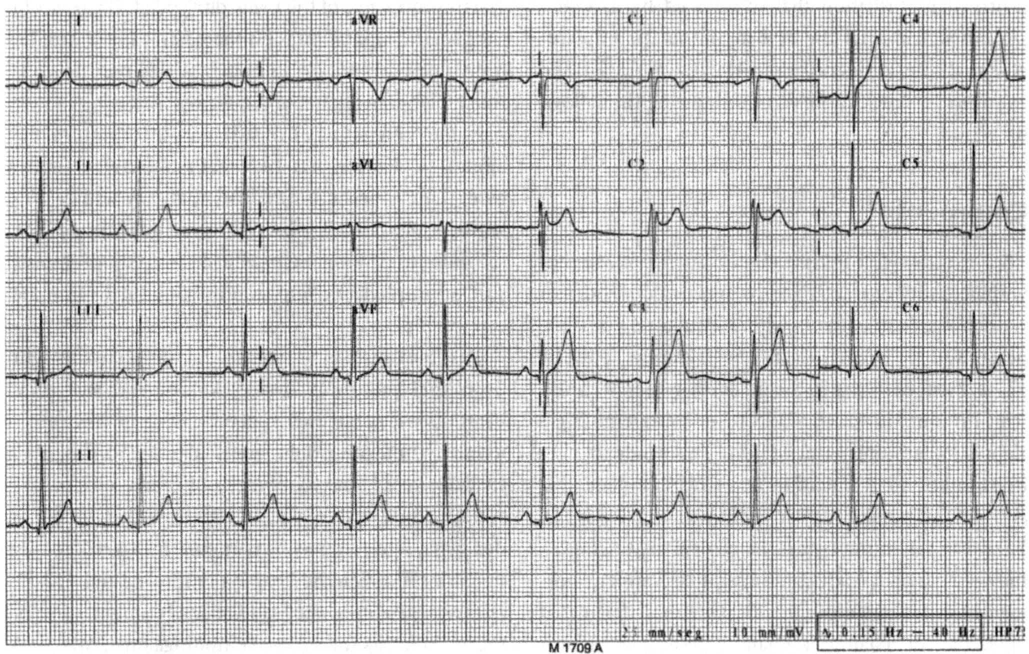

Figure 53.1 The patient's baseline electrocardiogram.

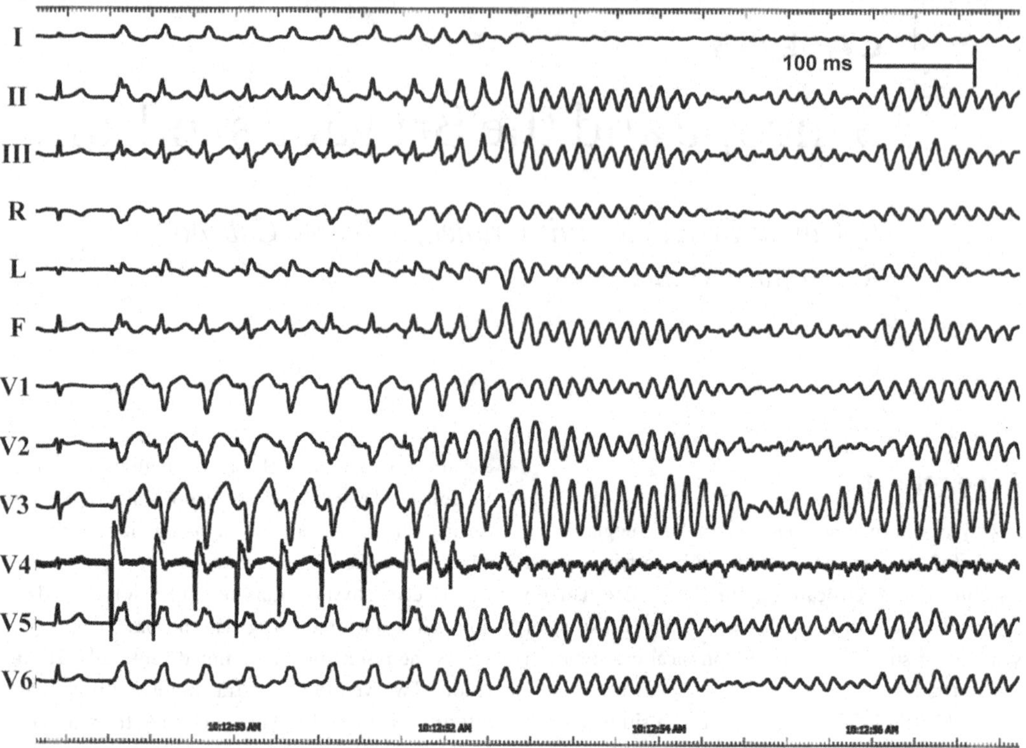

Figure 53.2 Programmed ventricular stimulation results in the induction of ventricular fibrillation.

ventricular fibrillation that was ended by a direct-current shock. After the EPS, an automatic implantable cardioverter-defibrillator (AICD) was placed, and appropriate shocks were observed during the follow-up period.

Comment

The Brugada syndrome is a clinical and electrocardiographic entity characterized by syncopal episodes or sudden death in patients with a structurally normal heart and a typical electrocardiographic pattern: ST-segment elevation in the precordial leads V_1 to V_3, with morphology of the QRS complex resembling a right bundle-branch block [1–3]. This syndrome has been linked to a mutation in *SCN5A*, a gene that encodes the human cardiac sodium channel [4]. The ECG features of the syndrome can vary over time in the same patient, leading to occasional transient normalization. In these cases, antiarrhythmic drugs that block the Na^+ channel (ajmaline, flecainide, or procainamide) can often reproduce the abnormal ECG.

The prevalence of the Brugada-type ECG pattern in the general population is estimated at 0.1% in healthy individuals and 0.22% in men, and the prevalence is much higher in Japan than in Europe [5].

In the presence of a Brugada-type ECG pattern, the clinical evaluation has two main objectives: firstly, to exclude other abnormalities that can lead to ST-segment elevation in the right precordial leads; and secondly, to detect patients who have a poor prognosis so that prophylactic implantation of an AICD can be carried out.

Possible causes of ST-segment elevation in the right precordial leads [6] include various types of structural heart disease [acute ischemia or infarction, myocarditis, arrhythmogenic right ventricular cardiomyopathy (ARVC), etc.] and also metabolic and electrolytic abnormalities (hyperkalemia, hypercalcemia, thiamine deficiency, etc.). It may be particularly difficult to differentiate between the Brugada syndrome and ARVC. In the present case, the “saddleback” configuration of the ST in lead V_2, the normal findings on cardiac imaging examinations (echocardiography and magnetic resonance imaging), and the induction of a polymorphic ventricular tachycardia fibrillation in the EPS argue against a diagnosis of ARVC.

Patients with the Brugada syndrome who have been resuscitated from near-sudden arrhythmic death have a high risk of recurrent ventricular fibrillation [1–3], and there is general agreement that an AICD should be implanted in these cases. However, the management in the remainder of patients with the ECG pattern of Brugada syndrome is controversial. Recently, Brugada *et al.* [7] analyzed a total of 547 patients with an ECG diagnostic of Brugada syndrome and no previous cardiac arrest. During a follow-up period of 24 ± 32 months, 8% of the patients suffered sudden cardiac death or presented with documented ventricular fibrillation. The multivariate analysis showed that inducibility of sustained ventricular arrhythmia and a history of syncope were predictive factors for events. The results of the study show that the patient in the present report, with a previous history of syncope, a spontaneously abnormal ECG, and inducible sustained ventricular arrhythmia, had a 27.2% probability of suffering sudden death or ventricular fibrillation during the following 2 years. Placement of the AICD therefore appears to be fully indicated in this patient.

References

1 Brugada P, Brugada J. Right bundle branch block, persistent ST segment elevation and sudden cardiac death: a distinct clinical and electrocardiographic syndrome. A multicenter report. *J Am Coll Cardiol* 1992; **20**: 1391–6.

2 Brugada J, Brugada P. Further characterization of the syndrome of right bundle branch block, ST segment elevation, and sudden cardiac death. *J Cardiovasc Electrophysiol* 1997; **8**: 325–31.

3 Brugada J, Brugada R, Brugada P. Right bundle-branch block and ST-segment elevation in leads V_1 through V_3: a marker for sudden death in patients without demonstrable structural heart disease. *Circulation* 1998: **97**: 457–60.

4 Chen Q, Kirsch GE, Zhang D, *et al.* Genetic basis and molecular mechanism for idiopathic ventricular fibrillation. *Nature* 1998; **392**: 293–6.

5 Sakurada H, Okazaki H, Tejima T. What is the prevalence, incidence and prognostic value of Brugada-type electrocardiogram in the general population? In: Raviele A, ed. *Cardiac Arrhythmias 2003: Proceedings of the 8th International Workshop on Cardiac Arrhythmias, Venice, 5–8 October 2003.* Springer, Milan, 2004: 331–4.

6 Wilde AAM, Antzelevitch C, Borggrefe M, *et al.* Proposed diagnostic criteria for the Brugada syndrome: consensus report. *Circulation* 2002; **106**: 2514–9.

7 Brugada J, Brugada R, Brugada P. Determinants of sudden cardiac death in individuals with the electrocardiographic pattern of Brugada syndrome and no previous cardiac arrest. *Circulation* 2003; **108**: 3092–6.

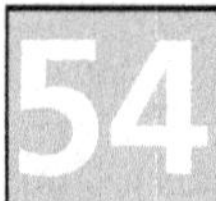

CASE 54

Two types of monomorphic ventricular tachycardia as a cause of syncope in Brugada syndrome

R. Ruiz Granell, S. Morell Cabedo, R. Sanjuán Mañez, R. García Civera

Case report

A 41-year-old man was admitted to our hospital for an electrophysiological examination due to recurrent syncope and presyncope during the previous 14 months, with four syncopal episodes in the 2 months before admission. The patient had no family history of syncope or sudden death. The patient had been examined at another institution a year before. The findings of this previous assessment [including clinical history, physical examination, baseline electrocardiogram (ECG), carotid sinus massage, postural blood-pressure testing, 24-h ambulatory monitoring, echocardiography, and magnetic resonance imaging] were normal. A head-up tilt-table test was negative. Despite a normal electroencephalogram, epilepsy had been suspected, and the patient had been treated with diphenylhydantoin. This did not lead to symptomatic relief, and the patient suffered a syncopal episode while driving, causing a car crash. The patient was then submitted to our hospital for evaluation. The tilt-table test with a nitroglycerin challenge was repeated, again with normal findings. An electrophysiological study was then scheduled.

The baseline 12-lead ECG at the time of the electrophysiological examination (Fig. 54.1) showed a sinus rhythm at 70 beats/min, a PR interval of 140 ms, a QRS width of 110 ms, and a QT interval of 400 ms. The QRS in leads V_1 and V_2 showed an rSR′ pattern and doubtful (less than 0.1 mV) ST-segment elevation. Tests of sinus and atrioventricular node function were within the normal ranges. The HV interval was 50 ms, and a sporadic infrahisian block of atrial premature beats was observed. Programmed right atrial and ventricular stimulation (with increasing heart rates and up to three extrastimuli at two basic cycles) did not induce significant arrhythmias. After intravenous administration of 50 mg ajmaline, the ECG showed a coved-type ST elevation in leads V_1 and V_2 (Fig. 54.2).

Despite a suspicion of syncope in Brugada syndrome, an implantable loop recorder (Reveal 9525; Medtronic, Inc., Minneapolis, Minnesota, USA) was implanted after the electrophysiological study in an attempt to further document the mechanism of the syncope. In the first week after implantation, the patient experienced two syncopal episodes and activated the device. The stored electrograms were retrieved by telemetry; a monomorphic regular ventricular tachycardia was detected during both activations, but the QRS polarity and morphology were different in each episode (Fig. 54.3).

A defibrillator was implanted, and during a follow-up period of more than 4 years, the device has delivered appropriate shocks, always in response to regular tachycardias.

Comment

The present case meets the diagnostic criteria for Brugada syndrome due to the presence of syncopal episodes and a type 1 ECG after ajmaline administration [1]. In addition, no structural heart disease was detected either at the initial evaluation or during the follow-up.

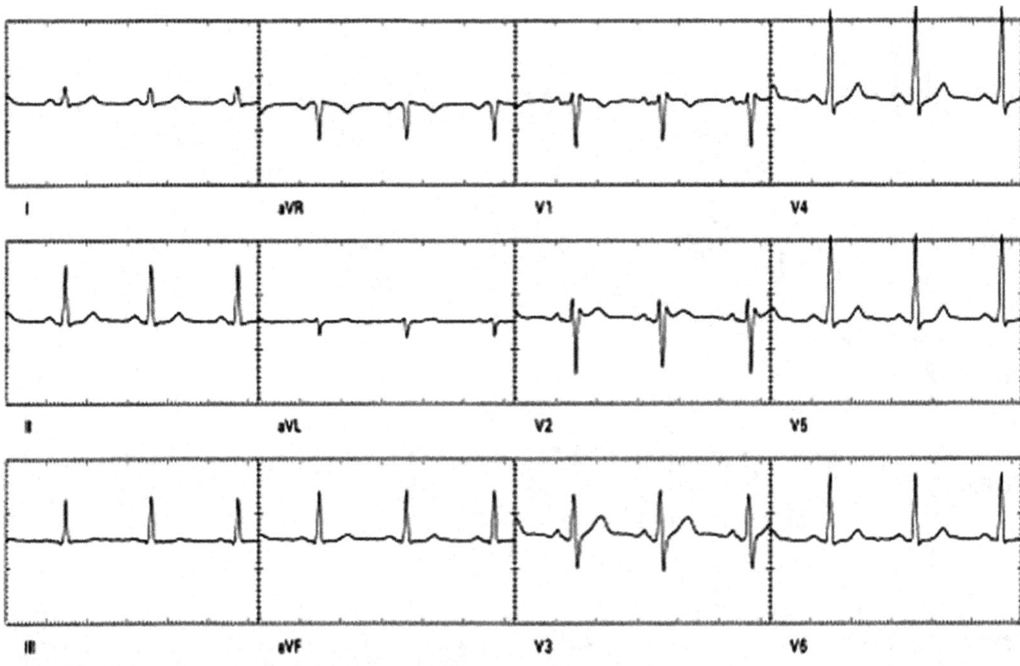

Figure 54.1 The baseline 12-lead electrocardiogram.

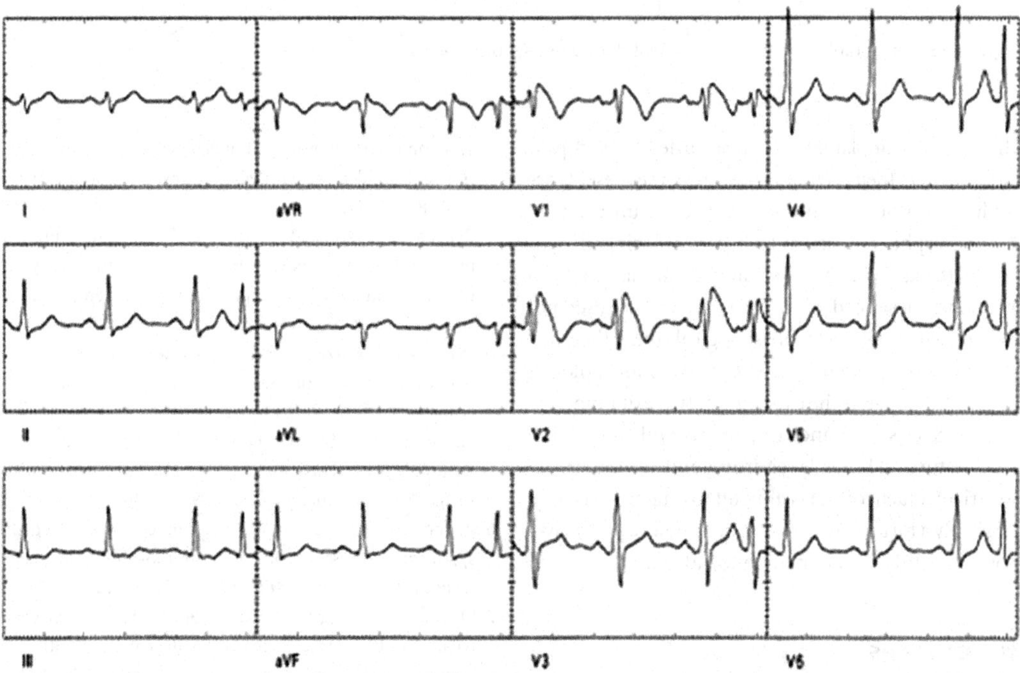

Figure 54.2 The electrocardiogram after ajmaline administration.

Syncopal attacks in Brugada syndrome are typically related to polymorphic ventricular tachycardia [2–5], but cases of monomorphic ventricular tachycardia have also been reported in the literature [6–8].

Nonsustained episodes of monomorphic regular ventricular tachycardia were the cause of the syncopal episodes in this patient. These arrhythmias could not be induced during the electrophysiological study, and only

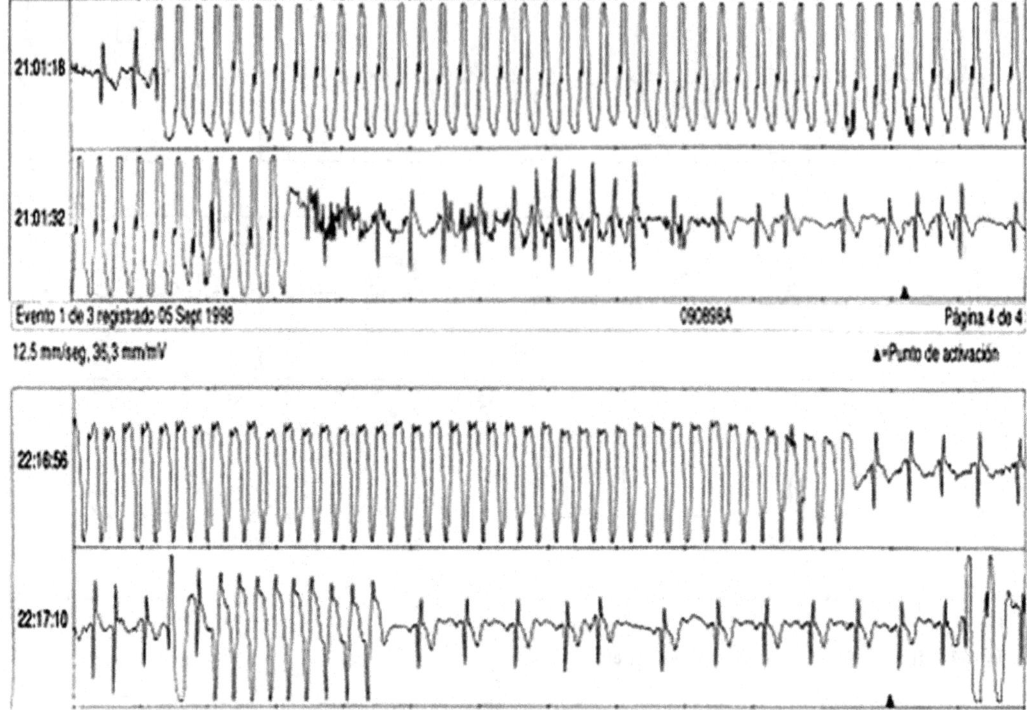

Figure 54.3 Implantable loop recorder tracings during two syncopal episodes.

the use of an implantable loop recorder made it possible to detect them. A unique feature of the present case is the detection of two distinct types of unsustained monomorphic ventricular tachycardia during the syncopal attacks. So far as we are aware, this has not been previously described. Since the tachycardias could not be induced in the electrophysiological study, their origin is uncertain, but the presence of two morphologies of the QRS suggests the existence of two exit points.

The exact significance of patients with the typical ECG features of Brugada syndrome and monomorphic ventricular tachycardia is difficult to establish. It could be simply a fortuitous association, or—more probably—could constitute a variant of the syndrome.

References

1 Brugada P, Brugada J. Right bundle branch block, persistent ST segment elevation and sudden cardiac death: a distinct clinical and electrocardiographic syndrome. A multicenter report. *J Am Coll Cardiol* 1992; **20**: 1391–6.

2 Brugada J, Brugada P. Further characterization of the syndrome of right bundle branch block, ST segment elevation, and sudden cardiac death. *J Cardiovasc Electrophysiol* 1997; **8**: 325–31.

3 Brugada J, Brugada R, Brugada P. Right bundle-branch block and ST-segment elevation in leads V_1 through V_3: a marker for sudden death in patients without demonstrable structural heart disease. *Circulation* 1998: **97**: 457–60.

4 Wilde AAM, Antzelevitch C, Borggrefe M, *et al.* Proposed diagnostic criteria for the Brugada syndrome: consensus report. *Circulation* 2002; **106**: 2514–9.

5 Shimada M, Miyazaki T, Miyosi S, *et al.* Sustained monomorphic ventricular tachycardia in a patient with Brugada's syndrome. *Jpn Circ J* 1996; **60**: 364–70.

6 Boersma LVA, Jaarsma W, Jessurun ER, *et al.* Brugada syndrome: a case report of monomorphic ventricular tachycardia. *Pacing Clin Electrophysiol* 2001; **24**: 112–5.

7 Ogawa M, Kumagai K, Saku K. Spontaneous right ventricular outflow tract tachycardia in a patient with the Brugada syndrome. *J Cardiovasc Electrophysiol* 2001; **12**: 838–40.

8 Mazur A, Iakobishvili Z, Kusniec J, Strasberg B. Bundle branch reentrant ventricular tachycardia in a patient with the Brugada electrocardiographic pattern. *Ann Noninvasive Electrocardiol* 2003; **8**: 352–5.

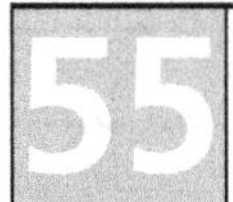

CASE 55

Syncope and Brugada-like electrocardiography pattern appearing during a febrile illness: neurally mediated or arrhythmic syncope?

J. García Sacristán, R. Ceres, C. Lafuente

Case report

A 32-year-old man with no pathological history presented at the emergency room in our hospital due to two syncopal episodes. He reported that he had awoken at 2 a.m. with throat pain, abdominal discomfort, sweating, and nausea. He went to the bathroom, where he had a syncopal episode with a rapid and complete recovery. Three hours later, he had another syncopal episode with the same characteristics, and he decided to come to the hospital.

In the emergency room, his physical examination was normal, with the exception of a temperature of 38.5 °C and throat congestion. The electrocardiogram (ECG) showed a sinus rhythm at 109 beats/min and an elevation of the ST segment of more than 2 mm in leads V_1 and V_2 (Fig. 55.1). Routine analytic tests, including troponin I, were normal. The patient was

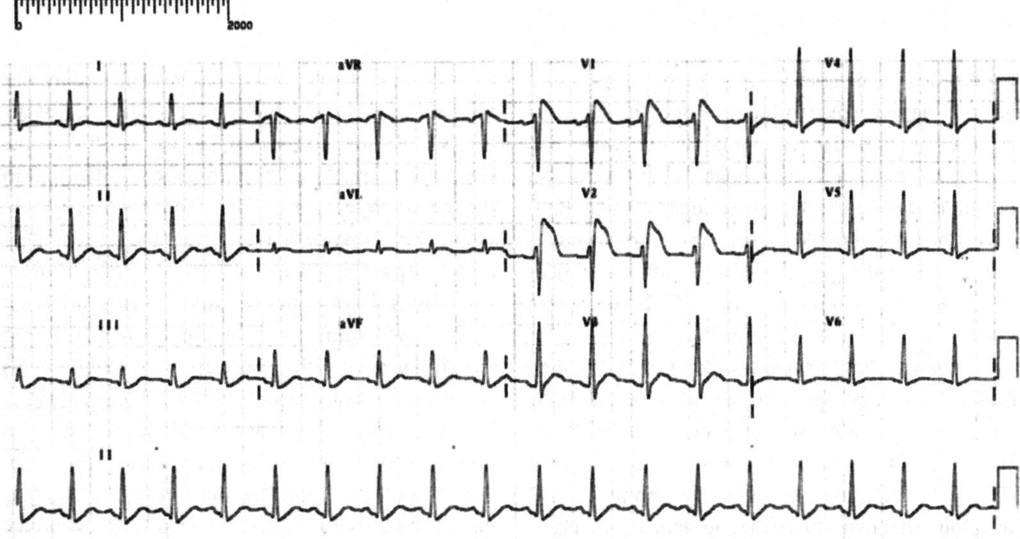

Figure 55.1 The electrocardiogram at admission, when the patient had a temperature of 38.5 °C.

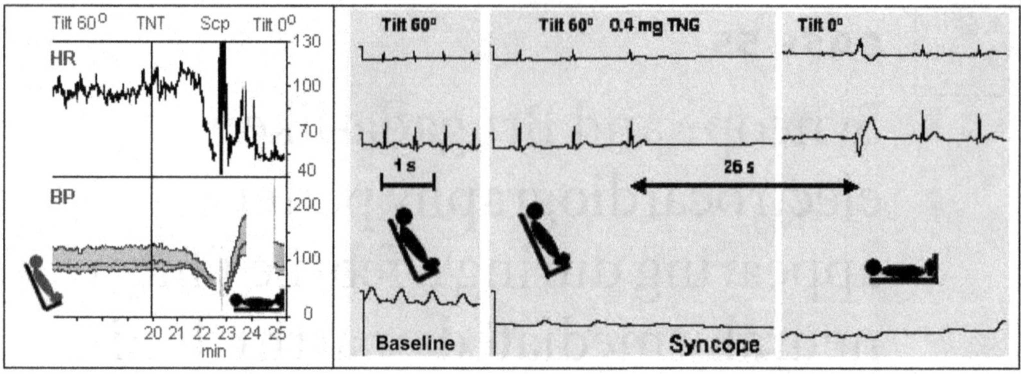

Figure 55.2 The positive tilt-table test (Vasovagal Syncope International Study type 2b). BP, blood pressure; HR, heart rate; Scp, syncope; TNG, trinitroglycerin.

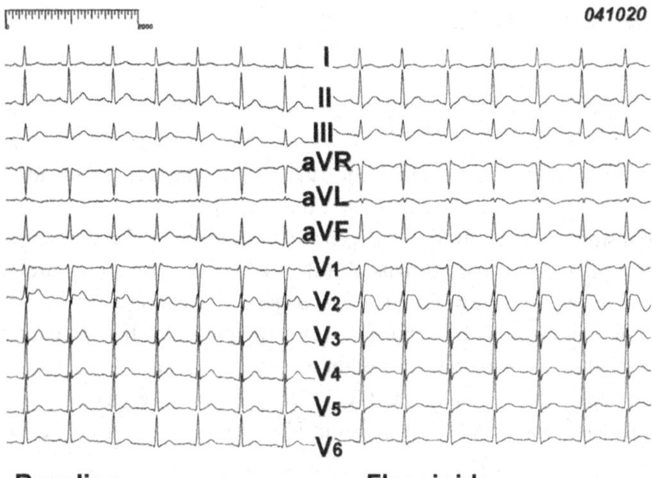

Figure 55.3 The positive flecainide test.

diagnosed as having vasovagal syncope during the course of a possible viral infection, but because of the abnormal ECG he was referred for cardiologic evaluation.

An echocardiogram was normal, and a tilt-table test, flecainide test, and electrophysiological study (EPS) were scheduled due to a suspicion of Brugada syndrome. The tests were carried out with the patient in an afebrile condition, and the ECG showed an ST saddleback abnormality in V_1 and V_2.

The tilt-table test was conducted using the "Italian protocol." After nitroglycerin administration, a classic vasovagal response (Vasovagal Syncope International Study type 2b) with a 26-s asystole was observed (Fig. 55.2). The patient had syncope with prodromal symptoms that reproduced the spontaneous attack.

Flecainide (2 mg/kg) was administered over 10 min by the intravenous route. The administration was interrupted when only 50 mg had been injected, as the test was already clearly positive (with a shift of the electrocardiography pattern from the "saddleback" to the "coved" type) (Fig. 55.3).

The EPS was carried out with the patient in a postabsorptive, unsedated state and free of cardiovascular drugs. The baseline atrioventricular conduction intervals were normal. During stimulation in the right ventricular apex with a basic cycle length of 500 ms and two ventricular extrastimuli, a polymorphic ventricular tachycardia/fibrillation was induced (Fig. 55.4). The arrhythmia was associated with a presyncopal episode and ceased spontaneously after 24 s, coinciding with a burst of pacing. No other attempts to induce the arrhythmia were made.

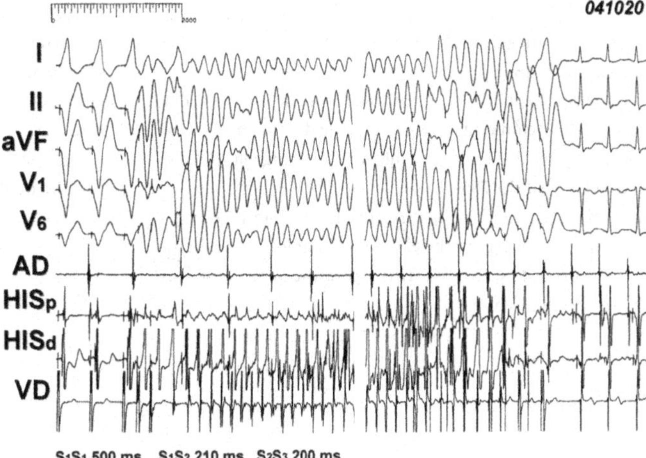

Figure 55.4 Induction of polymorphic ventricular tachycardia/fibrillation during the electrophysiological study. The arrhythmia ends spontaneously after 24 s, coinciding with a burst of pacing.

After the complete evaluation, the diagnosis was vasovagal syncope and Brugada syndrome. The risks of the Brugada syndrome were discussed with the patient, and implantation of an automatic cardioverter-defibrillator was eventually decided on and carried out. The patient has remained asymptomatic during a short follow-up period.

Comment

Since the classical description of vasovagal syncope by Sir Thomas Lewis, febrile illness has been recognized as a predisposing factor for vasovagal syncope [1]. However, recent reports have emphasized the importance of fever for unmasking or enhancing the electrocardiographic pattern of Brugada syndrome [2–4] and as a possible trigger for ventricular arrhythmias in this setting [4,5]. This effect of fever is probably due to the temperature dependence of the ionic mechanisms responsible for the electrocardiographic phenotype of the Brugada syndrome [6]. A new mutation of the *SCN5A* gene has recently been detected in a patient with Brugada syndrome that was unmasked by hyperthermia [7].

In the present case, therefore, fever is the common element predisposing the patient to a vasovagal faint and enhancing the electrocardiographic pattern of Brugada syndrome. The diagnosis of vasovagal syncope is suggested by the clinical features of the trigger (throat pain), predisposing factors (fever), and prodromal signs (abdominal discomfort, sweating, and nausea). In addition, a positive tilt-table test with a cardioinhibitory response confirms the susceptibility of the patient to vasovagal reactions. Equally, the presence of a Brugada syndrome is evident from the ECG pattern, the enhancement of this pattern by fever and flecainide administration, an absence of structural heart disease, and the response to programmed ventricular stimulation.

How should the patient be managed? A unique vasovagal syncope in the setting of a febrile illness does not require special treatment, but the presence of Brugada syndrome requires an evaluation of the risk. According to a recent study [8], the presence of syncope, a persistent ECG pattern, and induction of polymorphic ventricular tachycardia/fibrillation during the EPS is associated with a 27.2% probability of suffering sudden death or ventricular fibrillation during the following 2 years. Even if it is taken into account that the syncope is clearly vasovagal and it is excluded from the risk evaluation, the probability of a malignant event would still be 14%. Implantation of a defibrillator therefore seems an appropriate option.

References

1 Lewis T. Vasovagal syncope and the carotid sinus mechanism. *Br Med J* 1932; **i**: 873–6.

2 Saura D, García-Alberola A, Carrillo P, *et al.* Brugada-like electrocardiographic pattern induced by fever. *Pacing Clin Electrophysiol* 2002; **25**: 856–9.

3 Kum LCC, Fung JWH, Sanderson JE. Brugada syndrome unmasked by febrile illness. *Pacing Clin Electrophysiol* 2002; **25**: 1660–1.

4 Porres JM, Brugada J, Urbistondo V, *et al.* Fever unmasking the Brugada syndrome. *Pacing Clin Electrophysiol* 2002; **25**: 1646–8.

5 González Rebollo JM, Hernández Madrid A, García A, *et al.* Fibrilación ventricular recurrente durante un proceso febril en un paciente con síndrome de Brugada. *Rev Esp Cardiol* 2000; **53**: 755–7.

6 Dumaine R, Towbin JA, Brugada P, *et al.* Ionic mechanisms responsible for the electrocardiographic phenotype of the Brugada syndrome are temperature dependent. *Circ Res* 1999; **85**: 803–9.

7 Mock NS, Priori SG, Napolitano C, *et al.* A newly characterized *SCN5A* mutation underlying the Brugada syndrome unmasked by hyperthermia. *J Cardiovasc Electrophysiol* 2003; **14**: 407–11.

8 Brugada J, Brugada R, Brugada P. Determinants of sudden cardiac death in individuals with the electrocardiographic pattern of Brugada syndrome and no previous cardiac arrest. *Circulation* 2003; **108**: 3092–6.

56

CASE 56

Syncope in a case of acquired long QT syndrome

R. Sanjuán Mañez, R. García Civera, S. Morell Cabedo, R. Ruiz Granell

Case report

A 56-year-old woman presented to the emergency department due to two syncopal attacks during the previous few hours. The patient had a history of valvular heart disease and permanent atrial fibrillation. She was being treated with digitalis, diuretics, amiodarone, and acenocoumarin.

At the initial examination, the patient was conscious and oriented; she had an irregular pulse of around 90 beats/min and a blood pressure of 130/60 mmHg. The initial electrocardiogram (ECG) (Fig. 56.1) showed atrial fibrillation, narrow QRS complexes, and a prolonged QT interval (real QT = 0.60 s).

The patient was admitted to the intensive-care unit due to the prolonged QT interval. The ECG was monitored and electrolytes were assessed. In the intensive-care unit, the patient developed a new syncopal episode related to ventricular tachycardia of the *torsade de pointes* type (Fig. 56.2). The tests showed a serum K^+ of 3.5 mEq/L and digoxinemia of 2.06 ng/dL. A transvenous temporary electrocatheter was inserted, and ventricular pacing was started at an initial rate of 90 beats/min, which prevented the recurrence of ventricular arrhythmias. After withdrawal of the diuretics and amiodarone and correction of the hypokalemia, the patient was discharged with a normal QT interval.

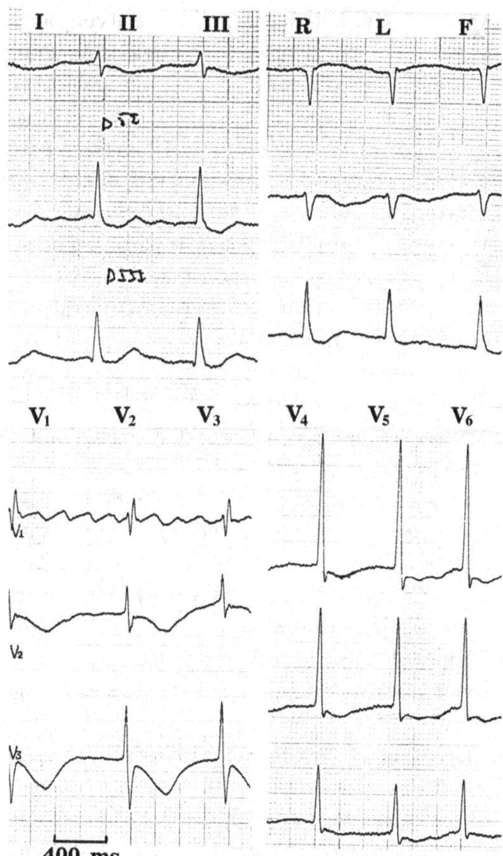

Figure 56.1 The electrocardiogram at admission.

Comment

Torsade de pointes (TdP) is a distinctive form of polymorphic ventricular tachycardia characterized by QRS complexes (*pointes*) of changing amplitude and contour that appear to rotate around the isoelectric line. TdP is usually a self-terminating form of arrhythmia, but it can occasionally degenerate into ventricular fibrillation, leading to sudden cardiac death. Frequently, TdP produces acute hemodynamic deterioration and syncope.

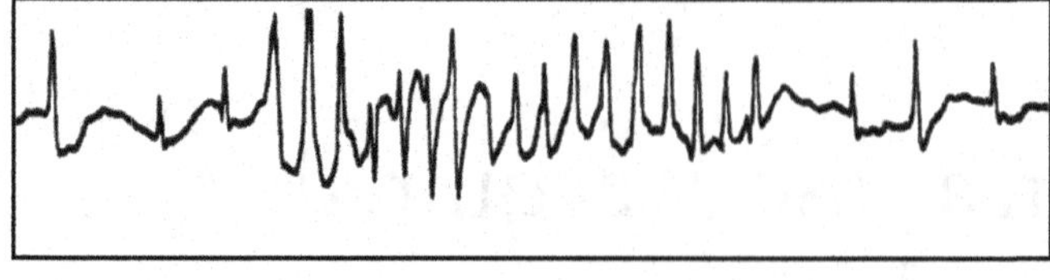

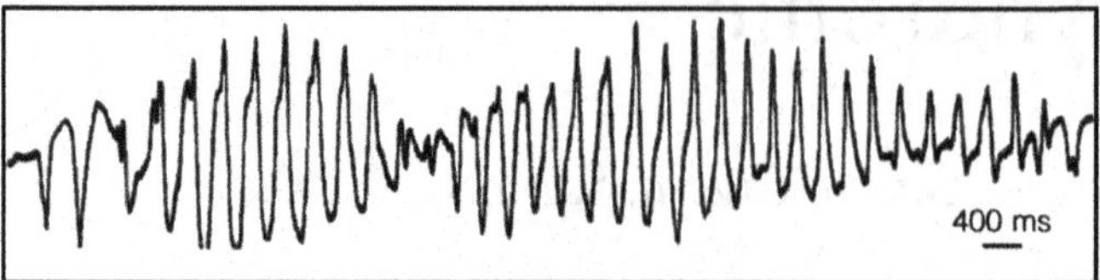

Figure 56.2 The electrocardiography tracing during a syncopal attack.

Torsade de pointes characteristically occurs in the setting of a prolonged QT interval [1]. The QT interval prolongation may be due to any of several congenital disorders (congenital long QT syndromes), or may be an acquired disorder due to drug toxicity and several other clinical conditions [1]. A large number of drugs are capable of prolonging the QT interval [1–3]. Severe bradycardia (due to sinus node dysfunction or atrioventricular block) and electrolyte abnormalities, including hypokalemia, hypomagnesemia, and hypocalcemia, may also prolong repolarization [4–6]. Other causes of QT interval prolongation include liquid protein diets [7], subarachnoid hemorrhage [8], and stroke.

In the present case, hypokalemia and treatment with amiodarone could have had a synergistic effect in prolonging the QT interval and precipitating the arrhythmia.

Various electrophysiological mechanisms have been proposed as the cause of the TdP associated with the acquired long QT syndrome, including dispersion of refractoriness and triggered activity due to early afterdepolarizations (EADs). Drugs that prolong the QT interval and cause TdP usually block cardiac K^+ channels and selectively block the rapidly activating delayed rectifier channel I_{Kr} [2].

Treatment of drug-induced TdP starts with the identification and immediate withdrawal of any potential offending drug and with the correction of any known risk factors. The goal of therapy is to shorten the QT interval, to reduce QT dispersion, and to suppress EADs. This can be achieved by increasing the heart rate (cardiac pacing, isoproterenol, atropine) and by intravenous administration of magnesium sulfate [9].

References

1 Roden DM, Lazzara R, Rosen M, Schwartz PJ, Towbin J, Vincent GM. Multiple mechanisms in the long QT syndrome. Current knowledge, gaps and future directions. *Circulation* 1996; **94**: 1996–2012.

2 Tamargo J. Drug-induced *torsade de pointes:* from molecular biology to bedside. *Jpn J Pharmacol* 2000; **83**: 1–19.

3 Haverkamp W, Breithardt G, Camm AJ, *et al.* The potential for QT prolongation and proarrhythmia by non-antiarrhythmic drugs: clinical and regulatory implications. Report on a policy conference of the European Society of Cardiology. *Eur Heart J* 2000: **21**: 1216–31.

4 Bens JL, Quiret JC, Lesbre JP. [Spike torsades with syncopal expression caused by hypokalemia; in French.] *Coeur Med Interne* 1972; **11**: 293–307.

5 Giustiniani S, Cuna FRD, Sardeo C, *et al. Torsade de pointes* induced by hypocalcemia. *G Ital Cardiol* 1982; **12**: 889–91.

6 Ramee SR, White CJ, Svinarich JT, *et al. Torsade de pointes* and magnesium deficiency. *Am Heart J* 1985; **109**: 164–8.

7 Singh BN, Gardner TD, Kanegae T, *et al.* Liquid protein diets and *torsade de pointes. J Am Med Assoc* 1978; **240**: 115–8.

8 Andreoli A, di Pascuale G, Pinelli G, *et al.* Subarachnoid hemorrhage: frequency and severity of cardiac arrhythmias. *Stroke* 1987; **18**: 558–61.

9 Tzivoni D, Banaii S, Schuger C, *et al.* Treatment of *torsade de pointes* with magnesium sulfate. *Circulation* 1988; **77**: 392–7.

CASE 57

Syncope due to *torsade de pointes* in an HIV-infected patient receiving methadone treatment

I. Anguera, M. Gil, M. Sala, O. Chapinal, M. Cervantes, J.R. Gumà, F. Segura, A. Martínez Rubio

Case report

A 36-year-old man who was a parenteral drug abuser receiving methadone replacement therapy, and who had stage C2 human immunodeficiency virus (HIV) infection, was hospitalized after three syncopal episodes. In the emergency room, a polymorphic ventricular tachycardia of the *torsade de pointes* (TdP) type was recorded. Two years previously, after a modification of the antiretroviral treatment, the patient had developed an abstinence syndrome to opiates, which led to an increase in the dosage of methadone from 65 mg/day to 275 mg/day. The electrocardiogram (ECG) showed sinus bradycardia at 40 beats/min, intermittent ventricular bigeminy, and QT prolongation up to 0.60 s (Fig. 57.1). Mild hypocalcemia (ionic calcium 4.3 mg/dL) and hypomagnesemia (1.4 mg/dL) were detected. Despite correction of the ionic values and perfusion with isoproterenol, a new episode of TdP occurred (Fig. 57.2), requiring electric cardioversion with 200 J.

A temporary pacemaker was implanted, after which the patient became asymptomatic. The echocardiogram showed a slightly dilated left ventricle, with contractile function in the lower limit of the normal range. After correction of the ionic disorders, the QTc was

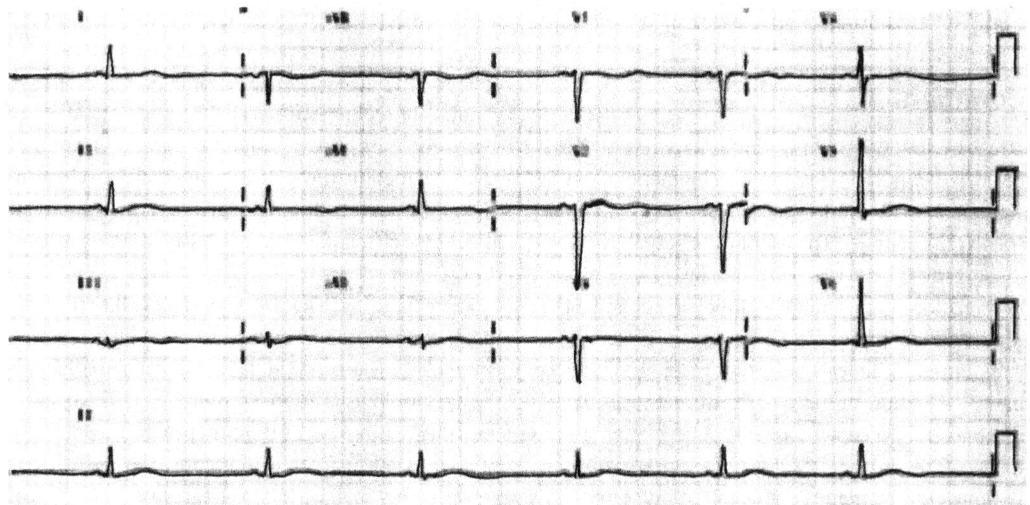

Figure 57.1 The electrocardiogram at admission.

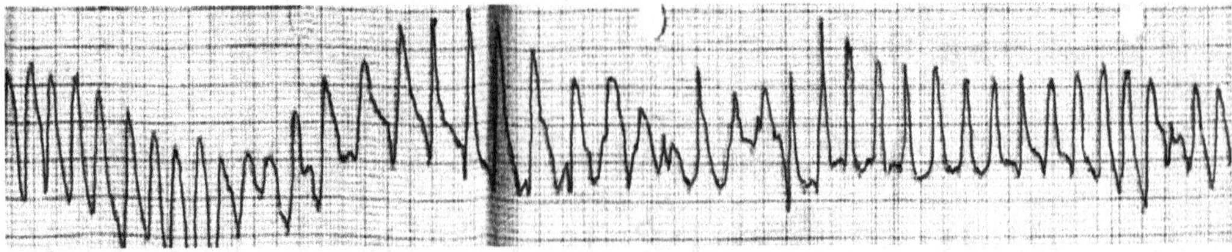

Figure 57.2 *Torsade de pointes.*

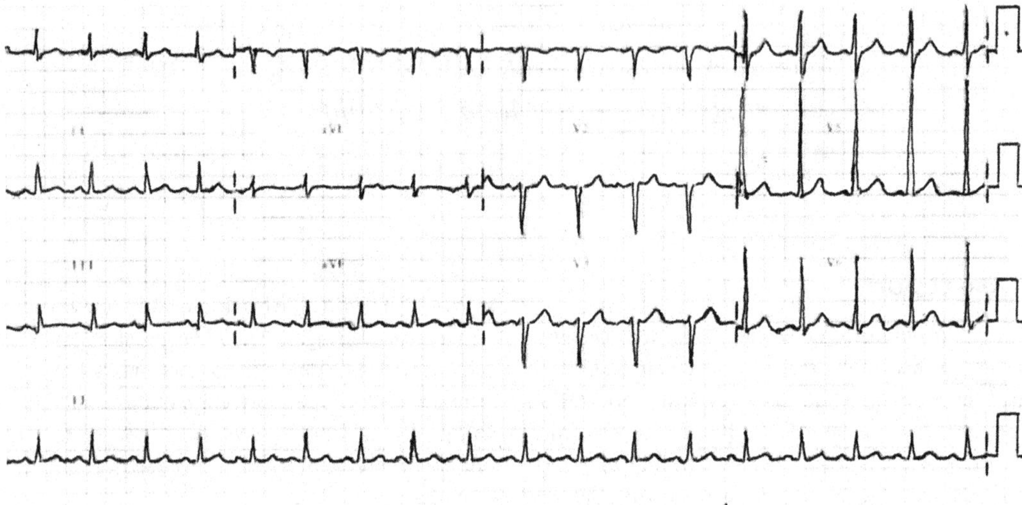

Figure 57.3 The electrocardiogram after a reduction in the methadone dosage.

0.53 s. After the dosage of methadone was reduced to 160 mg/day, the QTc shortened to normal values (Fig. 57.3). The patient was discharged and has remained asymptomatic during a 2-year follow-up period.

Comment

Drug-induced QT prolongation is a well-known predisposing condition for the development of severe ventricular arrhythmias (*torsade de pointes* and ventricular fibrillation). The list of drugs capable of prolonging the QT interval is continually being reviewed and includes both antiarrhythmic agents and other drugs with no cardiovascular action [1].

The present clinical case is that of an HIV-infected patient receiving antiretroviral treatment who developed several syncopal episodes while receiving high doses of methadone (> 200 mg/day). A significant prolongation of the QTc interval was detected, and several episodes of TdP were recorded.

High methadone doses have been found to affect heart function in experimental studies in guinea-pig heart-cell preparations [2]. Methadone dose-dependently potentiates the inotropic cardiac response to sympathetic nerve stimulation. Methadone also enhances the dose-inotropic response curve of exogenous norepinephrine. High concentrations of methadone are able to affect several parameters of cardiac function through a nonspecific mechanism different from the stimulation of opiate receptors, and all of these effects could account for a prolongation of the QT interval.

There is little evidence concerning the effect of methadone on the human heart. In a study of parenteral heroin abusers [3], ECG abnormalities including QT prolongation and prominent U waves were documented in 66% of the patients, and one case of sudden death occurred. Recently, an association between very high doses of methadone and a risk of TdP has been reported in a group of 17 patients from a methadone maintenance treatment program for opioid addiction and from a chronic pain clinic [4].

While a higher prevalence of acquired long QT has been described in HIV-infected patients [5], probably related to viral cardiomyopathies or autonomous neuropathy [6], QT prolongation in these patients is also frequently associated with drugs used in the treatment of opportunistic or other types of infection [1]. No association between a long QT and antiretroviral drugs has yet been described. In HIV-infected patients, electrolyte disorders caused or enhanced by the use of some of the drugs mentioned may prolong the QT interval. Although the present patient also had a number of nonpharmacological factors that might have prolonged the QT interval, it is interesting that shortening of the QT interval occurred when methadone doses were reduced.

In conclusion, there is experimental evidence supporting the possibility that methadone prolongs the QT interval through a dose-dependent mechanism. High-dose methadone may be responsible for prolongation of the QT interval in humans, with the subsequent arrhythmogenic risk probably boosted by electrolyte disorders, probable silent heart involvement due to HIV infection, and an association with other potentially arrhythmogenic drugs. The sequence of events in this case suggests that methadone caused QT prolongation and provided the substrate for TdP and syncope.

References

1 De Ponti F, Poluzzi E. Organising evidence of QT prolongation and occurrence of *torsades de pointes* with non-antiarrhythmic drugs: a call for consensus. *Eur J Clin Pharmacol* 2001; **57**: 185–209.

2 Mantelli L, Corti V, Bini R, Cerbai E, Ledda F. Effect of dl-methadone on the response to physiological transmitters and on several functional parameters of the isolated guinea-pig heart. *Arch Int Pharmacodyn Ther* 1986; **282**: 298–313.

3 Lipski J, Stimmel B, Donoso E. The effect of heroin and multiple drug abuse on the electrocardiogram. *Am Heart J* 1973; **86**: 663–8.

4 Krantz MJ, Lewkowiez L, Hays H, Woodroffe MA, Robertson AD, Mehler P. *Torsade de pointes* associated with very-high-dose methadone. *Ann Intern Med* 2002; **137**: 501–4.

5 Kocheril AG, Bokhari SA, Batsford WP, Sinisas AJ. Long QTc and *torsades de pointes* in human immunodeficiency virus disease. *Pacing Clin Electrophysiol* 1997; **20**: 2810–6.

6 Villa A, Foresti V, Confalonieri F. Autonomic neuropathy and prolongation of QT interval in human immunodeficiency virus infection. *Clin Auton Res* 1995; **5**: 48–52.

CASE 58

Congenital long QT syndrome

A. Solano, P. Donateo, M. Brignole, D. Oddone, F. Croci

Case report

A 31-year-old woman had six episodes of syncope preceded by palpitations over a 6-month period, three of them during the week before she was hospitalized in 1998. One of the syncope episodes had occurred during the night, just after the phone rang, awakening the patient suddenly; all of the other episodes had occurred after she had experienced strong emotions.

The electrocardiogram (ECG) in the emergency room showed a long QT interval (0.64 s) and some sequences of polymorphic ventricular tachycardia (Fig. 58.1). The clinical, radiographic, and echocardiographic examinations were normal. The blood count and electrolyte measurements were also within normal limits, with the exception of a slightly low potassium level (3.2 MEq/L). Her hypopotassemia was related to a chronic idiopathic diarrhea syndrome. The patient was initially treated with an intravenous potassium infusion, which led to rapid normalization of the blood potassium levels, but the QT prolongation continued unchanged.

A diagnosis of congenital long QT syndrome was made, and treatment with nadolol 80 mg b.i.d. was started. The diagnosis was confirmed by genetic analysis, which showed a mutation in the *KCNH2* gene (locus 7q35–q36). After 1 month, the patient underwent a left cardiac sympathetic denervation and implantation of an AAI pacemaker to correct the symptomatic bradycardia caused by beta-blocker therapy. As a collateral effect of surgical denervation, she developed persistent miosis and alterations of hemisomatic sensibility, which caused severe psychological complaints. In addition, the patient refused to accept the pacemaker psychologically and pretended to remove it 1 year later.

Afterwards, she had no symptoms until 2002, when she reported three episodes of unwitnessed loss of consciousness, all of which occurred during the night just after she was suddenly awoken by the phone ringing or by an unexpected noise. She declined further investigations. She died suddenly in March 2003.

Comment

This is a case of syncope, probably due to episodes of undocumented ventricular tachycardia or fibrillation, in a patient affected by congenital Romano–Ward syndrome (long QT syndrome). The long QT syndrome is a genetically transmitted disease. Mutations in the potassium-channel genes *KCNQ1* (locus 11p15.5) and *KCNH2* (locus 7q35–q36) and in the sodium-channel gene *SCN5A* (locus 3p21) are the most common

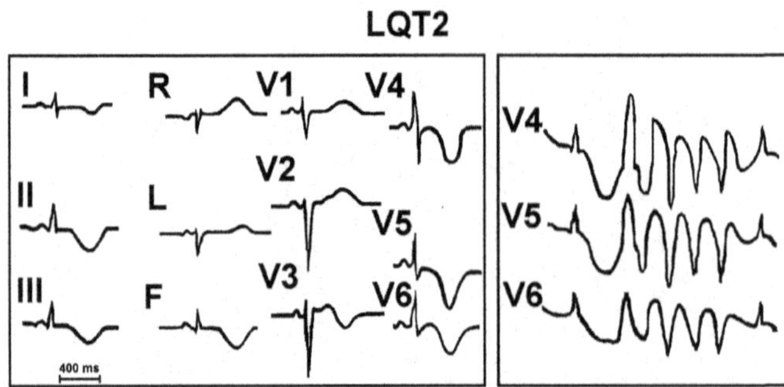

Figure 58.1 The electrocardiogram at admission.

causes of the syndrome. Ventricular repolarization is prolonged, predisposing carriers to develop life-threatening arrhythmias [1]. The initial manifestation of the condition may occur relatively late in life, and the cardiac events can be separated by long periods without symptoms [2]. Syncope is associated with a sudden increase in sympathetic activity, such as unexpected emotions or physical activity. In some patients, the trigger can be sudden wakening. Syncope is also possible at rest, especially in patients with mutations in the *KCNH2* and *SCN5A* genes [1]. Untreated patients have a 13% incidence of cardiac arrest or sudden death [2]. Patients with *KCNQ1* (locus 11p15.5) mutations have a lesser risk than those with the other two forms. Women with *KCNH2* (locus 7q35–q36) mutations and men with *SCN5A* (locus 3p21) mutations are more likely to develop symptoms before treatment and before the age of 40 [3]. The QT interval is affected by the gene mutation and strongly correlates with the probability of cardiac events [4].

Treatment is warranted: firstly, in *KCNQ1* (locus 11p15.5) patients with a QTc ≥ 500 ms; secondly, in all women with *KCNH2* (locus 7q35–q36) mutations, irrespective of QTc duration, and men with these mutations with a QTc ≥ 500 ms; and thirdly, in all patients with *SCN5A* (locus 3p21) mutations [2,5]. Treatment for primary prevention is based on lifestyle measures, including avoidance of strenuous physical exercise and of QT-prolonging agents and beta-blocker therapy. Placement of an implantable cardioverter-defibrillator (ICD) (plus full-dose beta-blocking therapy) is mandatory for secondary prevention [6].

In the era of the ICD, left cardiac sympathetic denervation is no longer indicated, with very few exceptions [7].

References

1 Schwartz PJ, Priori SG, Napolitano C. The long QT syndrome. In: Zipes DP, Jalife J, eds. *Cardiac Electrophysiology: from Cell to Bedside*, 3rd ed. Saunders, Philadelphia, 2000: 597–615.

2 Priori SG, Schwartz PJ, Napolitano C, *et al.* Risk stratification in the long QT syndrome. *N Engl J Med* 2003; **348**: 1866–74.

3 Locati EH, Zareba W, Moss AJ, *et al.* Age and sex-related differences in clinical manifestations in patients with congenital long QT syndrome: findings from the international LQTS registry. *Circulation* 1998; **97**: 2237–44.

4 Priori SG, Schwartz PJ, Napolitano C. Low penetrance in the long QT syndrome: clinical impact. *Circulation* 1999; **99**: 529–33.

5 Moss AJ, Schwartz PJ, Crampton RS, *et al.* The long QT syndrome: prospective longitudinal study of 328 families. *Circulation* 1991; **84**: 1136–44.

6 Priori SG, Aliot E, Blomstrom-Lundqvist C, *et al.* Task Force on Sudden Cardiac Death, European Society of Cardiology. *Europace* 2002; **4**: 3–18.

7 Priori SG, Aliot E, Blomstrom-Lundqvist C, *et al.* Task Force on Sudden Cardiac Death of the European Society of Cardiology. *Eur Heart J* 2001; **22**: 1374–450.

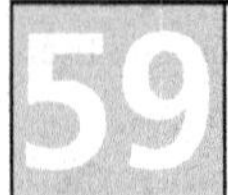

CASE 59

Long QT syndrome revealed by exercise

A.A.M. Wilde, T.A. Simmers

Case report

A 14-year-old boy died suddenly while playing soccer. He was in the middle of a sprint when he suddenly collapsed. Resuscitation efforts were unsuccessful. His family stated that he had had no previous symptoms and that the family history was unremarkable. However, his brother, who was 2 years older, remembered that he had also collapsed once while playing an exciting soccer match. This had occurred when he was 10, after which he had experienced no further events. His brother's death worried him (and his family) and he visited a cardiologist for medical advice.

The physical examination was unremarkable; the electrocardiogram (ECG) is shown in Fig. 59.1. The ECG shows a sinus rhythm (70 beats/min) with a normal QRS axis. The PQ interval and QRS width are normal. Repolarization is completely normal, and the QTc interval is 384 ms, well within normal limits. The ECG is therefore completely normal. An echocardiogram was also normal.

From the patient's history and from his family

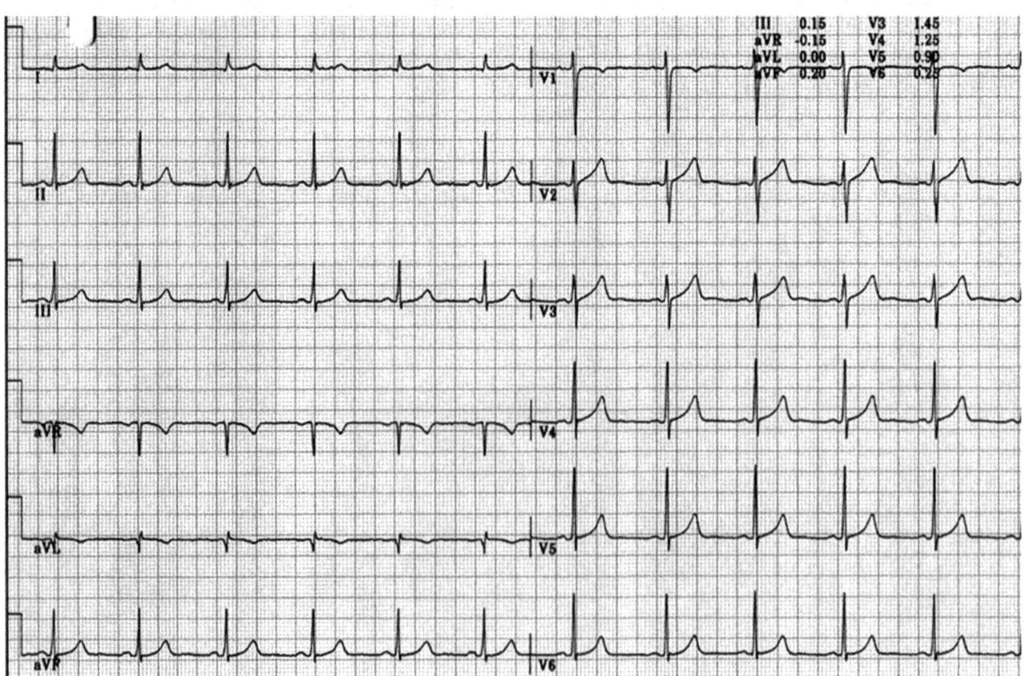

Figure 59.1 The baseline electrocardiogram.

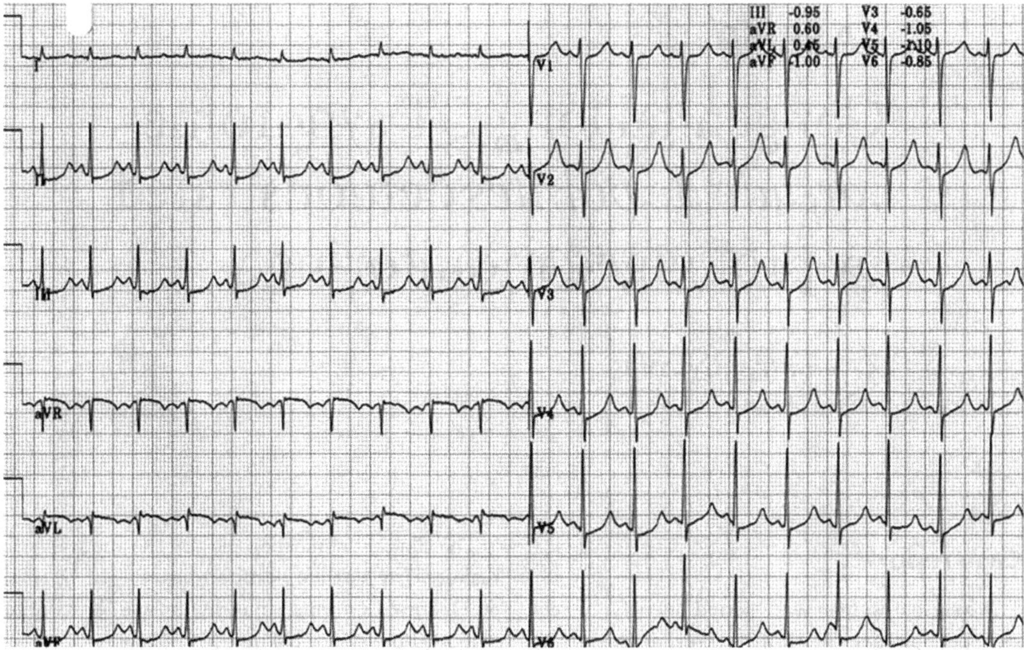

Figure 59.2 The electrocardiogram during the effort test.

history, it became clear that both events (his collapse and the circumstances of his brother's death) were triggered by exercise. An exercise test was therefore included in the cardiological work-up.

Figure 59.2 shows the ECG after 6 min of exercise. There is still a sinus rhythm, 130 beats/min, and the conduction intervals remain normal. The QT interval is now markedly prolonged, approaching 530 ms (QTc 527 ms). This response should raise a suspicion of a type 1 long QT syndrome, and in conjunction with the symptoms, beta-blockade therapy is warranted. Molecular-genetic screening did in fact reveal a mutation in the *KCNQ1* gene.

Comment

The congenital long QT syndrome (LQTS) is a genetically transmitted disease. Mutations causing LQTS have been identified in five genes, each encoding a cardiac ion channel and its regulatory subunit. LQT1 is caused by mutations in the *KCNQ1* gene, encoding one of the main repolarizing potassium currents [1].

Type 1 LQTS is characterized by QT prolongation, particularly during exercise. The QT interval fails to adapt to an increase in rate and therefore becomes inappropriately prolonged. In conjunction with this, events (dizziness, syncope, and sudden death) are typically triggered by adrenergic stimuli, including exercise. Other typical triggers are diving and swimming; the age of onset of symptoms is usually around 5 years. A careful family history should be taken. The treatment of choice is a beta-blocker, titrated in symptomatic patients up to the highest possible tolerated dose. Asymptomatic young patients should receive prophylactic treatment, but asymptomatic individuals over the age of 20 with a QTc interval < 500 ms appear to be at low risk. Molecular-genetic screening is mandatory [2].

Acknowledgment

This case was previously published in Netherlands Heart Journal. We are grateful to Bohn Stafleu van Loghum for granting permission to reprint.

References

1 Schwartz PJ, Priori SG, Napolitano C. The long QT syndrome. In: Zipes DP, Jalife J, eds. *Cardiac Electrophysiology: from Cell to Bedside*, 3rd ed. Saunders, Philadelphia, 2000: 597–615.

2 Priori SG, Aliot E, Blomstrom-Lundqvist C, *et al.* Task Force on Sudden Cardiac Death of the European Society of Cardiology. *Eur Heart J* 2001; **22:** 1374–450.

3 Wilde AAM, Simmers TA. 'Just one collaps during soccer'. *Neth Heart J* 2004; **12:** 355–357.

CASE 60

Congenital long QT syndrome: *torsade de pointes* demonstrated by prolonged monitoring

X. Sabaté, J. Nicolás

Case report

A 28-year-old woman was referred due to recurrent syncopal episodes. She had no previous history of other diseases, and she stated that her mother had also had recurrent syncopal episodes. Her syncopal episodes usually occurred in the morning and were usually related to emotional stress. There were no clear prodromal signs before the syncope, and she never had seizures or sphincter incontinence. She reported a total of two to four syncopal episodes per year, but in the previous year they had increased in frequency, with seven episodes.

The clinical examination did not show any abnormalities. The baseline electrocardiogram (ECG) (Fig. 60.1) showed a normal sinus rhythm at 67 beats/min, with a QT interval of 470 ms (QTc 480 ms).

A head-up tilt test was performed, which was positive after sublingual nitroglycerin administration, with a mixed response. The patient recognized her response to the tilt test as similar to the spontaneous symptoms.

Treatment with oral bisoprolol at 5 mg daily was initiated. After the start of bisoprolol treatment, she had a few syncopal episodes, but they became less frequent.

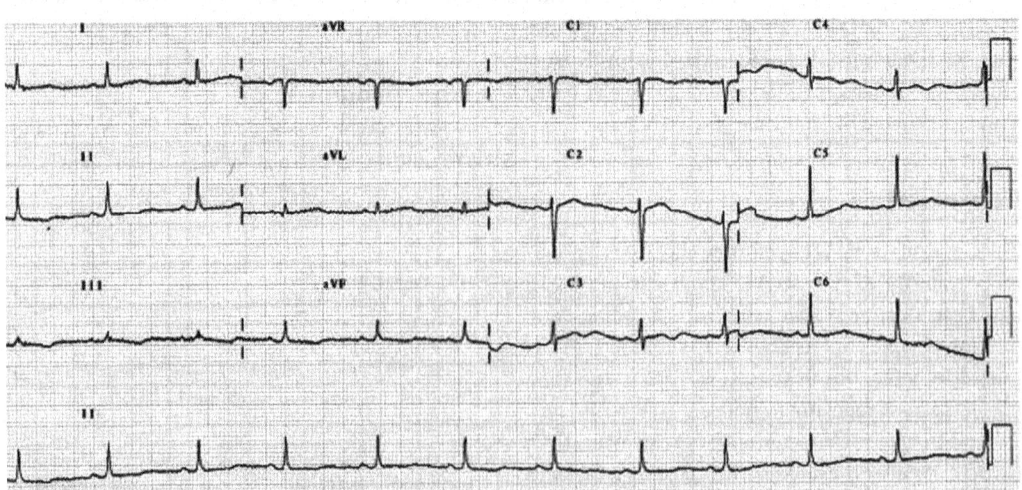

Figure 60.1 The baseline electrocardiogram. There is a normal sinus rhythm at 65 beats/min, with a normal PR interval and QRS configuration, and with a QT interval of 470 ms.

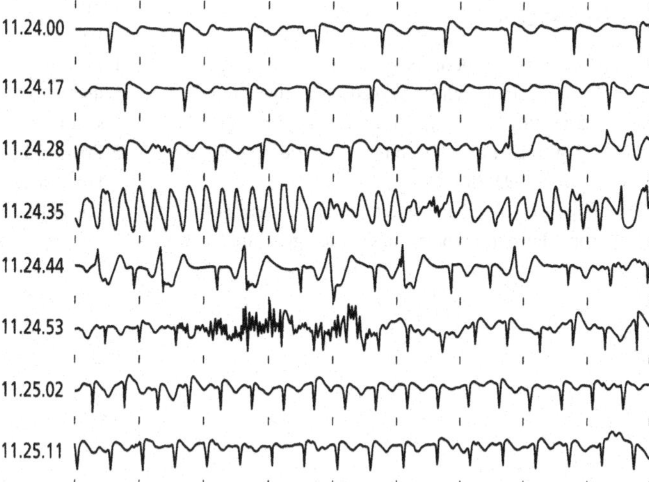

Figure 60.2 At the beginning of the tracing, the patient is in sinus rhythm at 60 beats/min. There is a premature ventricular beat, followed by a sinus beat and a second premature ventricular beat, in a short–long–short sequence, that initiates a nonsustained polymorphic ventricular tachycardia. The patient activated the device 27 s after the arrhythmia.

At a follow-up examination, she reported that her mother had died suddenly. After this, an implantable loop recorder was placed. Five months after implantation, she developed presyncope, similar to previous episodes, and activated the device. The tracing showed self-limited polymorphic ventricular tachycardia (Fig. 60.2). After this observation, an implantable cardioverter-defibrillator was implanted.

Comment

This case illustrates the difficulties of ascertaining the etiology of syncope in some patients, as the patient had a few data suggesting various mechanisms of syncope, but the data did not initially meet the criteria sufficiently to be considered diagnostic. The patient had had syncope since she was a teenager, and syncopal episodes had recurred over a long period—a finding that is characteristic of reflex syncope [1].

The baseline ECG showed a slightly prolonged QT interval [2], strongly suggesting congenital long QT syndrome but not permitting a definitive diagnosis in the absence of other data [3]. In addition, the syncopal episodes in this patient were triggered by emotional stress—a symptom that can be present in both reflex syncope [1,3] and also syncope due to a congenital long QT interval.

This case also illustrates the difficulty of interpreting the results of the tilt test. The tilt test was positive in this patient, and she reported that the symptoms during tilt-induced syncope were similar to those of her spontaneous syncope. According to the guidelines, a tilt test must be considered diagnostic when there is a positive response in the absence of structural heart disease and with a normal ECG or, in the presence of structural heart disease or an abnormal ECG, when cardiac causes of syncope have been excluded [3]. In this patient, an arrhythmic cause of syncope was not excluded before the presyncopal episode documented with the implantable loop recorder. Due to the ECG finding of a prolonged QT interval, the possibility of a congenital long QT interval was considered and beta-blocker therapy was consequently initiated, as this is recommended as the first-line treatment in such patients [4].

Although data on the predictive value of a family history of sudden cardiac death are not conclusive, there are a few data suggesting that, within selected families, a previous occurrence of sudden cardiac death can have a strong positive predictive value and increases the risk [5]. When this patient was seen initially, she stated that there was no family history of sudden death, but her mother died suddenly during the follow-up period. This established an indication for placement of an implantable loop recorder in order to rule out an arrhythmic origin of her syncopal episodes. The data obtained from the loop recorder showed that the cause of her syncopal episodes was a nonsustained polymorphic ventricular tachycardia, characteristic of *torsade de pointes*.

As the patient had polymorphic ventricular tachycardia despite beta-blocker treatment, an implantable cardioverter-defibrillator was placed and treatment with beta-blockers continued [5].

References

1 Wieling W, Ganzeboom KS, Saul JP. Reflex syncope in children and adolescents. *Heart* 2004; **90**: 1094–100.

2 Schwartz PJ, Moss AJ, Vincent GM, Crampton RS. Diagnostic criteria for the long QT syndrome: an update. *Circulation* 1993; **88**: 782–4.

3 Brignole M, Alboni P, Benditt D, *et al.* Task Force on Syncope, European Society of Cardiology. Guidelines on management (diagnosis and treatment) of syncope. Task Force Report. *Eur Heart J* 2001; **22**: 1256–1306.

4 Moss AJ, Zareba W, Hall WJ, *et al.* Effectiveness and limitations of beta-blocker therapy in congenital long-QT syndrome. *Circulation* 2000; **101**: 616–23.

5 Priori SG, Aliot E, Blomstrom-Lundqvist C, *et al.* Task Force on Sudden Cardiac Death of the European Society of Cardiology. *Eur Heart J* 2001; **22**: 1374–450.

CASE 61

Short-coupled variant of *torsade de pointes*

R. García Civera, R. Ruiz Granell, S. Morell Cabedo, R. Sanjuán Mañez

Case report

A 37-year-old woman was referred to the hospital due to suspected arrhythmic syncope. A few days previously, she had suffered three consecutive syncopal episodes without warning. She had been admitted to another hospital, where polymorphic ventricular tachycardias were detected on Holter monitoring, and was treated with beta-blockers and referred to our hospital's arrhythmia unit. She had no previous diseases and no family history of heart disease or sudden death. The physical examination and echocardiogram were normal. The baseline electrocardiogram (ECG) (Fig. 61.1) showed a normal sinus rhythm at 53 beats/min, a PR interval of 0.16 s, a normal QRS, and a QT interval of 0.44 s (a corrected QT interval of 0.42 s).

A 24-h Holter recording showed the presence of multiple sequences of polymorphic ventricular tachycardia of the *torsade de pointes* type (Fig. 61.2). These short runs of tachycardia (3–15 beats) were more prevalent during the daytime and were not perceived by the patient. At the beginning of the episodes, a very short coupling interval between the last sinus beat and the first beat of the tachycardia was noted (coupling intervals between 0.26 and 0.30 s).

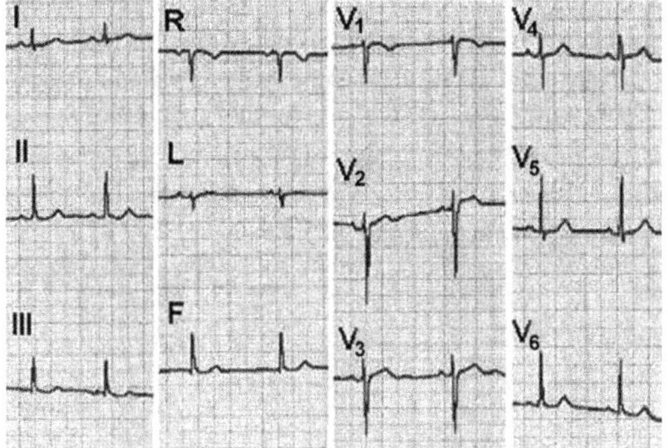

Figure 61.1 The baseline electrocardiogram.

Cardiac catheterization and magnetic resonance imaging did not disclose any cardiac anomalies, and the laboratory values (Na^+, K^+, Ca^{2+}, Mg^{3+}, catecholamines, and thyroid hormones) were in the normal range. An electrophysiological study was also normal.

An idiopathic short coupling interval *torsade de pointes* syndrome was diagnosed. Because of concern regarding the prognosis of this case, it was decided in agreement with the patient and her family to implant a defibrillator and to continue with beta-blocker treatment. No new syncopal episodes or activations of the implantable cardioverter-defibrillator occurred during a follow-up period of 7 years. Short runs of *torsade de pointes* continued to appear in successive Holter recordings.

Comment

Torsade de pointes (TdP) is a distinctive type of polymorphic ventricular tachycardia that characteristically occurs in the setting of a prolonged QT interval [1]. The presence of persistent runs of TdP in a patient with no structural heart disease, no detectable metabolic abnormalities, and a normal QT interval on the ECG is exceptional.

In 1994, Leenhardt *et al.* [2] described a new electrocardiographic entity in the spectrum of idiopathic

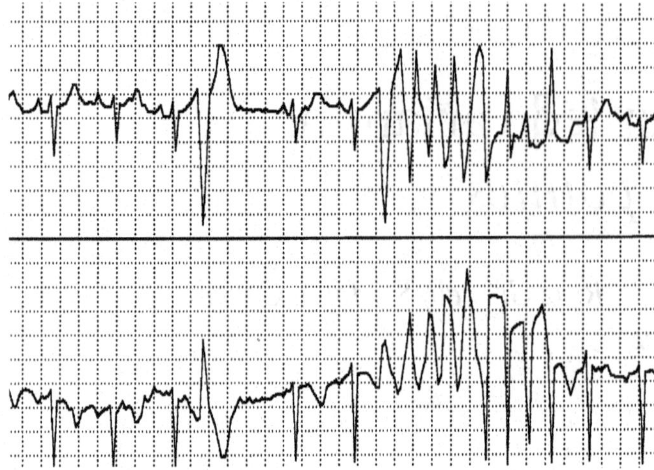

Figure 61.2 *Torsade de pointes*, with a short-coupled interval, on Holter monitoring.

ventricular tachycardias. The report included 14 patients with no structural heart disease who presented with syncope related to tachycardia with the typical ECG pattern of TdP. However, there was no evidence of a long QT syndrome, and TdP had the unusual characteristic of an extremely short coupling interval in the first beat of the tachycardia or of isolated premature beats. In 10 cases in this initial report, ventricular tachycardia degenerated into ventricular fibrillation. After a mean follow-up period of 7 years, there had been five deaths (four sudden) and nine patients were still alive (three with defibrillators and six with verapamil treatment).

The short coupling variant of TdP appears to be a very rare entity; only isolated cases have been published since the initial description [3–6]. The present case matches the characteristics of Leenhardt's description—a normal QT, *torsade de pointes* ventricular tachycardia, and a very short coupling interval in the initial beats of the tachycardia. Interestingly, the patient has been asymptomatic since the beginning of treatment with beta-blockers, although short TdP sequences continue to appear in successive Holter recordings.

Shiga *et al.* have suggested two possible mechanisms for this type of tachycardia: triggered activity due to late afterdepolarizations, or reentry due to a short and heterogeneous QT interval [4].

References

1 Roden DM, Lazzara R, Rosen M, Schwartz PJ, Towbin J, Vincent GM. Multiple mechanisms in the long QT syndrome: current knowledge, gaps and future directions. *Circulation* 1996; **94**: 1996–2012.

2 Leenhardt A, Glaser E, Burguera M, Nurnberg M, Maison-Blanche P, Coumel P. Short-coupled variant of *torsade de pointes:* a new electrocardiographic entity in the spectrum of idiopathic ventricular tachyarrhythmias. *Circulation* 1994; **89**: 206–15.

3 Cheng TO. Short-coupled variant of *torsade de pointes* with normal QT interval and risk of sudden death. *Am J Cardiol* 1996; **77**: 1028–9.

4 Shiga T, Shoda M, Matsuda N, *et al.* Electrophysiological characteristics of a patient exhibiting the short-coupled variant of *torsade de pointes. J Electrocardiol* 2001; **34**: 271–5.

5 Durand-Dubief A, Burri H, Chevalier P, Toubul P. Short-coupled variant of *torsades de pointes* with intractable ventricular fibrillation: lifesaving effect of cardiopulmonary bypass. *J Cardiovasc Electrophysiol* 2003; **14**: 329.

6 Takeuchi T, Sato N, Kawamura Y, *et al.* A case of a short-coupled variant of *torsades de pointes* with electrical storm. *Pacing Clin Electrophysiol* 2003; **26**: 632–6.

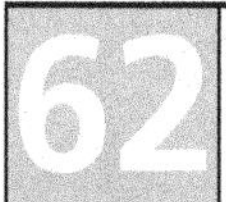

CASE 62

Syncope in a patient with a short QT interval

C. Giustetto, F. Gaita

Case report

A healthy 20-year-old man experienced a syncopal episode without any prodromal symptoms soon after jogging on the beach. He rapidly recovered consciousness and there were no sequelae.

Since the age of 18, he had had sporadic episodes of presyncope and suffered from palpitations, with documented atrial fibrillation (Fig. 62.1) and common atrial flutter. The peculiarity of the atrial flutter was a very short FF interval, of 150–170 ms, with 4 : 1 atrioventricular conduction. On the baseline electrocardiogram (ECG) (Fig. 62.2), he had sinus bradycardia with a heart rate of 52 beats/min, a PR interval of 0.10 s, a QRS duration of 0.06 s, left axis deviation, and, above all, tall and peaked T waves, particularly in the right precordial leads, with an almost absent ST interval. The QT interval was 280 ms, with a QTc of 260 ms. All of the ECGs recorded throughout his life had shown QT intervals ranging between 240 and 280 ms, with the QTc never exceeding 280 ms.

The physical examination, blood laboratory tests, echocardiogram, and stress test were all normal. The tilt test did not evoke vagal symptoms. He reported that his father had died suddenly one morning at the age of 39, while taking a cup of coffee with his wife. He had been healthy, and the autopsy ruled out any cardiac disease.

At this point, our diagnosis was syncope and atrial fibrillation of vasovagal origin in a patient with a normal heart and short QT interval on the ECG. Due to the frequent episodes of atrial fibrillation, flecainide

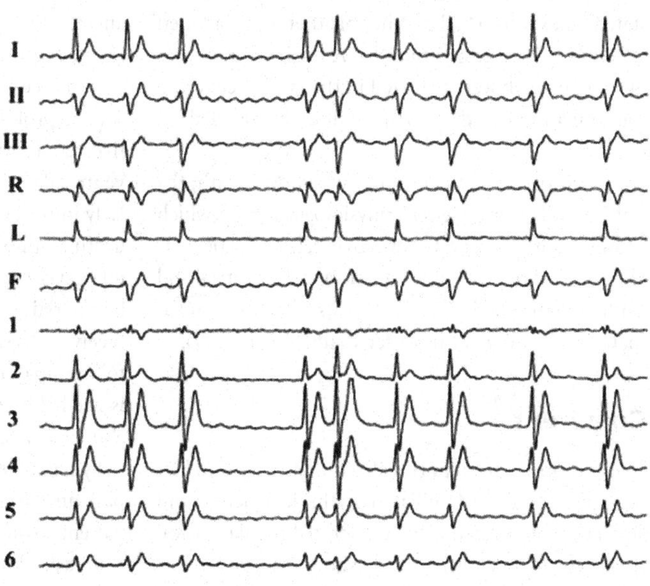

Figure 62.1 Atrial fibrillation.

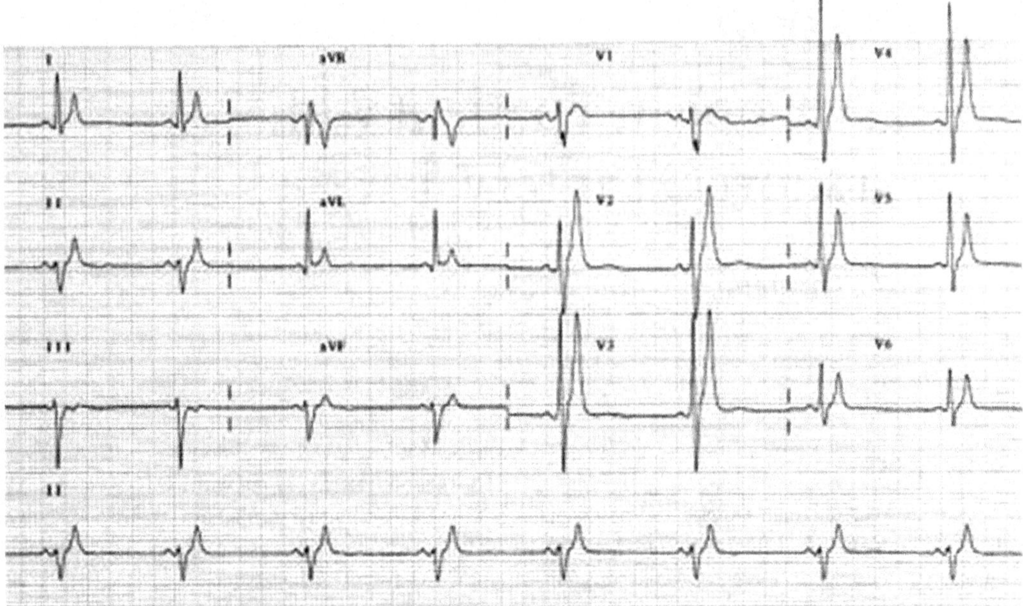

Figure 62.2 Electrocardiogram in sinus rhythm.

treatment was started, and an annual follow-up examination was suggested. The patient did well and was later lost to follow-up.

Fifteen years later, he came to medical attention again as he had a sister with similar symptoms of dizziness and palpitations, whose ECG also showed a short QT interval, of 220 ms (QTc 280 ms). She had a 6-year-old son who had had a cardiac arrest at the age of 8 months, with severe neurological sequelae. She stated that she also had another brother who had died suddenly at the age of 3 months. A further three cases of sudden death were reported in the family, covering four generations and occurring in individuals aged 39, 49, and 62.

In view of the familial history of sudden death, the siblings underwent an electrophysiological study, which showed short atrial and ventricular refractory periods and easy and reproducible induction of both atrial and ventricular fibrillation. Both patients received an automatic implantable cardioverter-defibrillator (ICD).

Comment

The authors of this report realized that they were facing a new cause of familial arrhythmic syncope and sudden death, related to an accelerated repolarization time, which they termed the "short QT syndrome" [1]. This is a genetic disease, the prevalence of which has yet to be determined, caused by a mutation in *KCNH2* (*HERG*), the gene encoding for the rapidly activating delayed rectifier potassium current (I_{Kr}), causing a functional gain in this channel [2], or by a mutation in *KCNQ1* (*KvLQT1*), which causes a functional gain in I_{Ks}, the slowly activating delayed rectifier potassium current [3].

Due to the high incidence of sudden cardiac death and the absence of a known pharmacological treatment, the implantation of an ICD is at present the first-choice therapy. Quinidine, but not flecainide or sotalol, prolongs the QT interval and ventricular effective refractory period and prevents the induction of ventricular arrhythmias [4]. This finding is particularly important, as these patients are at risk of sudden death from birth, and implanting an ICD is not feasible in very young children. Quinidine therapy can also be offered to patients who refuse an ICD or to those receiving frequent shocks from the device. Long-term follow-up of patients with ICD who receive quinidine is needed in order to clarify whether the drug may be able to serve as an alternative to ICD implantation.

Syncopal episodes are present in about 30% of patients with short QT. As it is easy to identify these patients from an ECG, this is a cause of syncope that can easily be ruled out and must be considered in particular if there is a history of familial sudden death or of atrial fibrillation at a young age.

References

1 Gaita F, Giustetto C, Bianchi F, *et al.* Short QT syndrome: a familial cause of sudden death. *Circulation* 2003; **108**: 965–70.

2 Brugada R, Hong K, Dumaine R, *et al.* Sudden death associated with short QT syndrome linked to mutations in *HERG*. *Circulation* 2004; **109**: 30–5.

3 Bellocq C, van Ginneken A, Bezzina C, *et al.* Mutation in the *KCNQ1* gene leading to the short QT-interval syndrome. *Circulation* 2004; **109**: 2394–7.

4 Gaita F, Giustetto C, Bianchi F, *et al.* Short QT syndrome: pharmacological treatment. *J Am Coll Cardiol* 2004; **43**: 1494–9.

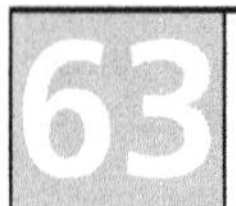

CASE 63

Syncope in a woman with no heart disease, a normal electrocardiogram, and a family history of sudden death

R. Ruiz Granell, S. Morell Cabedo, R. Sanjuán Mañez, R. García Civera

Case report

A 54-year-old woman was admitted for an electrophysiological study due to a history of recurrent syncope and presyncope during the previous 18 years, with two syncopal episodes in the last year. She reported that she did not experience palpitations or any other warning symptoms before losing consciousness. The patient had a family history of sudden death. A sister had died suddenly at the age of 26, a son of her sister at the age of 15, and two of the patient's own children at 28 months and 15 years of age, respectively. No heart disease had been detected in any of the family cases. At the age of 40, the patient was diagnosed with epilepsy on the basis of her repeated losses of consciousness. She had received anticonvulsant treatment for 2 years, without any improvement in her condition.

A month before admission, the patient had undergone a cardiological assessment at another institution. The results of this assessment [including clinical history, physical examination, a baseline electrocardiogram (ECG), carotid sinus massage, postural blood-pressure testing, 24-h ambulatory monitoring, exercise stress test, echocardiography, and cardiac magnetic resonance] were normal. A head-up tilt-table test was negative. The patient was then referred to our hospital for electrophysiological and hemodynamic studies.

The baseline 12-lead ECG at the time of the electrophysiological study (Fig. 63.1) showed a sinus rhythm at 61 beats/min, a PR interval of 160 ms, a QRS width of 100 ms, and a QT interval of 360 ms. The electrophysiological study (with the patient off medication) showed normal values for sinus and atrioventricular node function. The HV interval was 55 ms, and the programmed right atrial and ventricular stimulation (two basic cycles, two sites, and up to three extrastimuli) did not induce significant arrhythmias. No diagnostic changes in the ECG were observed after intravenous administration of procainamide 10 mg/kg (Fig. 63.2), and repeated ventricular stimulation did not induce any arrhythmia. The hemodynamic assessment showed normal ventricular (right and left) morphology and function, a left ventricular ejection fraction of 70%, and normal coronary angiography.

After this negative work-up, an insertable loop recorder (Reveal Plus, Medtronic, Inc., Minneapolis, Minnesota, USA) was implanted. Six months after implantation, the patient experienced a syncopal episode with no apparent triggers, and the family activated the device. The recorded ECG showed a long-lasting (25 s) self-limited polymorphic ventricular tachycardia that started with a ventricular ectopic beat with a very short coupling interval (Fig. 63.3). A defibrillator was implanted, and several adequate

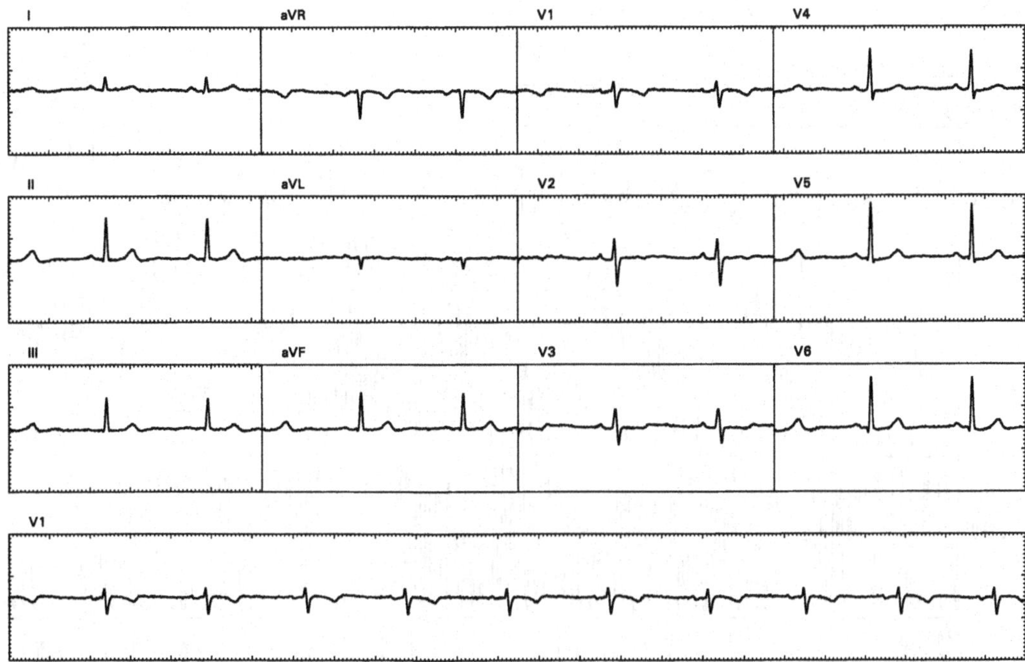

Figure 63.1 The baseline electrocardiogram.

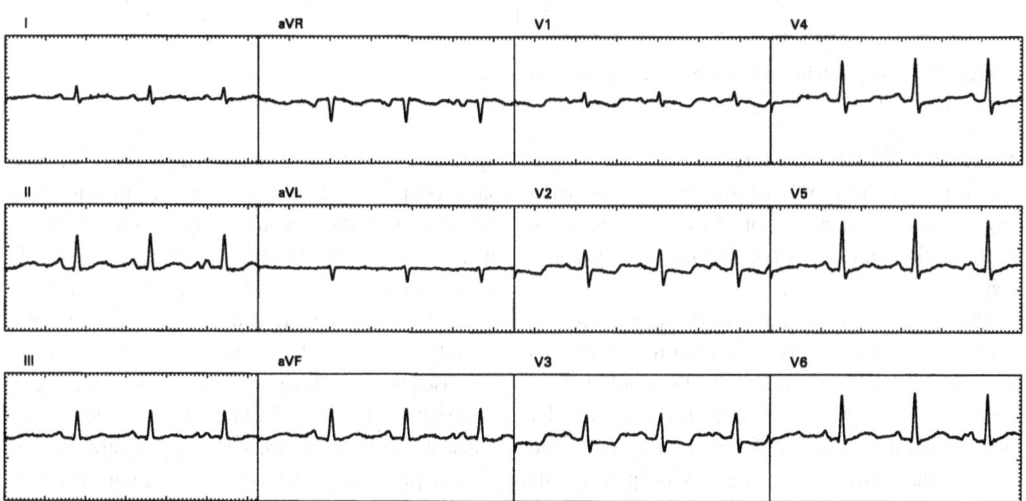

Figure 63.2 The electrocardiogram after intravenous administration of procainamide 10 mg/kg.

activations have been observed during a follow-up period of 3 years.

Comment

A family history of sudden death is an independent predictor of mortality in patients with or without structural heart disease [1,2]. When familial antecedents of sudden death are present in a patient who has suffered a syncopal episode, a complete cardiological evaluation is mandatory [3]. In the present case, the extensive investigations carried out made it quite reasonable to exclude structural heart disease. Attempts to demonstrate any known primary arrhythmogenic

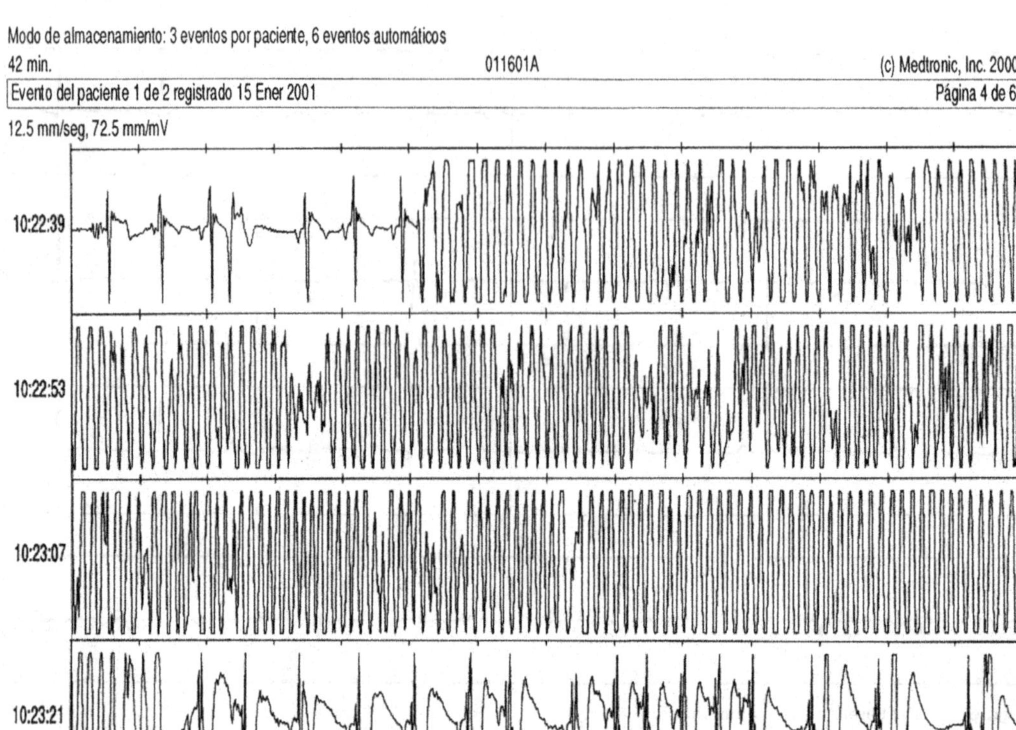

Figure 63.3 The implantable loop recorder tracing during syncope.

disease also failed. No QT interval prolongation was detected, and the procainamide test did not elicit any ECG change suggestive of Brugada syndrome. In addition, the effort stress test and the electrophysiological study were negative.

After this full but negative work-up, the authors decided to place an implantable loop recorder (ILR) and wait and see. Six months later, the result was the detection of a syncopal polymorphic ventricular tachycardia. After this, a defibrillator was implanted [4]. The diagnosis of the cause of syncope certainly appears to be evident, but another important question remains unresolved—what was the electrophysiological substrate of this form of tachycardia? Some interesting findings are derived from the ILR recording. Firstly, before the start of the tachycardia, an ST elevation was noted on the registered lead; secondly, a previous ventricular ectopic beat and the ventricular premature beat that triggered the tachycardia had a very short coupling interval; thirdly, after the end of the tachycardia, a significant T wave inversion was apparent, and new ventricular ectopic beats with very short coupling interval were present. Any interpretation of these findings is inevitably speculative. Nevertheless, three principal possible explanations can be offered: firstly, the case could represent a familial form of the *torsade de pointes* with short coupling interval condition described by Leenhardt *et al.* [5]; secondly, the case could represent an atypical form of Brugada syndrome without an ECG response to drugs that block the sodium channels [6]; and finally, the case could represent an unknown form of idiopathic polymorphic ventricular tachycardia.

References

1 Friedlander Y, Siskovick DS, Weinmann S, *et al.* Family history as a risk factor for primary cardiac arrest. *Circulation* 1988; **97**: 155–60.

2 Jouven X, Desnos M, Guerot C, Ducimetière P. Predicting sudden death in the population: the Paris prospective study. *Circulation* 1999; **99**: 1978–83.

3 Consensus Statement of the Joint Steering Committees of the Unexplained Cardiac Arrest Registry of Europe and of the Idiopathic Ventricular Fibrillation Registry of the United States. Survivors of out-of-hospital cardiac arrest with apparently normal heart: need for definition and standardized clinical evaluation. *Circulation* 1997; **95**: 265–72.

4 Brugada J, Brugada P. What to do in patients with no structural heart disease and sudden arrhythmic death? *Am J Cardiol* 1996; **78** (5A): 69–75.

5 Leenhardt A, Glaser E, Burguera M, Nurnberg M, Maison-Blanche P, Coumel P. Short-coupled variant of *torsade de pointes*: a new electrocardiographic entity in the spectrum of idiopathic ventricular tachyarrhythmias. *Circulation* 1994; **89**: 206–15.

6 Remme CA, Weber EFD, Wilde AMM, *et al.* Diagnosis and long-term follow-up of the Brugada syndrome in patients with idiopathic ventricular fibrillation. *Eur Heart J* 2001; **22**: 400–9.

CASE 64

Palpitations and syncope: an unusual case of bradycardia–tachycardia syndrome

R. García Civera, R. Sanjuán Mañez, S. Morell Cabedo

Case report

In September 1979, a 75-year-old woman was admitted to hospital due to an episode of palpitations. During a 2-year period before admission, she had had several episodes of paroxysmal palpitation, followed in some instances by syncope. The electrocardiogram (ECG) on admission (Fig. 64.1A) showed regular tachycardia at 150 beats/min, with a narrow QRS complex. Spontaneous termination of the tachycardia was followed by a junctional rhythm at 48 beats/min, QT interval prolongation (QT 0.56 s), and frequent ventricular ectopic beats. This situation led to ventricular tachycardia, which showed a QRS morphology suggesting *torsade de pointes* ventricular tachycardia (Fig. 64.1B). During the ventricular tachycardia, the patient lost consciousness and recovered after a 100-J direct-current shock. The junctional rhythm persisted, and the patient suffered two more self-limited episodes of ventricular tachycardia while a temporary electrocatheter was being inserted. Once the electrocatheter had been positioned in the right ventricular

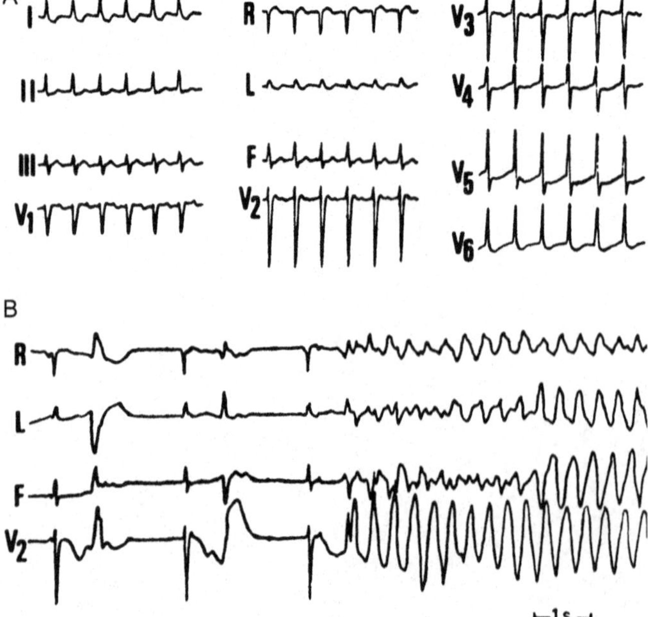

Figure 64.1 A. The electrocardiogram at admission, showing a paroxysmal supraventricular tachycardia. **B.** After spontaneous termination of the tachycardia, a junctional rhythm with QT interval prolongation and frequent ventricular ectopic beats gives place to a polymorphic ventricular tachycardia.

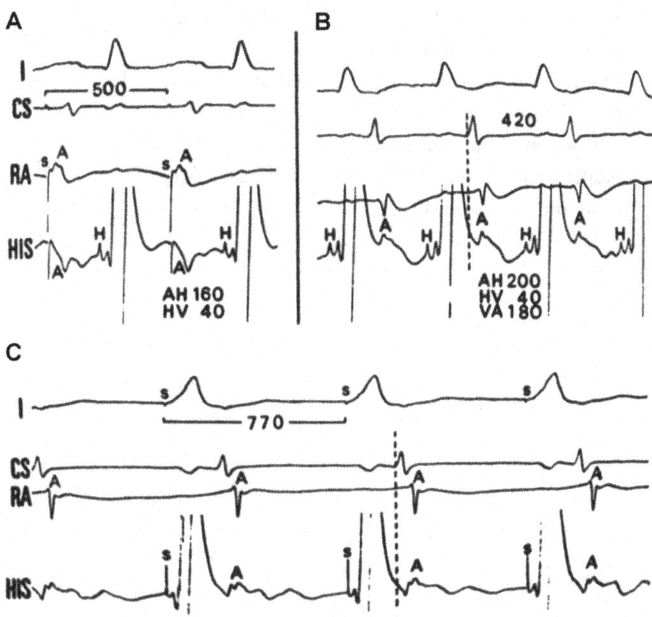

Figure 64.2 The electrophysiological study. **A.** Atrial pacing. **B.** Supraventricular tachycardia. **C.** Ventricular pacing.

apex, pacing at an initial rate of 90 beats/min prevented the recurrence of ventricular arrhythmias.

Clinical, radiographic, and echocardiographic examinations failed to detect structural heart disease. The blood count and electrolytic determinations were also within the normal limits.

An electrophysiologic study was carried out on the fourth day of hospitalization. His bundle recordings in sinus rhythm revealed an AH interval of 85 ms and an HV interval of 40 ms. No ventricular preexcitation was demonstrated with atrial pacing (Fig. 64.2A). Cessation of atrial overdrive pacing resulted in a cardiac pause of 1.9 s, which terminated with a junctional escape beat. A supraventricular tachycardia at a cycle length of 420 ms was induced by two atrial extrastimuli or one ventricular extrastimulus. During the tachycardia, atrial activation occurred after the QRS and the atrial activation sequence was eccentric, the activation of the left atrium (coronary sinus lead) preceding low septal activation (Fig. 64.2B). The retrograde activation sequence of the atria during ventricular pacing was identical to that of the tachycardia, confirming the presence of a concealed left accessory pathway (Fig. 64.2C).

In summary, the patient presented with a bradycardia –tachycardia syndrome due to sinus node dysfunction and atrioventricular reciprocating tachycardia, utilizing a concealed left accessory pathway as the retrograde arm of the circuit. In addition, the bradycardia led to QT interval prolongation and *torsade de pointes* ventricular tachycardia with syncope. Following the electrophysiological study, a permanent pacemaker was implanted, and the patient started treatment with oral amiodarone. No episodes of recurrent syncope were observed during the follow-up.

Comment

The term "alternating bradycardia–tachycardia syndrome" was introduced in 1954 by Short [1] and implies the coexistence of pathological bradycardia and tachycardia. Although there are multiple possible mechanisms for the bradycardia–tachycardia syndrome, the coexistence of sick sinus syndrome and circus movement tachycardia with retrograde utilization of a concealed accessory pathway is very unusual.

Syncope is not rare in the bradycardia–tachycardia syndrome and is generally due to ventricular pauses following the termination of the tachycardia. However, in the present case, syncope was related to a polymorphic ventricular tachycardia (*torsade de pointes* ventricular tachycardia)—a form of arrhythmia typically triggered by bradycardia and QT prolongation.

In the present case, the electrophysiological study made it possible to identify the tachycardia mechanism and was helpful in selecting the appropriate therapy. This is quite an old case, dating from 1979 [2]. Nowadays, the appropriate therapy would be transcatheter radiofrequency ablation of the accessory pathway and implantation of a DDD pacemaker.

References

1 Short DS. The syndrome of alternating bradycardia and tachycardia. *Br Heart J* 1951; **16**: 208–12.
2 Garcia Civera R, Segui Bonin J, Sanjuan Mañez R, *et al.* Bradycardia–tachycardia syndrome due to sinus node disease and concealed Wolff–Parkinson–White syndrome. *Pacing Clin Electrophysiol* 1982; **5**: 517–22.

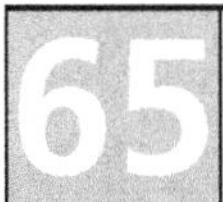

CASE 65

Arrhythmic syncope in a child: catecholaminergic ventricular tachycardia

J.M. Ormaetxe, M.F. Arkotxa, R. Sáez, J.D. Martínez Alday

Case report

A 5-year-old boy had an 18-month history of frequent stress-induced or emotion-induced presyncopal and syncopal episodes. There was no family history of syncope or sudden cardiac death, and the physical examination, chest radiography, 12-lead electrocardiogram (ECG; including the corrected QT interval), two-dimensional echocardiography, stress test (Bruce protocol), and Holter monitoring were normal. The result of an electroencephalogram had led his neurologist to treat him with valproic acid; the treatment was unsuccessful and was therefore stopped. An ECG and exercise test conducted for his parents were absolutely normal. He had no brothers or sisters.

Due to the relationship between stress or emotion and the episodes, as well as our previous experience with the device in adults with syncope of unknown origin, it was decided to place an implantable loop recorder (ILR) (Reveal 9525, Medtronic, Inc., Minneapolis, Minnesota, USA). With the patient under sedation, the device was implanted in the subcutaneous area of the left anterior thorax, with no complications. Twenty days after the implantation, and while the patient was practicing sport (karate), he suffered a syncopal episode similar to the recurrent episodes previously experienced. His parents activated the device, and the stored electrogram, which was retrieved by telemetry, showed an episode of very fast and sustained, irregular, wide QRS complex tachycardia (Fig. 65.1). After this, an electrophysiological examination was conducted, which was negative. Accessory pathways and an atrioventricular node reentry substrate were not found, nor was it possible to induce supraventricular or ventricular arrhythmias with rapid trains and with up to three extrastimuli introduced in the right atrium and in two points on the right ventricle, either in baseline conditions or during isoproterenol infusion. Administration of intravenous flecainide also failed to demonstrate the Brugada syndrome. The patient is still asymptomatic 20 months later, receiving beta-blocker treatment. In addition, testing of the device has not shown any automatically detected events.

Comment

Six types of polymorphic ventricular tachycardia have been described in patients with "apparently normal hearts":

- *Torsade de pointes*, in the long QT syndrome.
- Polymorphic ventricular arrhythmias, associated with the Brugada syndrome.
- The short-coupled variant of *torsade de pointes.*
- Polymorphic ventricular arrhythmias associated with the short QT syndrome.
- Catecholaminergic polymorphic ventricular tachycardia (CPVT).
- Idiopathic ventricular fibrillation.

In the present case, the 5-year-old boy presented with stress-induced or emotion-induced syncopal episodes, and prolonged monitoring with an ILR disclosed polymorphic ventricular tachycardia as the cause of syncope. Clinical evaluation in this case excluded long or short QT syndromes and Brugada syndrome, and the examination of the ILR recording suggested CPVT.

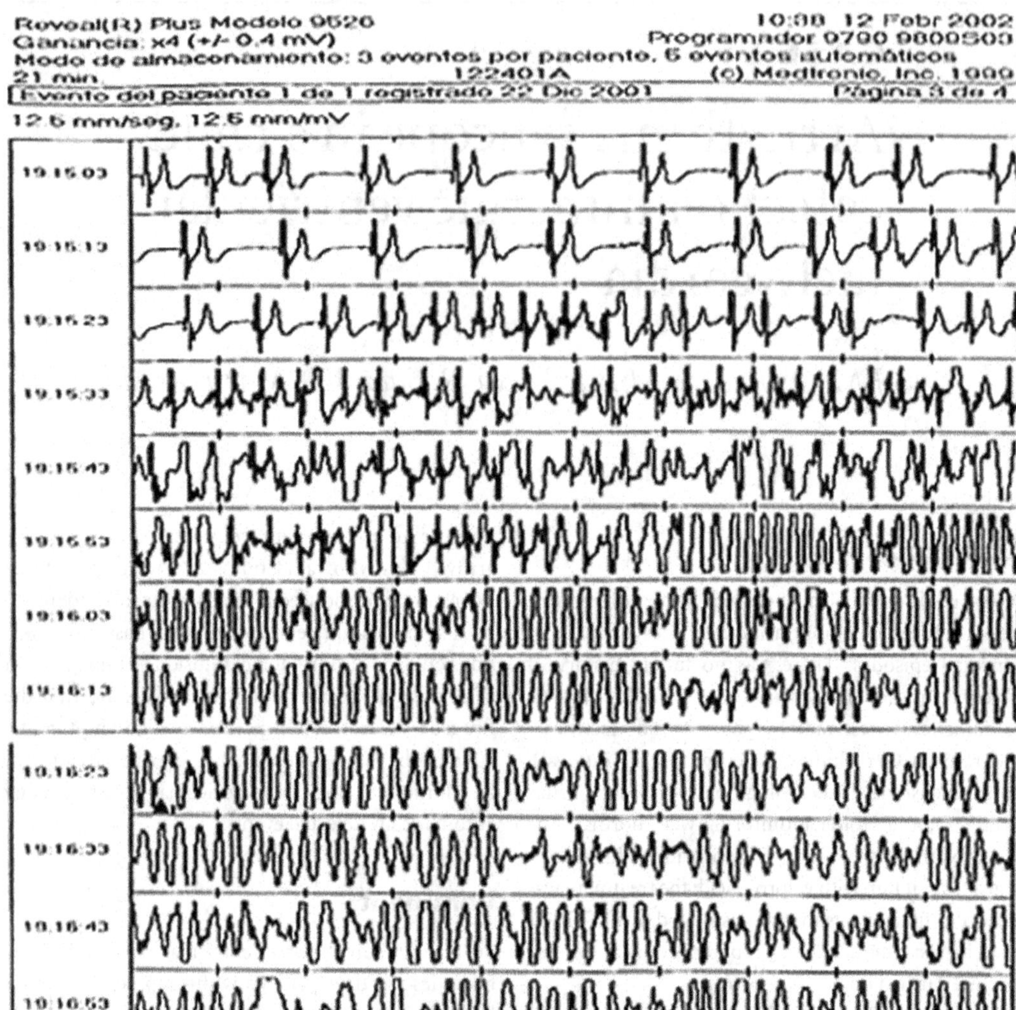

Figure 65.1 The electrogram recorded during the syncopal episode retrieved by telemetry from the patient's implantable loop recorder. A 75-s episode of polymorphic ventricular tachycardia is recorded. The small black triangle (in the ninth line of the figure) shows the moment at which the parents activated the recording. Note the sinus tachycardia before and after the episode. The device was programmed to C-storage mode, allowing separate recording of three patient-activated events 6 min before and 1 min after activation. (Reprinted from [8] with kind permission of Springer Science and Business Media.)

CPVT is an uncommon form of arrhythmogenic disease occurring in children and adolescents with a structurally normal heart [1,2]. Typically, the tachycardia is induced by situations associated with the release of catecholamines, such as effort or emotion. The arrhythmia, consisting of isolated polymorphic ventricular extrasystoles followed by salvoes of bidirectional and polymorphic ventricular tachycardia, is liable to degenerate into ventricular fibrillation [1,2].

The electrophysiological substrate for CPVT has not been clearly identified, but Leenhardt *et al.* [1] and Nakajima *et al.* [3] have suggested that triggered activity may be the mechanism involved.

Familial occurrence of catecholaminergic polymorphic ventricular tachycardia is common, but there are also isolated cases. Mutations in the cardiac ryanodine receptor gene (*RYR2*) [4,5] and in the calsequestrin 2 gene (*CASQ2*) [6] have been described in familial cases.

Beta-blockers are the treatment of choice for CPVT [1]. The dosage has to be titrated carefully in order to prevent the heart rate from exceeding 120–130 beats/min, and the success of the treatment in the present case was assessed by the disappearance of symptoms and the absence of ventricular tachycardia on monitoring.

Interestingly, in the present case, the tachycardia was not induced during the effort test or isoproterenol infusion. This case therefore demonstrates the value of implantable loop recordings for diagnosing arrhythmic events in patients with primary arrhythmogenic diseases associated with recurrent syncope [7].

References

1 Leenhardt A, Lucet V, Denjoy I, Grau N, Ngoe DD, Coumel P. Catecholaminergic polymorphic ventricular tachycardia in children: a 7-year follow-up of 21 patients. *Circulation* 1995; **91**: 1512–9.

2 Priori SG, Napolitano C, Memmi M, *et al.* Clinical and molecular characterization of patients with catecholaminergic polymorphic ventricular tachycardia. *Circulation* 2002; **106**: 69–74.

3 Nakajima T, Kanedo Y, Taniguchi Y, *et al.* The mechanism of catecholaminergic polymorphic ventricular tachycardia may be triggered activity due to delayed afterdepolarization. *Eur Heart J* 1997; **18**: 530–1.

4 Laitinen PJ, Brown KM, Piippo K, *et al.* Mutations of the cardiac ryanodine receptor (*RyR2*) gene in familial polymorphic ventricular tachycardia. *Circulation* 2001; **103**: 485–90.

5 Priori SG, Napolitano C, Tiso N, *et al.* Mutations in the cardiac ryanodine receptor gene (*hRyR2*) underlie catecholaminergic polymorphic ventricular tachycardia. *Circulation* 2001; **103**: 196–200.

6 Lahat H, Eldar M, Levy-Nissenbaum E, *et al.* Autosomal recessive catecholamine- or exercise-induced polymorphic ventricular tachycardia: clinical features and assignment of the disease gene to chromosome 1p13-21. *Circulation* 2001; **103**: 2822–7.

7 Hasdemir C, Priori SG, Overholt E, Lazzara R. Catecholaminergic polymorphic ventricular tachycardia, recurrent syncope, and implantable loop recorder. *J Cardiovasc Electrophysiol* 2004; **15**: 729.

8 Ormaetxe JM, Saez R, Arkotxa MF, Martinez-Alday JD. Catecholaminergic polymorphic ventricular tachycardia detected by an insertable loop recorder in a pediatric patient with exercise syncopal episodes. *Pediatr Cardiol* 2004; **25** (6): 693–5.

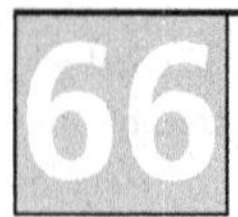

CASE 66

Adenosine triphosphate-sensitive paroxysmal atrioventricular block

R. Maggi, M. Brignole, P. Donateo, A. Solano, D. Oddone, F. Croci, E. Puggioni

Case report

A 51-year-old woman with recurrent episodes of presyncope and two episodes of syncope preceded by blurring vision was hospitalized because 24-h electrocardiography (ECG) monitoring showed a paroxysmal atrioventricular (AV) block with asystolic pauses (maximum pause of 6 s) during the presyncopal symptoms.

Apart from syncope, her history was negative. The physical examination, basic laboratory tests, standard ECG, and two-dimensional echocardiographic Doppler examination were normal. Right and left carotid sinus massage was performed with the patient in both the supine and upright positions and showed a normal response. A head-up tilt-table test with sublingual nitroglycerin challenge was also carried out.

During in-hospital telemetric monitoring, several asystolic pauses (maximum 4 s) due to paroxysmal AV blocks were recorded (Fig. 66.1).

Adenosine triphosphate (ATP) was injected into a brachial vein as a rapid (< 2 s) bolus of 20 mg. The drug caused an AV block, with ventricular asystole of 9.4 s and presyncope.

On the day after this, an electrophysiological study was conducted. Normal nodal and infrahisian AV conduction was found at the baseline, during incremental atrial pacing, and after ajmaline. Sinus node function was also normal—sinus node recovery time (SNRT) 1190 ms, corrected SNRT 220 ms. The ATP test was repeated during the electrophysiological study, again inducing an asystolic pause due to an AV block located inside the AV node, with a maximum pause of 11.5 s (Fig. 66.2) and a drop in systolic blood pressure from 120 mmHg to 70 mmHg (Fig. 66.3). Finally, the ATP test was repeated after theophylline infusion (the receptor antagonist for ATP); in this case, the AV block was not induced and blood pressure showed a mild asymptomatic decrease.

A diagnosis of adenosine-sensitive AV block was made, and treatment with oral slow-release theophylline (600 mg b.i.d.) was started. Blood theophylline levels reached the therapeutic range (8–20 mg/L), and the patient was discharged.

There were no syncopal or presyncopal events during the following 15 months while the patient was continuing theophylline therapy. Nevertheless, a 24-h ECG recording carried out after 14 months showed persistence of asymptomatic episodes of paroxysmal AV block with a maximum pause of 3.3 s.

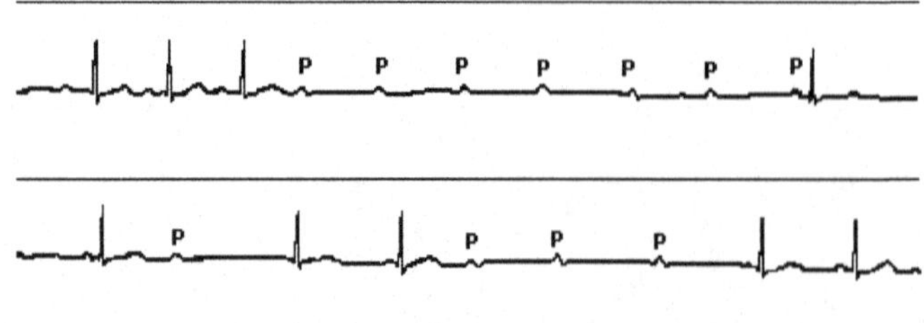

Figure 66.1 Paroxysmal atrioventricular block during in-hospital telemetric monitoring.

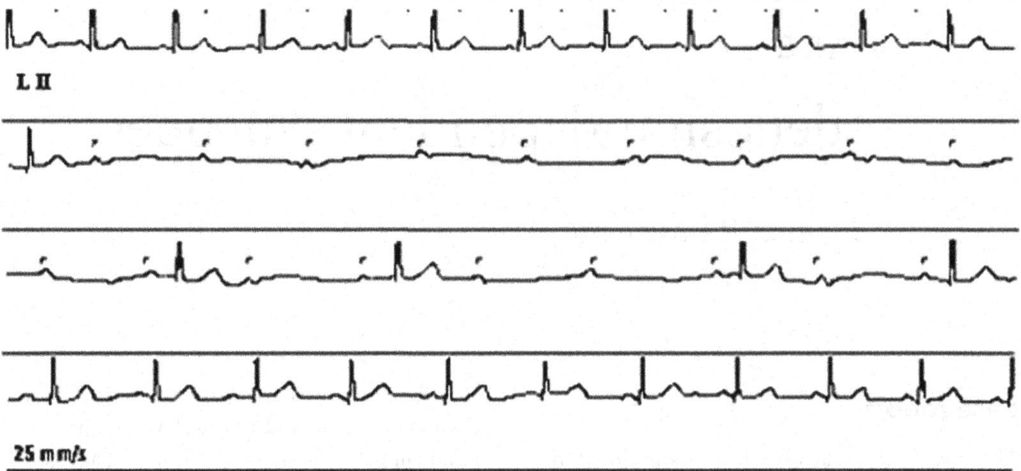

Figure 66.2 Injection of adenosine triphosphate caused an atrioventricular block, with a maximum pause of 11.5 s.

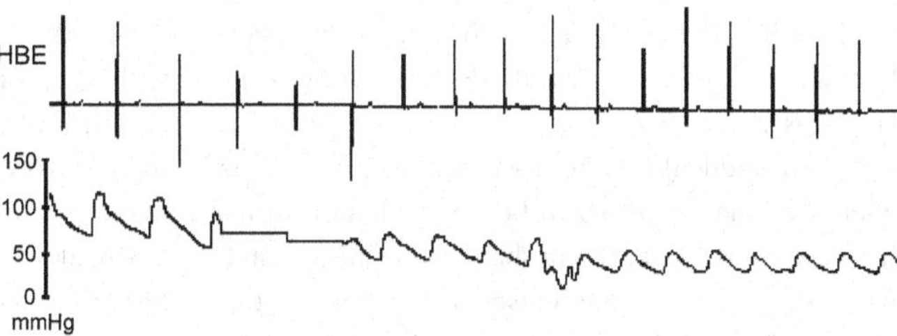

Figure 66.3 The adenosine triphosphate test after theophylline infusion did not cause an atrioventricular block. There was a fall in systolic blood pressure from 120 mmHg to 70 mmHg. HBE, His bundle electrogram.

Comment

In general, symptomatic third-degree AV block is regarded as a manifestation of intrinsic disease of the AV conduction system, either at the level of the AV node or the His–Purkinje system. A permanent pacemaker is therefore usually indicated. In this specific case, however, several features argued against this pathophysiological mechanism. The patient's young age, the long history of presyncopal attacks since youth, the absence of structural heart disease, the normal AV conduction properties as evaluated during the electrophysiological study, combined with a hypersensitive ATP response, did not suggest an organic disease of the AV node or His–Purkinje system, but rather a functional disorder [1–3].

A minority of patients with unexplained syncope show increased susceptibility to ATP injection. In these "hypersensitive" patients, endogenous adenosine, released in physiological and pathological conditions, can trigger bradycardia and/or hypotension and cause syncope, due to the agent's powerful cardiac and hypotensive effects. This hypothesis still needs to be proved. However, there is some evidence that the ATP test identifies a group of patients with otherwise unexplained syncope with definite clinical features, an absence of structural heart disease, and a benign prognosis—although the mechanisms of syncope involved are heterogeneous.

An adenosine-mediated paroxysmal AV block is regarded as a more specific mechanism of syncope in this group of patients, but this finding is observed only in a minority of these cases. The favorable outcome of adenosine-sensitive syncope in this case suggested the strategy of postponing pacemaker therapy and starting with a milder and more pathophysiology-guided form of treatment with theophylline.

References

1 Brignole M, Donateo P, Menozzi C. The diagnostic value of ATP testing in patients with unexplained syncope. *Europace* 2003; **5**: 425–8.

2 Donateo P, Brignole M, Menozzi C, *et al.* Mechanism of syncope in patients with positive adenosine triphosphate tests. *J Am Coll Cardiol* 2003; **41**: 93–8.

3 Brignole M, Gaggioli G, Menozzi C, *et al.* Adenosine-induced atrioventricular block in patients with unexplained syncope: the diagnostic value of ATP test. *Circulation* 1997; **96**: 3921–7.

CASE 67

Adenosine-dependent syncope?

J.J. Blanc, P. Castellant

Case report

An active 80-year-old woman was admitted during the summer due to a typical syncopal episode. She was receiving long-term treatment for hypertension (amlodipine 10 mg/day and bisoprolol 10 mg/day), but had no other cardiovascular or extracardiovascular disease.

She fell suddenly, without any warning symptoms, while washing the dishes in her kitchen, and hit her head against the sink. Her husband came immediately while she regained consciousness. He noticed that she remained confused for a few minutes and that she reported nausea. When she reached the emergency room, the only immediate abnormal finding was a cut on her scalp, which needed four or five stitches. Computed tomography did not show any pathological findings.

History-taking revealed that she had had three identical episodes within the two previous years, but she had not consulted her physician, as she had had no trauma. There was no orthostatic hypotension, and the physical examination was normal. Electrocardiography showed a sinus rhythm with normal QRS complexes and a PR interval lasting 180 ms.

Carotid sinus massage with the patient in the upright position induced a slight slowing in heart rate and no fall in blood pressure. Tilt testing at baseline and after a drug challenge with nitroglycerin remained negative.

An adenosine test was carried out in accordance with the usual protocol and proved to be highly abnormal, with a long ventricular pause (8 s) following an atrioventricular block (Fig. 67.1). A dual pacemaker was implanted, and the patient did not report any recurrences of syncope during a follow-up period of 12 months.

Comment

In this 80-year-old woman with repeated syncopal episodes, the initial clinical evaluation was normal. The normal physical evaluation and electrocardiography suggested an absence of structural heart disease, and carotid sinus massage and the tilt-table test were not diagnostic.

In accordance with the European Society of Cardiology guidelines [1], an adenosine triphosphate test can be carried out in these cases to identify a subset of patients with adenosine-sensitive syncope [2,3]. In the

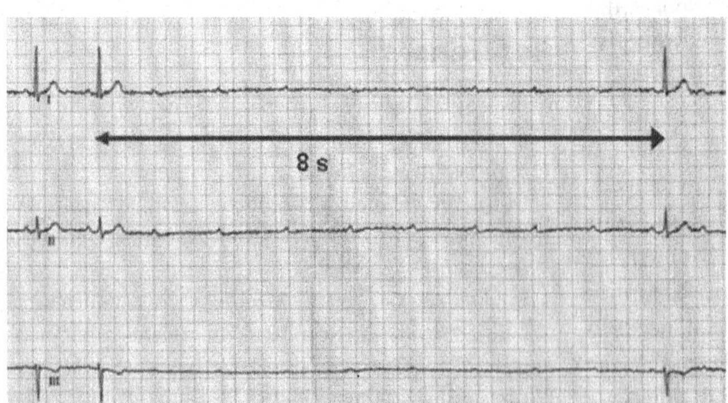

Figure 67.1 The result of the adenosine test.

present case, a ventricular asystolic pause of 8 s due to atrioventricular block was observed after the intravenous injection of adenosine; pauses longer than 6 s are considered to be abnormal.

There is at present no consensus with regard to the treatment of adenosine-sensitive syncope. Some authors have treated these patients with theophylline [3], while others have obtained good results with permanent pacemaker implantation [4]. In the present case, in view of the number of recurrences over a relatively short period of time, the patient's age, and the traumatic consequences of the syncope, the authors decided to implant a dual pacemaker. During a 12-month follow-up period, the patient did not report any recurrent episodes of syncope. However, this is only a case report, and well-designed trials are certainly needed before it can be considered that pacing is a definitive treatment for this condition.

References

1 Brignole M, Alboni P, Benditt DG, *et al.* Task Force on Syncope, European Society of Cardiology. Guidelines on management (diagnosis and treatment) of syncope. *Eur Heart J* 2001; **22**: 1256–306.

2 Flammang D, Church T, Waynberger M, Chassing A, Antiel M. Can adenosine-5′-triphosphate be used to select treatment in severe vasovagal syndrome? *Circulation* 1997; **26**: 1201–8.

3 Brignole M, Gaggioli G, Menozzi C, *et al.* Adenosine-induced atrioventricular block in patients with unexplained syncope: the diagnostic value of ATP testing. *Circulation* 1997; 96: 3921–7.

4 Flammang D, Antiel M, Church T, *et al.* Is a pacemaker indicated for vasovagal patients with severe cardioinhibitory reflex as identified by the ATP test? A preliminary randomized trial. *Europace* 1999; **1**: 140–5.

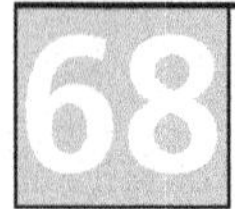

CASE 68

Syncope due to paroxysmal junctional tachycardia

R. García Civera, S. Morell Cabedo, R. Sanjuán Mañez, R. Ruiz Granell

Case report

A 54-year-old man was referred to the electrophysiology laboratory for evaluation of a syncopal paroxysmal supraventricular tachycardia. He had had a long history of paroxysmal palpitations, occasionally associated with syncope. The episodes had been electrocardiographically documented as supraventricular tachycardia. Four years before, he had been diagnosed with arterial hypertension and treated with vasodilators and diuretics. In the previous 6 months, the patient had experienced five episodes of tachycardia, with syncope developing immediately after the beginning of the palpitations on three occasions. The baseline electrocardiogram was normal, and an echocardiogram showed mild left ventricular hypertrophy with preserved systolic ventricular function (with a left ventricular ejection fraction of 70%).

An electrophysiological study was carried out without sedation and with the patient in the supine position. In addition to the usual electrocatheters (located in the right ventricular apex, right atrium, His bundle region, and coronary sinus), an arterial catheter was inserted into the femoral artery for continuous monitoring of blood pressure. Supraventricular tachycardia at 240 beats/min was repeatedly induced and terminated by programmed atrial and ventricular stimulation. Atrioventricular reentry using a concealed left accessory pathway as the retrograde limb of the circuit was shown to be the mechanism of the tachycardia. A sudden drop in arterial pressure from 200/95 to 75/50 mmHg was observed when the tachycardia was induced (Fig. 68.1), and the patient developed presyncope (with light-headedness, blurred vision, and pallor), associated with palpitations, despite his recumbent position. Figure 68.2 shows the changes in arterial

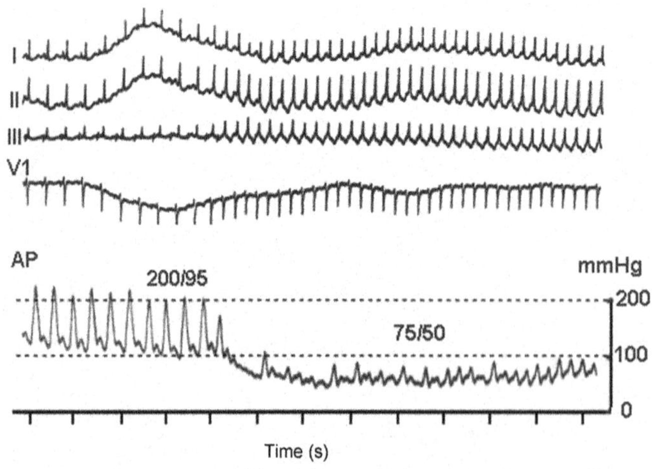

Figure 68.1 With induction of tachycardia, there is a sudden drop in blood pressure and development of presyncopal symptoms. AP, arterial pressure.

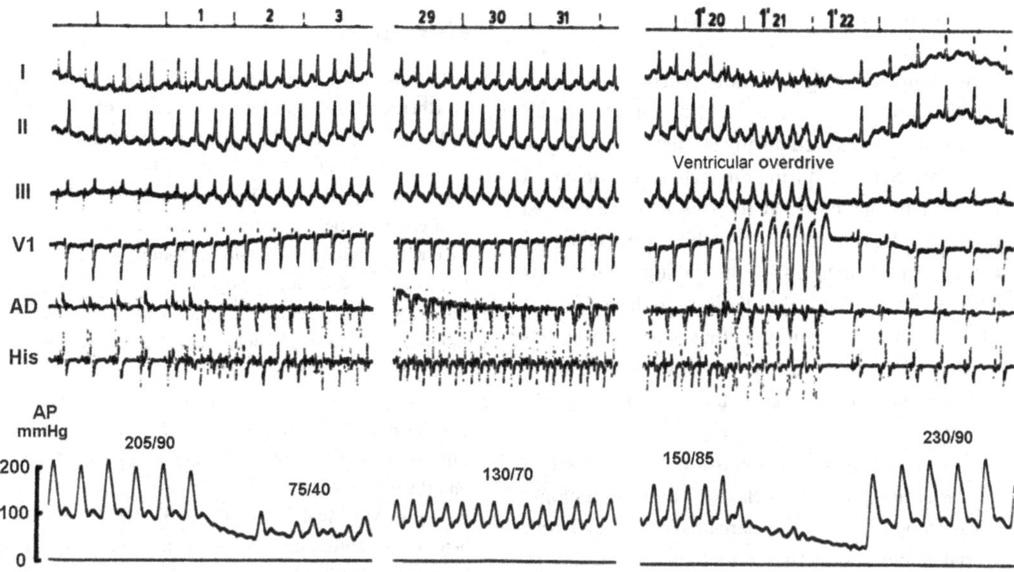

Figure 68.2 Changes in blood pressure during the tachycardia.

pressure during the course of the tachycardia. After the first 8 s, blood pressure begins to rise slowly (132/72 at 30 s, 150/85 at 80 s) and termination of the tachycardia by ventricular overdrive pacing results in a blood-pressure overshoot (230/92 mmHg).

In this case, therefore, the initial hypotension and delayed vasomotor compensatory response appeared to be the mechanism for the syncopal attacks associated with tachycardia.

Comment

Paroxysmal junctional tachycardia is a common form of arrhythmia, due to intranodal reentry or atrioventricular reentry using a concealed accessory pathway as the retrograde limb of the circuit. Palpitation is the most common symptom in paroxysmal supraventricular tachycardias, but syncope or presyncope has been found to be associated with palpitation in 18% of cases [1].

The mechanism of syncope associated with paroxysmal supraventricular tachycardia is multifactorial. Fundamental mechanisms include hemodynamic derangement, vasomotor compensatory responses, and possible induction of vasovagal reactions. Other factors that may be important include the body position during the tachycardia, the patient's previous hemodynamic state, and the use of medications (antiarrhythmic drugs, vasodilators, etc.).

The purely hemodynamic response to tachycardia mainly depends on the ventricular rate, the timing of the P wave, and previous ventricular function [2]. Several studies have failed to show differences in heart rate between supraventricular tachycardias associated or not associated with syncope [1,3,4]. Waxman *et al.* [5] have studied the hemodynamic effect of P-wave timing during tachycardia simulated by DDD pacing. They found that the decrease in blood pressure and increase in central venous pressure were significantly lower during simulated long RP tachycardia (atrial tachycardia) than during tachycardia with simultaneous atrial and ventricular systole (intranodal tachycardia) or during short RP tachycardia (atrioventricular reentry tachycardia).

Hypotension at the onset of tachycardia activates the baroreceptor system, and increased sympathetic tone develops [5,6]. The increase in sympathetic tone results in peripheral vasoconstriction and increased cardiac inotropism. An increase in blood pressure is consequently observed. After this initial compensatory phase, activation of cardiac mechanoreceptors during the tachycardia results in withdrawal of sympathetic tone and enhanced vagal tone [6]. At this point, the vagal discharge can be responsible for spontaneous termination of the supraventricular tachycardia [6], and, in certain cases, for producing a vasovagal reaction with further hypotension and syncope [1,4].

In the study by Leitch *et al.* [4], supraventricular tachycardia was induced during 60° head-up tilting in 22 patients. Syncope during the tachycardia occurred in seven patients, either at the onset of tachycardia or 1–2 min later, after initial stabilization of blood pressure. The mean heart rate during supraventricular tachycardia was identical in patients with or without syncope. It was hypothesized that syncope was related to inadequate compensation of vasoconstriction mechanisms or to the development of a late vasovagal response.

In the present case, hypotension at the onset of tachycardia and probably a delayed vasomotor response appear to be the main mechanisms for the syncope. Arterial hypertension may also have played a role. Chronic hypertension can affect the peripheral vasoconstriction capacity and reduce the baroreflex sensitivity [7], contributing to the delayed or blunted vasomotor response. There have also been concerns regarding the response of the cerebral circulation, about which little is known. Grubb *et al.* recently showed that, in some patients with chronic arterial hypertension, a sudden drop in blood pressure may result in derangement of cerebral autoregulation, with vasoconstriction and syncope even at normal blood pressures [8].

In any case, elimination of the tachycardia by accessory pathway ablation is the treatment of choice in this patient.

References

1 Brembilla-Perrot B, Beurrier D, Houriez P, Claudon O, Wertheimer J. Incidence and mechanism of presyncope and/or syncope associated with paroxysmal junctional tachycardia. *Am J Cardiol* 2001; **88**: 134–8.

2 Insa Pérez L, Llopis R, Sayegh JM, Sáez JM, Cosín J. Consecuencias hemodinámicas de las arritmias. In: García Civera R, Sanjuán R, Cosín J, López Merino V, eds. *Síncope*. MCR, Barcelona, 1989: 221–42.

3 Yee R, Klein GJ. Syncope in the WPW syndrome: incidence and electrophysiologic correlates. *Pacing Clin Electrophysiol* 1984; **7**: 381–8.

4 Leitch JW, Klein GJ, Yee R, Leather RA, Kim YH. Syncope associated with supraventricular tachycardia: an expression of tachycardia rate or vasomotor response? *Circulation* 1992; **85**: 1064–71.

5 Waxman MB, Wald RW, Cameron DA. Interactions between the autonomic nervous system and tachycardias in man. *Cardiol Clin* 1982; **1**: 143–85.

6 Waxman MB, Sharma AD, Cameron DA, *et al.* Reflex mechanism responsible for early spontaneous termination of paroxysmal supraventricular tachycardia. *Am J Cardiol* 1982; **49**: 259–72.

7 Bristow JD, Honour AJ, Pickering JW, *et al.* Diminished baroreflex sensitivity in high blood pressure. *Circulation* 1969; **39**: 48–54.

8 Grubb BP, Kanjwal Y, Kosinsky D. Hypertensive syncope: loss of consciousness in hypertensive patients in absence of systemic hypotension [abstract]. *Heart Rhythm* 2004; **1**: S258–S259.

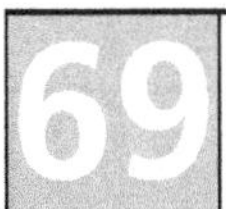

CASE 69

Syncope in a patient with atrioventricular nodal reentry tachycardia: reflex hypotension?

A. Del Rosso

Case report

A 79-year-old woman was referred to the syncope unit due to recurrent episodes of syncope during the previous year. Loss of consciousness was preceded by diaphoresis and occurred when she was in the standing position. The patient had mild hypertension, which was being treated with enalapril. The physical examination was normal. The baseline electrocardiogram (ECG) showed sinus tachycardia at 110 beats/min, a PR interval of 140 ms, and isolated ventricular ectopic beats. Carotid sinus massage was negative. A head-up tilt (HUT) test with sublingual nitroglycerin administration was carried out. In the fourth minute after nitroglycerin administration, the patient experienced syncope with hypotension (a Vasovagal Syncope International Study type 3 positive response). Treatment was limited to providing the usual counseling information for vasovagal syncope and withdrawal of the antihypertensive drug.

However, the patient experienced three further syncopal episodes, with severe head trauma on the last occasion. To ascertain the mechanism underlying the spontaneous episodes, a Reveal implantable loop recorder (ILR) (Medtronic, Inc., Minneapolis, Minnesota, USA) was placed. After 1 month, the patient had a new episode of syncope. The ILR recording showed a regular narrow complex tachycardia (mean rate 187 beats/min) (Fig. 69.1).

An electrophysiological study (EPS) was carried out. With programmed atrial stimulation, a dual atrioventricular nodal physiology was demonstrated, and atrioventricular nodal reentry tachycardia (AVNRT) was induced (Fig. 69.2). Radiofrequency catheter ablation of the slow pathway was carried out, and the arrhythmia was no longer inducible.

The patient remained free of symptoms during a 24-month follow-up period. The ILR showed no recurrences of AVNRT.

Comment

Syncope occurs in up to 8.5% of patients with AVNRT [1]. The rate of the tachycardia, the patient's volume status and posture at the time of onset of the arrhythmia, the presence of associated cardiopulmonary disease, and the integrity of reflex peripheral vascular compensation are key factors determining whether hypotension of sufficient severity to cause syncope occurs. A neural reflex component and drugs may play an important role, especially when the heart rate is not particularly high [2]. This patient was in fact being treated with an antihypertensive drug and showed a propensity for vasodepressor syncope during the HUT test.

Syncope that is preceded by palpitations is highly suggestive of tachyarrhythmia as the cause [3], but a lack of palpitations does not exclude tachycardia, especially in elderly patients. Palpitations are present in 63% of younger patients with tachyarrhythmic syncope, but only in 21% of those over the age of 65 [4]. The decision to implant an ILR in this patient instead of doing an electrophysiological study was based on two considerations: firstly, the severity of syncope, requiring tailored treatment; and secondly, the absence of clinical data suggestive of cardiac syncope.

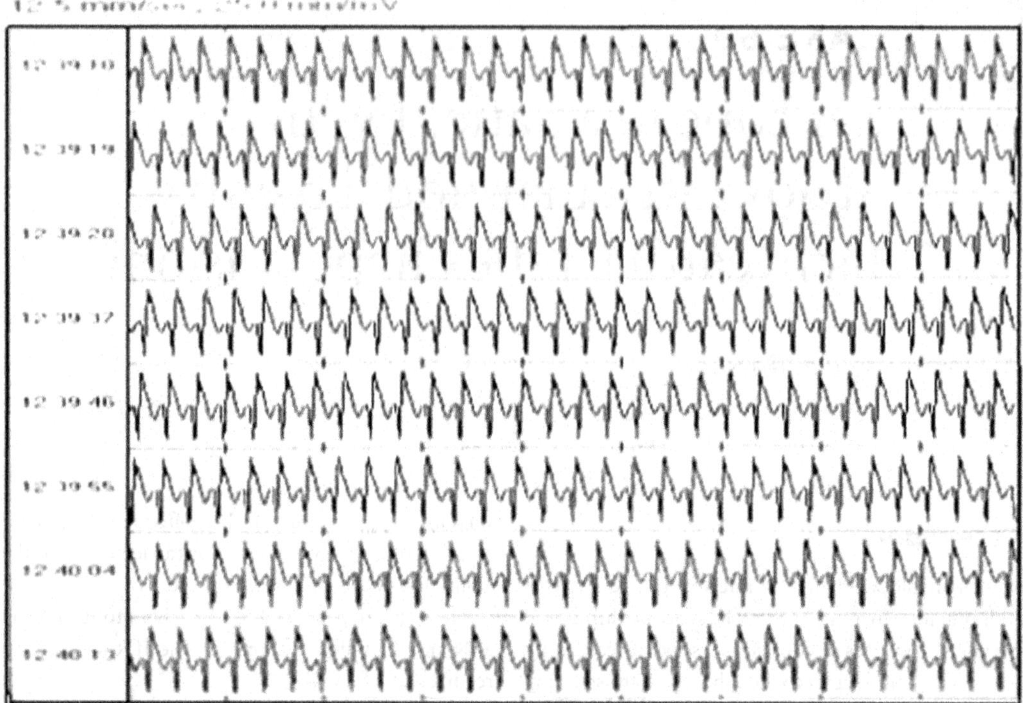

Figure 69.1 The implantable loop recorder tracing during a syncopal episode.

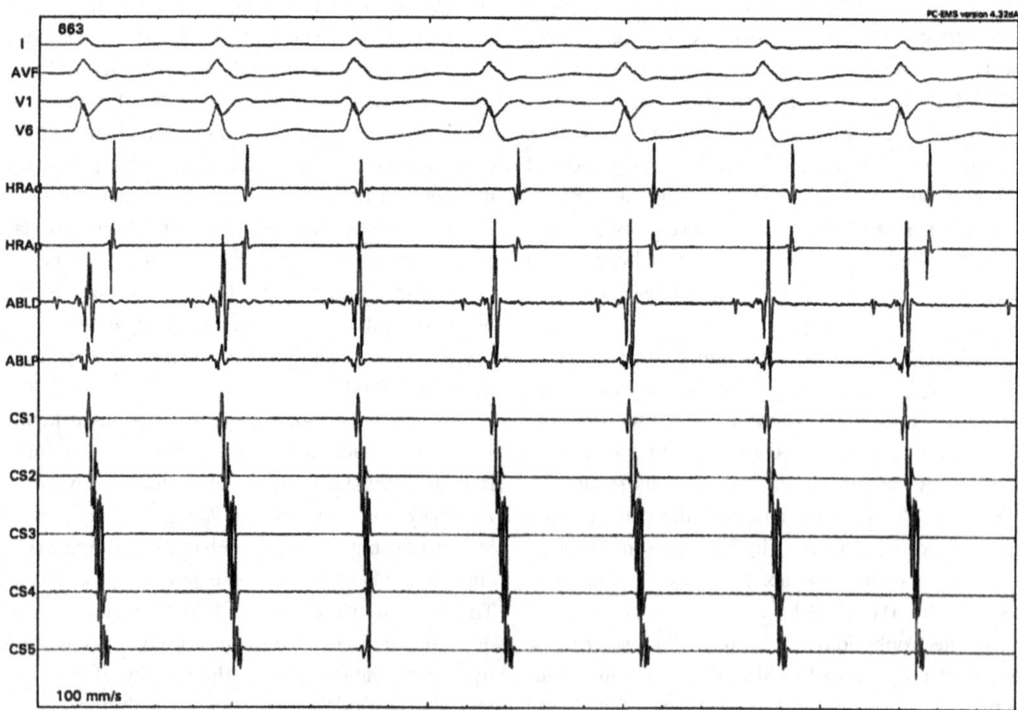

Figure 69.2 The electrophysiological study recording during tachycardia.

Dual atrioventricular nodal pathways may be detected and supraventricular tachycardia can be incidentally induced in up to 10% of patients undergoing electrophysiological testing. Additional criteria are usually required before it can be considered the cause of syncope—a high rate (> 180 beats/min) or hypotensive tachycardia. The arrhythmia induced in the electrophysiology laboratory did not meet these criteria in the present case, but the correlation between tachycardia and symptoms during ILR monitoring was diagnostic.

Transcatheter ablation is a very cost-effective therapeutic option in patients with recurrent supraventricular tachycardia, and is probably the treatment of choice when AVNRT is the cause of syncope.

References

1 Wellens JJ. Supraventricular tachycardia with reentry in the atrioventricular node. In: Kastor JA, ed. *Arrhythmias.* Saunders, Philadelphia, 1994: 250–61.

2 Leitch JW, Klein GJ, Yee R, Leather RA, Kim YH. Syncope associated with supraventricular tachycardia: an expression of tachycardia rate or vasomotor response? *Circulation* 1992; **85**: 1064–71.

3 Alboni P, Brignole M, Menozzi C, *et al.* The diagnostic value of history in patients with syncope with or without heart disease. *J Am Coll Cardiol* 2001; **37**: 1921–8.

4 Del Rosso A, Alboni P, Brignole M, Menozzi C, Raviele A. Relation of clinical presentation of syncope to the age of patients. *Am J Cardiol* 2005; **96**: 1431–5.

CASE 70

Arrhythmic and neuromediated syncope in a young woman

R. Peinado, J.L. Merino, M. Gnoatto, M. González Vasserot

Case report

An 18-year-old woman with recurrent syncopal episodes was referred to our outpatient clinic for evaluation. She had no family history of syncope or sudden cardiac death. Her medical history was unremarkable, except for a high number of presyncopal and syncopal episodes since she was 15.

She had been examined at another hospital, where a tilt-table test was carried out, during which the patient developed presyncope with bradycardia and hypotension (a Vasovagal Syncope International Study type 1 response). Reassurance and information about the nature of the condition were provided, but she continued to have frequent presyncopal and syncopal episodes.

A detailed clinical history revealed that rapid-onset palpitations, accompanied by a pounding sensation in the neck, preceded many of the syncopal episodes. After recovering consciousness, the patient did not feel palpitations, but polyuria was almost always present. In addition to this, dizziness, blurred vision, and sweating, but not palpitations, preceded other episodes that occurred after prolonged standing or stress.

The physical examination, 12-lead electrocardiography (ECG), and chest radiograph were normal.

Due to the presence of rapid-onset palpitations at the start of many of the syncopal episodes, an electrophysiological study was performed. Baseline conduction intervals were normal. The absence of VA conduction and the presence of anterograde dual atrioventricular node physiology were demonstrated. No tachycardias were induced in the baseline state. After infusion of isoproterenol, a focal atrial tachycardia was reproducibly induced by atrial pacing. Termination of atrial tachycardia was observed either spontaneously or after continuous atrial pacing (Fig. 70.1). When tachycardia was induced, the patient experienced dizziness, coinciding with a marked decrease in blood pressure (50 mmHg). During tachycardia, spontaneous changes in the AH interval and cycle length, related to anterograde conduction through the fast or slow pathway, were observed (Fig. 70.2). The tachycardia was mapped and successfully ablated at the crista terminalis, under the sinus node area (Fig. 70.3).

The patient improved significantly after ablation, but after a few weeks she presented again with recurrent episodes of presyncope during standing, not preceded by rapid-onset palpitations. Increased dietary salt and electrolyte intake, moderate exercise training, and counterpressure maneuvers were strongly recommended. Despite these, the patient presented again with several syncopal episodes. A second electrophysiological study was conducted without induction of tachycardia at the baseline or after isoproterenol infusion. Pharmacological therapy with paroxetine 20 mg/day was started.

Comment

Two different possible causes of syncope were found during evaluation of this case—vasovagal fainting and atrial tachycardia.

Vasovagal syncope was suggested by the presence of episodes triggered by prolonged standing or emotional stress, with vegetative prodromal symptoms without palpitation and a positive head-up tilt test. Atrial tachycardia was induced during the electrophysiological study, and its involvement is suggested by the

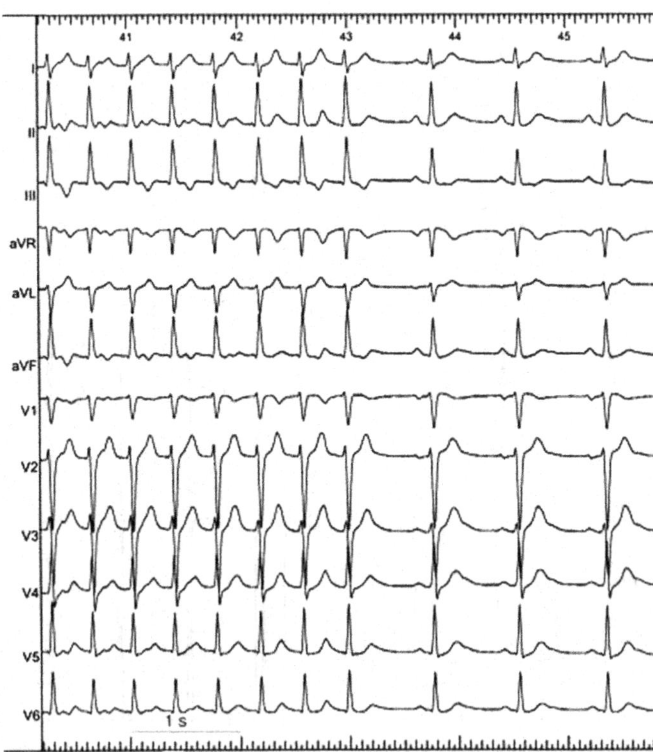

Figure 70.1 The 12-lead electrocardiography tracing during atrial tachycardia, with spontaneous termination of the tachycardia in the electrophysiological study.

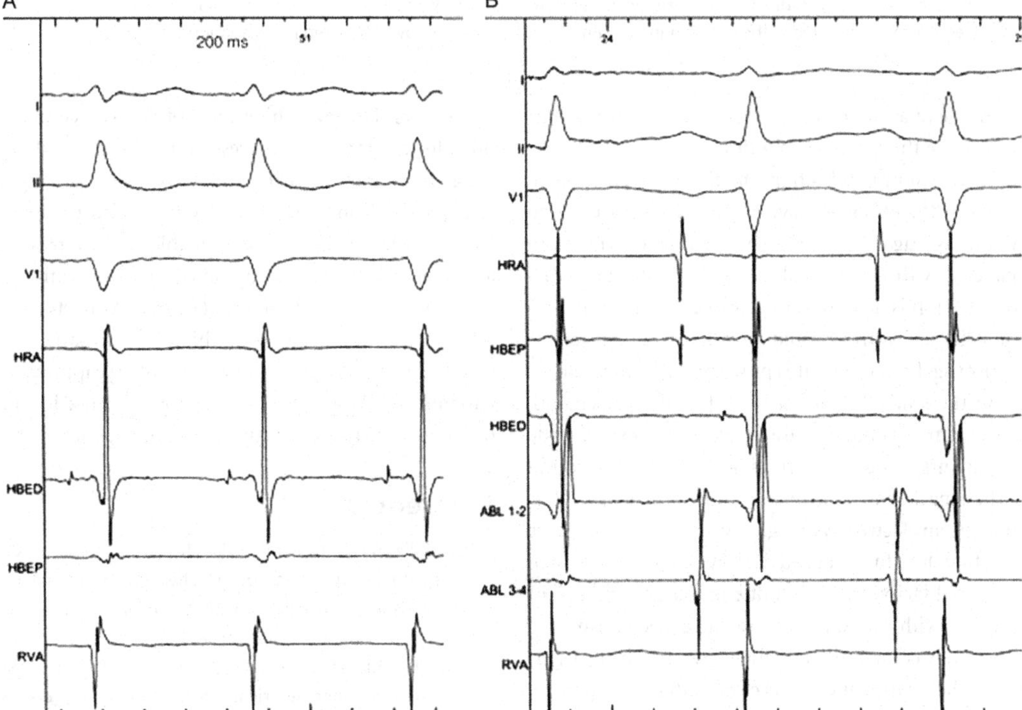

Figure 70.2 Surface leads I, II, and V_1 are shown along with intracardiac recordings from the high right atrium (HRA), distal and proximal His bundle region (HBED and HBEP), and right ventricular apex. Two different AH intervals and tachycardia cycle lengths were observed, depending on the anterograde conduction through the slow (A) or fast (B) pathway. The ablation catheter was located at the proximal coronary sinus.

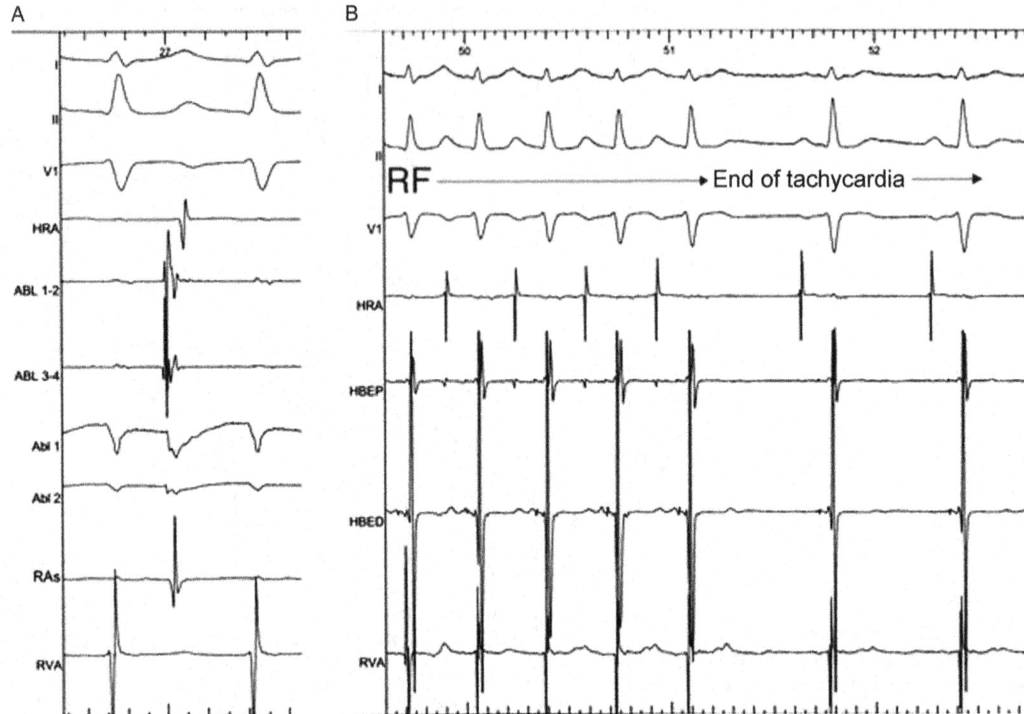

Figure 70.3 **A.** Bipolar (ABL 1–2 and ABL 3–4) and unipolar (Abl 1 and Abl 2) recordings obtained from the ablation catheter at the successful radiofrequency application point. RAs: electrograms recorded in the septal right atrium underneath the His bundle area. **B.** Termination of the tachycardia shortly after the onset of radiofrequency (RF) application. Recordings from the ablation catheter have been removed to avoid radiofrequency artifacts.

presence of a sudden onset of palpitations at the start of some of the syncopal episodes.

It is possible that both mechanisms played a role in some of the episodes. Several studies have suggested that a vasovagal reaction can be the cause of syncope in patients with paroxysmal supraventricular tachycardia [1–3]. It is therefore conceivable that the initiation of atrial tachycardia could have been the trigger for a vasovagal reaction in this predisposed individual.

In the study by Alboni *et al.* [4], the presence of paroxysmal palpitation during the syncopal episode in patients without structural heart disease was found to be a marker for a cardiologic cause of syncope. Conducting an electrophysiologic study in the present case was therefore fully indicated. However, the ablation of the atrial tachycardia did not eliminate the recurrent syncope with a presumably vasovagal mechanism.

In the vast majority of patients with vasovagal syncope, the treatment consists of providing reassurance, information about the nature of the condition, and general measures including training in counterpressure maneuvers. However, high rates of recurrence make other forms of treatment necessary in some cases. Many drugs have been used in the treatment of vasovagal syncope, but long-term placebo-controlled prospective trials have generally been unable to demonstrate any benefit with active drugs in comparison with the placebo [5]. In a placebo-controlled trial, paroxetine—a selective serotonin reuptake inhibitor—was shown to be effective in a large number of highly symptomatic patients [6]. However, further trials are needed in order to confirm the effectiveness of this agent.

References

1 Brembilla-Perrot B, Beurrier D, Houriez P, Claudon O, Wertheimer J. Incidence and mechanism of presyncope and/or syncope associated with paroxysmal junctional tachycardia. *Am J Cardiol* 2001; **88**: 134–8.

2 Leitch JW, Klein GJ, Yee R, Leather RA, Kim YH. Syncope associated with supraventricular tachycardia: an expression of tachycardia rate or vasomotor response? *Circulation* 1992; **85**: 1064–71.

3 Waxman MB, Wald RW, Cameron DA. Interactions between the autonomic nervous system and tachycardias in man. *Cardiol Clin* 1982; **1**: 143–85.
4 Alboni P, Brignole M, Menozzi C, *et al.* Diagnostic value of the history in patients with syncope with and without heart disease. *J Am Coll Cardiol* 2001; **37**: 1921–8.
5 Brignole M, Alboni P, Benditt DG, *et al.* Guidelines on management (diagnosis and treatment) of syncope: update 2004. *Europace* 2004; **6**: 467–537.
6 Di Girolamo E, Di Iorio C, Sabatini P, Leonzio L, Barbone C, Barsotti A. Effects of paroxetine hydrochloride, a selective serotonin reuptake inhibitor, on refractory vasovagal syncope: a randomized, double-blind, placebo-controlled study. *J Am Coll Cardiol* 1999; **33**: 1227–30.

CASE 71

Syncope and Wolff–Parkinson–White syndrome: atrial fibrillation with rapid ventricular response

C. Alonso, A. Moya i Mitjans

Case report

A 16-year-old patient was admitted to the emergency room. He had started feeling dizzy and had experienced a loss of consciousness with spontaneous recovery while playing football. While recovering, he reported palpitations. In the emergency room, his blood pressure was 90/65 mmHg, and an electrocardiogram (ECG) showed irregular tachycardia at about 200–250 beats/min with variations in the QRS duration and morphology, ranging from narrow normal QRS complexes to very wide complexes with a QRS duration of up to 140 ms (Fig. 71.1).

Direct-current electrical cardioversion was successfully carried out with the patient under sedation. After cardioversion, the ECG showed a normal sinus

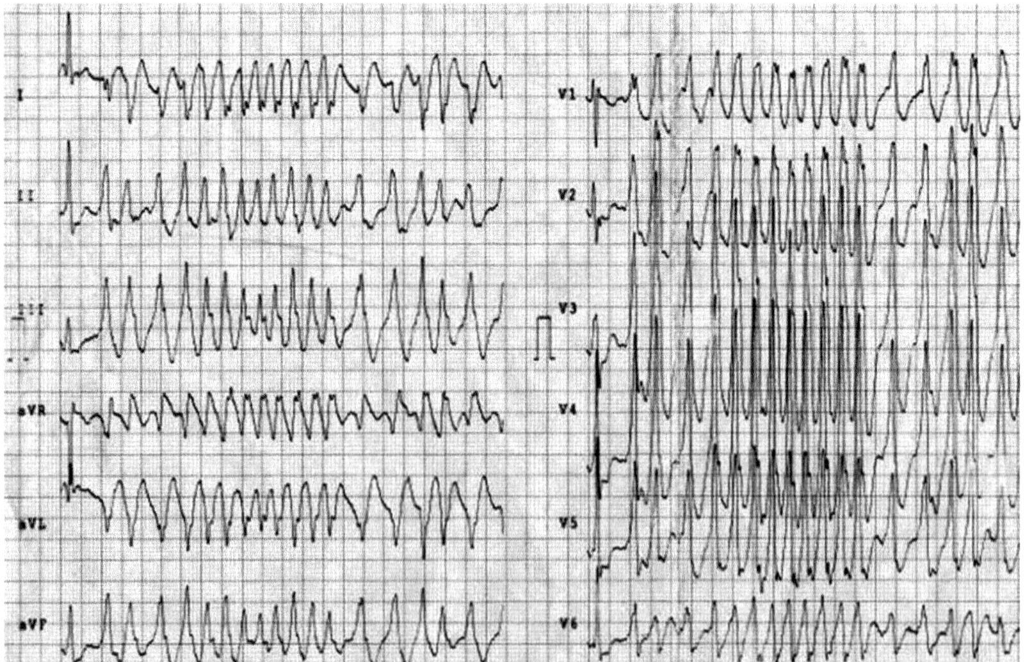

Figure 71.1 The 12-lead electrocardiogram recorded in the emergency room. This tracing shows irregular tachycardia, with a heart rate of approximately 250 beats/min, with wide variation in the QRS—ranging from the first complex, which is narrow and almost normal but with minimal preexcitation, to very broad complexes.

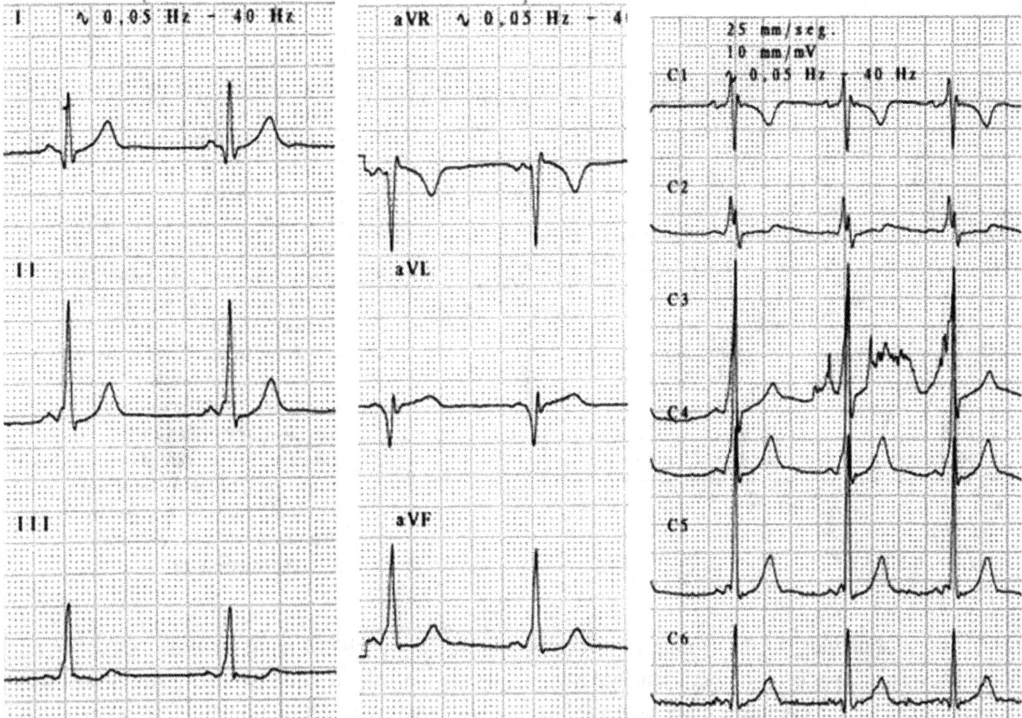

Figure 71.2 Electrocardiography in sinus rhythm after direct-current electrical cardioversion. A short PR interval is seen, with a delta wave that is negative in DI and aVL and positive in the inferior as well as precordial leads—diagnostic of Wolff–Parkinson–White syndrome, with a left posterolateral free wall accessory pathway.

rhythm, with a PR interval of 0.12 s and a delta wave, which was negative on DI and L and positive in the inferior as well as precordial leads—diagnostic of Wolff–Parkinson–White syndrome, with an accessory pathway located in the free left posterolateral wall (Fig. 71.2).

The patient had no history of palpitations or syncope. The physical examination was unremarkable, and an echocardiogram was also normal.

Due to the presence of a syncopal episode in the context of rapid atrial fibrillation in a patient with Wolff–Parkinson–White syndrome, he was referred to the arrhythmia unit.

An electrophysiological study was carried out, and the presence of an accessory pathway located in the posterolateral left free wall was confirmed. During the procedure, orthodromic reciprocating tachycardia was induced. The effective refractory period of the accessory pathway was 240 ms. The accessory pathway was ablated via a transaortic retrograde approach (Fig. 71.3). After ablation of the accessory pathway, a complete electrophysiological study was repeated, and no other accessory pathways were identified. There were no complications, and the patient was discharged 24 h after the procedure.

After a 1-year follow-up period, the patient is still asymptomatic, with a normal ECG.

Comment

This patient illustrates one of the characteristic situations of potentially fatal but curable arrhythmic syncope.

The Wolff–Parkinson–White syndrome is defined as the presence of an ECG with ventricular preexcitation and supraventricular tachyarrhythmias [1]. The preexcitation indicates the presence of an accessory pathway with anterograde conduction. The most frequent form of arrhythmia in these patients is orthodromic atrioventricular (AV) reciprocating tachycardia, which uses the AV node as the anterograde limb and the accessory pathway as the retrograde limb, resulting in an ECG with a narrow complex during the tachycardia

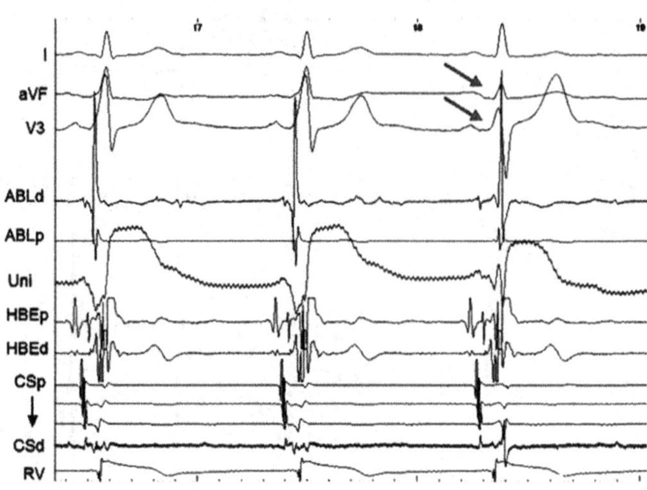

Figure 71.3 Intracavitary recordings and three electrocardiography leads during radiofrequency ablation. The first two complexes are preexcited. The distal bipolar electrogram of the mapping catheter (ABLd) shows continuous atrial and ventricular activity, as well as premature activation of the ventricular electrogram in comparison with the delta wave. The unipolar electrogram shows an initially positive deflection, corresponding to atrial activation, followed by a rapid and negative deflection, indicating that the catheter is at the origin of the ventricular activation. The third beat shows disappearance of delta wave on the electrocardiogram, as well as lengthening of the AV interval in the bipolar and unipolar electrograms, with an initial "r" wave in the unipolar electrogram.

[2]. In these situations, hemodynamic tolerance is normally good, and patients only occasionally develop syncope, usually at the beginning of the tachycardia—probably due to poor hemodynamic adaptation in the context of a neuromediated reflex and not related to the tachycardia itself [3]. This mechanism of syncope is not specific for paroxysmal reciprocating tachycardias mediated by an accessory pathway, but has also been described in other types of supraventricular tachycardia [4].

However, some patients with an accessory pathway can develop atrial fibrillation, which—due to the conduction properties of the accessory pathway—can allow very fast conduction to the ventricle, with the characteristic pattern observed in this case, in which different morphologies of QRS are present due to different degrees of conduction by both the AV node and the accessory pathway [5]. This very fast and irregular tachycardia can lead to hemodynamic compromise, producing a transient loss of consciousness, as in this case, and can even potentially trigger a ventricular fibrillation that causes sudden death [6].

Atrial fibrillation can appear as a primary arrhythmia or—more commonly, and as the probable mechanism in this case—can be triggered during rapid orthodromic reciprocating AV tachycardia, usually facilitated by an increased adrenergic tone, as probably happened in this case, in which syncope appeared while the patient was playing football.

Due to the risk of rapid atrial fibrillation or ventricular fibrillation, radiofrequency catheter ablation is considered a class I indication for ablation in patients with Wolff–Parkinson–White Syndrome and episodes of tachycardia or unexplained syncope [7–9]. The indication for ablation in asymptomatic patients is a matter of debate [9,10].

Radiofrequency catheter ablation is a curative approach, with a success rate of more than 95% and with a low rate of complications. No other treatment is needed in patients in whom syncope can be attributed to rapid preexcited atrial fibrillation.

References

1 Olgin JE, Zipes DP. Specific arrhythmias: diagnosis and treatment. In: Zipes DP, Libby P, Bonow RO, Braunwald E, eds. *Braunwald's Heart Disease.* Elsevier/Saunders, Philadelphia, 2004: 803–63.

2 Akhtar M, Lehmann MH, Denker ST, Mahmud R, Tchou P, Jazayeri M. Electrophysiologic mechanisms of orthodromic tachycardia initiation during ventricular pacing in the Wolff–Parkinson–White syndrome. *J Am Coll Cardiol* 1987; **9**: 89–100.

3 Leitch JW, Klein GJ, Yee R, *et al.* Syncope associated with supraventricular tachycardia: an expression of tachycardia or vasomotor response. *Circulation* 1992; **85**: 1064–71.

4 Brignole M, Gianfranchi L, Menozzi C, *et al.* Role of autonomic reflexes in syncope associated with paroxysmal atrial fibrillation. *J Am Coll Cardiol* 1993; **22**: 1123–9.

5 Bauernfeind RA, Wyndham CR, Swiryn SP, *et al.* Paroxysmal atrial fibrillation in the Wolff–Parkinson–White syndrome. *Am J Cardiol* 1981; **47**: 562–9.
6 Klein GJ, Bashore TM, Sellers TD, Pritchett EL, Smith WM, Gallagher JJ. Ventricular fibrillation in the Wolff–Parkinson–White syndrome. *N Engl J Med* 1979; **301**: 1080–5.
7 Almendral Garrote J, Marin Huerta E, Medina Moreno O, *et al.* [Practice guidelines of the Spanish Society of Cardiology on cardiac arrhythmias; in Spanish.] *Rev Esp Cardiol* 2001; **54**: 307–67.
8 Blomstrom-Lundqvist C, Scheinman MM, Aliot EM, *et al.* ACC/AHA/ESC guidelines for the management of patients with supraventricular arrhythmias: executive summary. A report of the American College of Cardiology/American Heart Association Task Force on practice guidelines and the European Society of Cardiology Committee for Practice Guidelines (Writing Committee to Develop Guidelines for the Management of Patients with Supraventricular Arrhythmias). *J Am Coll Cardiol* 2003; **42**: 1493–531 and *Circulation* 2003; **108**: 1871–909 (also available at http://www.acc.org/clinical/guidelines/arrhythmias/sva_index.pdf).
9 Almendral Garrote J, Gonzalez Torrecilla E, Atienza Fernandez F, Vigil Escribano D, Arenal Maiz A. [Treatment of patients with ventricular preexcitation; in Spanish.] *Rev Esp Cardiol* 2004; **57**: 859–68.
10 Pappone C, Santinelli V, Manguso F, *et al.* A randomized study of prophylactic catheter ablation in asymptomatic patients with the Wolff–Parkinson–White syndrome. *N Engl J Med* 2004; **351**: 1197–205.

72

CASE 72

Wolff–Parkinson–White syndrome with inapparent preexcitation in sinus rhythm: atrial flutter with 1 : 1 atrioventricular conduction

R. Ruiz Granell, R. García Civera, S. Morell Cabedo, R. Sanjuán Mañez

Case report

A 46-year-old man was admitted to the emergency department due to a syncopal episode with palpitations. The patient reported having had self-terminating paroxysms of palpitation during the previous 4 years, but an electrocardiogram (ECG) had never been recorded during these, and he had not previously experienced any syncopal attacks. Two hours before admission, while he had been sitting in his office, he had felt the start of rapid palpitations, followed immediately by syncope. The loss of consciousness had been brief (one or two minutes) and, after he recovered from it, without sequelae, the palpitations persisted.

In the emergency room, the patient was conscious and oriented. A feeble regular pulse at 300 beats/min was noted, and his arterial blood pressure was 100/60 mmHg. The initial ECG (Fig. 72.1) showed regular wide QRS complex tachycardia at 300 beats/min. The QRS was 0.14 s wide and the morphology suggested a right bundle-branch block with extreme deviation of the frontal axis to the right. In addition, close inspection of leads III and aVF suggested the presence of an atrial flutter wave. After sedation, direct-current shock cardioversion was carried out in the emergency room, allowing the restoration of sinus rhythm with a normal QRS complex (Fig. 72.2). Standard laboratory tests, cardiac enzymes, and an echocardiogram were all normal.

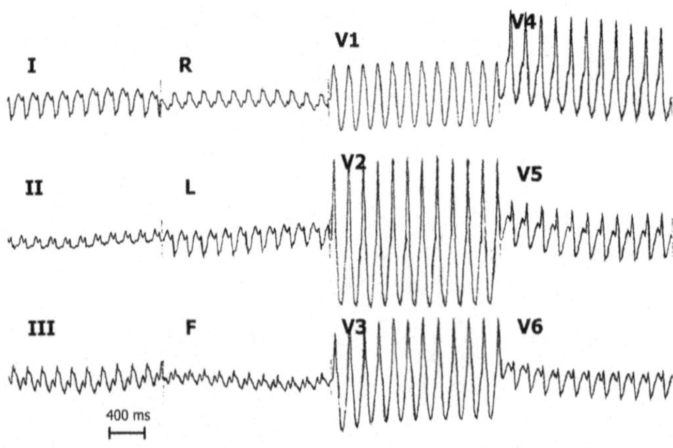

Figure 72.1 The electrocardiogram at admission.

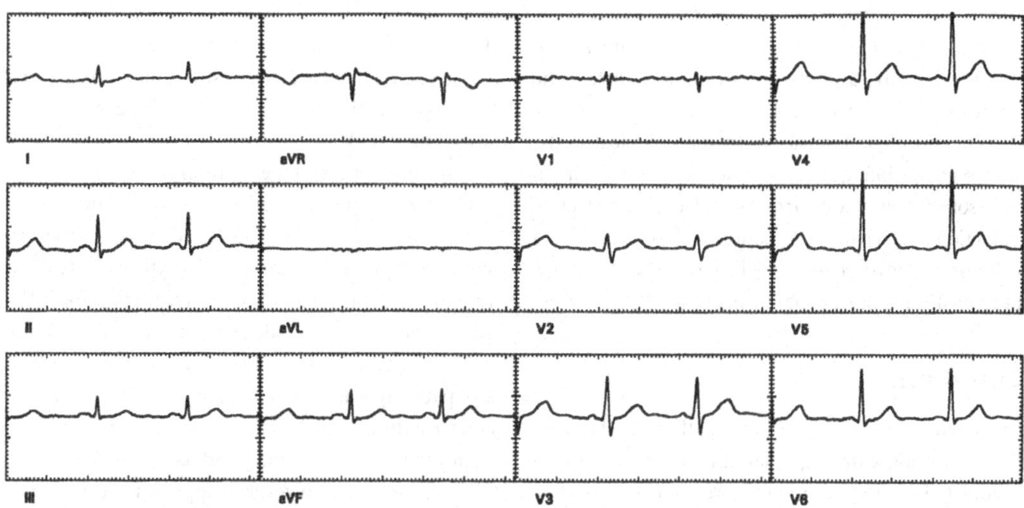

Figure 72.2 Electrocardiogram in sinus rhythm.

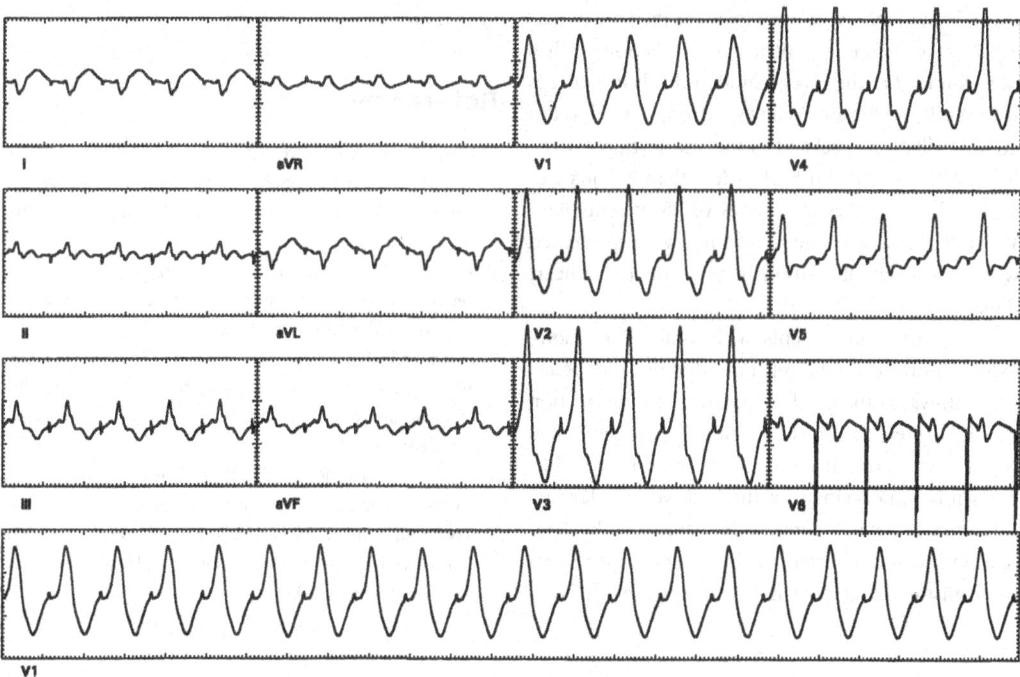

Figure 72.3 Electrocardiogram during coronary sinus stimulation.

The patient was referred for electrophysiological testing. Despite the normal baseline ECG, atrial pacing from coronary sinus showed ventricular preexcitation due to atrioventricular (AV) conduction through a left lateral accessory pathway. The preexcited QRS complex had a morphology similar to that observed during the tachycardia at admission (Fig. 72.3). At a baseline cycle length of 500 ms, the anterograde refractory period of the accessory pathway was less than 210 ms. Orthodromic supraventricular tachycardia with a normal QRS and a heart rate of 170 beats/min was induced with programmed atrial and ventricular stimulation. The accessory AV pathway was used as the retrograde limb of the reentry circuit during the tachycardia. No atrial flutter was induced during the electrophysiological testing.

After completion of the electrophysiological study, successful radiofrequency ablation of the left lateral accessory pathway was carried out. Despite the lack of induction of atrial flutter, ablation of the cavotricuspid isthmus was also performed. The patient has been free of palpitations and syncope during the follow-up period.

Comment

In patients with AV accessory pathways, the ventricular response during atrial fibrillation or flutter is modulated by the anterograde refractory period of the accessory pathway. Accessory pathways with a short anterograde refractory period can show 1 : 1 conduction at rates faster than 300 beats/min, resulting in hemodynamic compromise for the patient and a risk of developing ventricular fibrillation. It has been found that the risk of sudden death in patients with Wolff–Parkinson–White syndrome who develop atrial fibrillation is related to the shortest preexcited RR (SRR) interval. An SRR of less than 250 ms was observed in all cases in a series of 25 patients with Wolff–Parkinson–White syndrome who presented with ventricular fibrillation in the absence of heart disease [1].

Atrial flutter in patients with Wolff–Parkinson–White syndrome is relatively rare. In those with accessory pathways capable of supporting 1 : 1 conduction during flutter, as in the present case, preexcited regular tachycardia at about 300 beats/min is possible. Sudden commencement of the high ventricular rate can produce hemodynamic derangement with hypotension and syncope before vasomotor compensatory mechanisms can increase the blood pressure [2]. Other factors that can contribute to the hemodynamic alteration are abnormal ventricular activation during the preexcited tachycardia, posture, medications, etc. Vasovagal reactions during tachycardia have also been demonstrated [3].

In the present case, preexcitation was absent in sinus rhythm but appeared during coronary sinus pacing (near the atrial insertion of the accessory pathway). Inapparent preexcitation in sinus rhythm is related to differences between the time of conduction from the sinus node to the AV node and to the atrial end of the accessory pathway. In this case, the left lateral accessory pathway was far from the sinus node, so that, in sinus rhythm, ventricular activation was produced mainly through the normal conducting system and the QRS was normal. However, inapparent preexcitation in sinus rhythm can be associated with a short anterograde refractory period in the accessory pathway, leading to high-risk cases of Wolff–Parkinson–White syndrome [4].

References

1 Klein GJ, Bashore TM, Sellers TD, Pritchett EL, Smith WM, Gallagher JJ. Ventricular fibrillation in the Wolff–Parkinson–White syndrome. *N Engl J Med* 1979; **301**: 1080–5.

2 Waxman MB, Wald RW, Cameron DA. Interactions between the autonomic nervous system and tachycardias in man. *Cardiol Clin* 1983; **1**: 143–85.

3 Leitch JW, Klein GJ, Yee R, Leather RA, Kim YH. Syncope associated with supraventricular tachycardia: an expression of tachycardia rate or vasomotor response? *Circulation* 1992; **85**: 1064–71.

4 García Civera R, Ruiz Granell R, Morell Cabedo S, *et al.* Electrofisiologia de las vías accesoria AV comunes. In: Garcia Civera R, Ruiz R, Morell S, *et al.*, eds. *Electrofisiología Cardiaca Clínica y Ablación.* McGraw-Hill Interamericana, Madrid, 1999: 181–203.

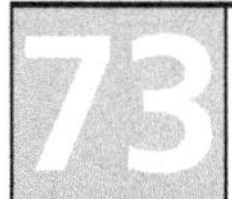

CASE 73

Syncope in a patient with atrial fibrillation: reflex hypotension?

F. Giada, A. Raviele

Case report

A 56-year-old man was referred to the syncope unit due to recurrent syncopes (three episodes in the previous 6 months), which were preceded and followed by palpitations. The syncopes occurred while the patient was standing and were associated with mild trauma. The patient had mild hypertension and hypercholesterolemia, and was taking enalapril (20 mg/day) and pravastatin (40 mg/day).

The physical examination was negative, as were carotid sinus massage and the orthostatic stress test, and he had no evidence of structural heart disease (normal electrocardiogram and echocardiogram). Holter monitoring showed a normal sinus rhythm with frequent supraventricular ectopic beats, and tilt testing with sublingual nitroglycerin administration proved negative.

Since the origin of the syncope was unexplained and there was a high probability of an arrhythmic cause, the patient underwent implantation of a Reveal loop recorder (Medtronic, Inc., Minneapolis, Minnesota, USA). During the follow-up period, the patient had an episode of recurrent syncope and effectively activated the device, which showed an episode of paroxysmal atrial fibrillation with a fast ventricular rate (Fig. 73.1).

To evaluate the role of autonomic reflexes in the genesis of his syncope and to guide the therapeutic approach, the patient underwent a transesophageal electrophysiological study in the upright position at 60° on the tilt table. Blood pressure was monitored continuously during the test. With short atrial bursts, atrial fibrillation was easily induced, and after a few seconds the patient's blood pressure significantly decreased and syncope occurred (Fig. 73.2).

Comment

Syncope is a quite unusual presentation of paroxysmal atrial fibrillation [1], and the ventricular rate at the onset of the arrhythmia is not always the main factor responsible. It has been shown that patients with paroxysmal atrial fibrillation who present with syncope

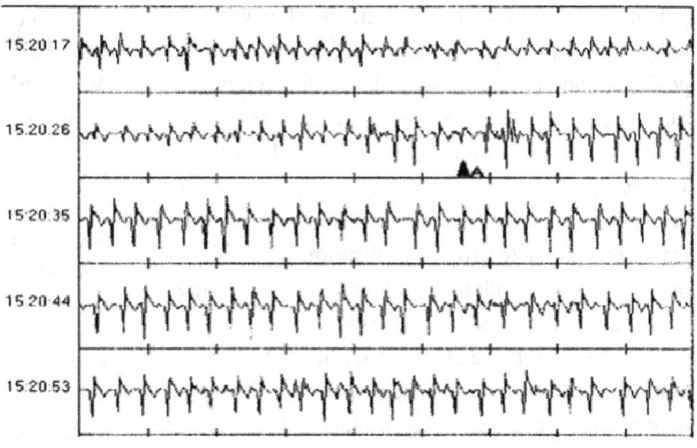

Figure 73.1 The rhythm strip from the implantable loop recorder during spontaneous syncope. Note the paroxysmal atrial fibrillation.

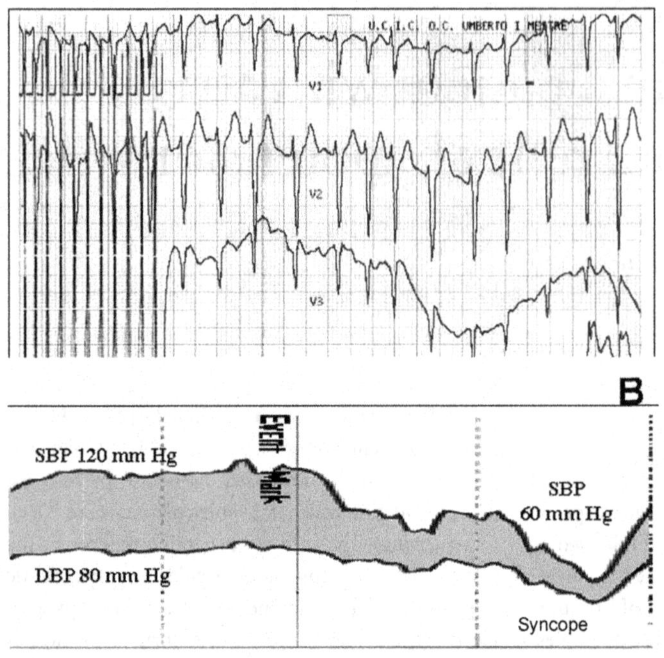

Figure 73.2 The electrocardiographic (A) and noninvasive blood-pressure (B) recordings during induction of atrial fibrillation using transesophageal stimulation with the patient in the upright position at 60° on the tilt table. DBP, diastolic blood pressure; SBP, systolic blood pressure.

may be predisposed to a disturbance of the autonomic nervous system, leading to loss of consciousness [2,3], and these data have had a strong impact on the management of such patients.

In some cases, as in the present report, the electrophysiological study demonstrates that atrial fibrillation is the cause of syncope. In the present patient, the onset of atrial fibrillation triggered a neurally mediated reflex and syncope, probably through the same mechanism suggested for tilt-induced syncope [4]. It can be postulated that the reduced cardiac output induced by atrial fibrillation, together with the reduced ventricular volume caused by the upright position, may activate the neurally mediated reflex. In these cases, treatment should be aimed first of all at preventing the recurrence of atrial fibrillation [3]. This patient underwent isolation of the pulmonary veins using transcatheter radiofrequency ablation, which effectively led to the prevention of both paroxysmal atrial fibrillation and syncope recurrences during a 12-month follow-up period.

It is also possible that the atrial fibrillation could have a vagal-dependent mechanism, secondary to intense vagal stimulation occurring at the time of neurally mediated syncope [5]. In such cases, the therapeutic approach should be aimed at preventing the neurally mediated reflex [3].

References

1 Brignole M, Alboni P, Benditt D, *et al.* Guidelines on management (diagnosis and treatment) of syncope. *Eur Heart J* 2001; **22:** 1256–306.

2 Leitch JW, Klein GJ, Yee R, *et al.* Syncope associated with supraventricular tachycardia: an expression of tachycardia rate or vasomotor response? *Circulation* 1992; **85:** 1064–71.

3 Brignole M, Gianfranchi L, Menozzi C, *et al.* Role of autonomic reflexes in syncope associated with paroxysmal atrial fibrillation. *J Am Coll Cardiol* 1993; **22:** 1123–9.

4 Raviele A, Giada F, Brignole M, *et al.* Diagnostic accuracy of sublingual nitroglycerin test and low-dose isoproterenol test in patients with unexplained syncope. *Am J Cardiol* 2000; **85:** 1194–8.

5 Coumel P, Leclercq JF, Attuel P, *et al.* Autonomic influences in the genesis of atrial fibrillation: atrial flutter and fibrillation of vagal origin. In: Narula OS, ed. *Cardiac Arrhythmias: Electrophysiology, Diagnosis and Management.* Williams & Wilkins, Baltimore, 1979: 243–55.

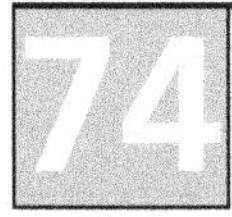

CASE 74

Neuromediated syncope inducing atrial fibrillation

R. García Civera, R. Ruiz Granell, S. Morell Cabedo, R. Sanjuán Mañez

Case report

A 68-year-old woman was admitted to the emergency department due to an episode of syncope followed by persistent irregular palpitations. She had a history of mild hypertension treated with beta-blockers and diuretics. Two months previously, she had suffered a similar episode of syncope followed by palpitations that ended spontaneously (after approximately half an hour) and had not sought medical assistance.

The physical examination showed an irregular pulse with a mean heart rate of 120 beats/min and a blood pressure of 160/75 mmHg. No signs of cardiac failure were found, and the standard analytical tests were normal. The electrocardiogram (ECG) confirmed the presence of atrial fibrillation with a mean ventricular rate of 110 beats/min and normal QRS morphology (Fig. 74.1).

A successful electrical cardioversion was performed, and the patient remained in sinus rhythm with a heart rate around 60 beats/min and a blood pressure of 175/70 mmHg. An echocardiographic examination did not detect any significant anomalies.

A head-up tilt-table test was carried out due to the presence of syncope with a normal baseline ECG and an absence of structural heart disease. Figure 74.2 shows the results of the tilt-table test. The baseline heart rate was 52 beats/min, rising to 60 beats/min

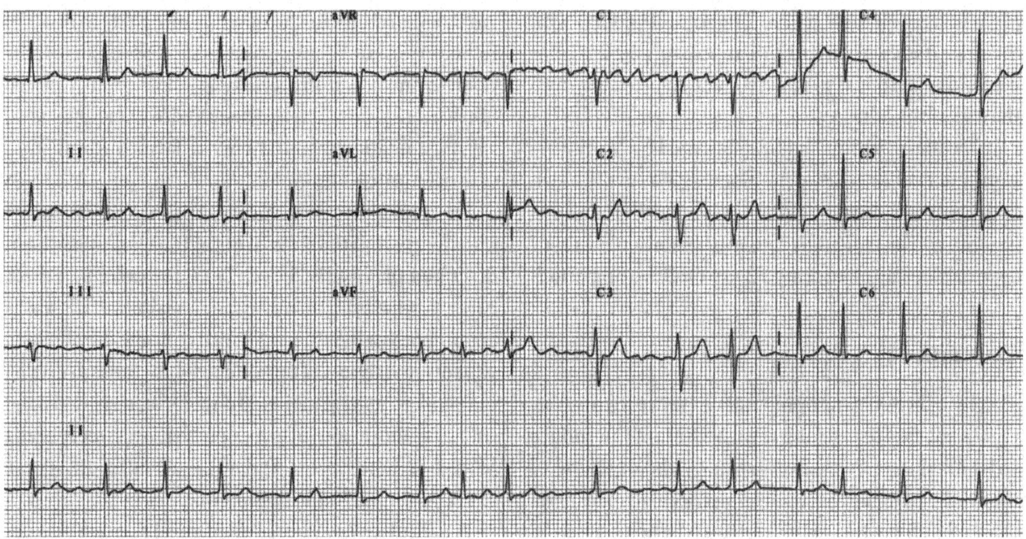

Figure 74.1 The electrocardiogram at admission.

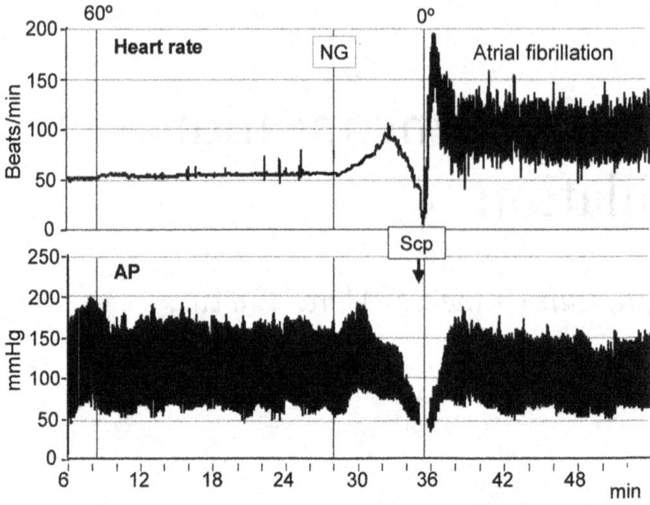

Figure 74.2 The head-up tilt-table test. AP, arterial pressure (noninvasive tonometric measurements; 60° and 0° represent the tilting points); NG, nitroglycerin administration (400 μg sublingual); Scp, syncope.

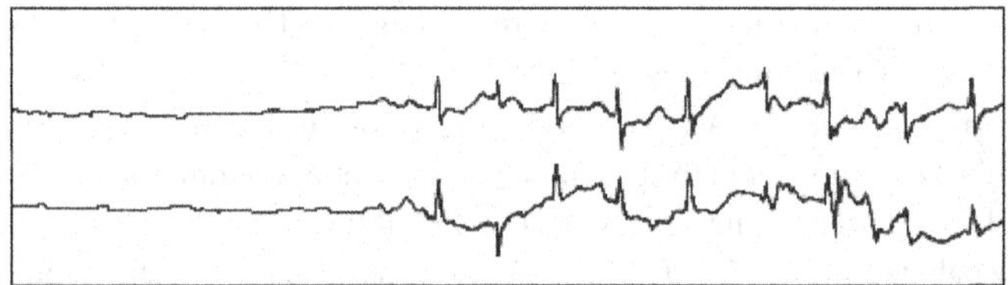

Figure 74.3 The asystole ended with the appearance of atrial fibrillation with an irregular ventricular response.

with tilting without any significant change in blood pressure. This blunted effect on the heart rate was probably due to the beta-blocker effect. Administration of 400 μg of sublingual nitroglycerin initially produced an increase in the heart rate, followed 2 min later by a fall in blood pressure and heart rate that gave place to asystole lasting 22 s. The asystole ended with the appearance of atrial fibrillation with an irregular ventricular response (Fig. 74.3), which persisted until the end of the test.

After sinus rhythm had been restored by cardioversion, medication with beta-blockers was withdrawn and replaced with angiotensin-converting enzyme inhibitors. The patient had no further episodes of syncope or palpitations during a 2-year follow-up period.

Comment

There are three separate points of relevance in this case. Firstly, the fact that strong vagal activation can induce atrial fibrillation is clearly shown by the outcome of the head-up tilt test. Secondly, this mechanism can become clinically active, giving rise to a type of bradycardia–tachycardia syndrome that could be termed "neuromediated syncope-induced atrial fibrillation." Thirdly, in this subset of patients, preventing vasovagal syncope would prevent paroxysms of atrial fibrillation.

In 1921, Lewis *et al.* showed that vagal stimulation caused atrial fibrillation in dogs [1]. Subsequently, experimental studies demonstrated that an increase in vagal tone results in shortening of the effective atrial refractory period, an increase in dispersion of the refractoriness, and an increase in vulnerability to atrial fibrillation [1–3]. The electrophysiological effects of vagal stimulation would therefore favor the induction of atrial fibrillation.

The possibility that vasovagal syncope can occasionally elicit paroxysms of atrial fibrillation has been described previously. Leitch *et al.* [4] described three patients with syncope in whom atrial fibrillation was documented after the syncopal episode. In all three patients, syncope was reproduced during head-up tilting, and in two patients atrial fibrillation occurred with the induction of syncope that was temporally related to bradycardia and vagal stimulation. These cases are similar to the present one.

The incidence of induction of atrial fibrillation during tilt-table testing is not well known. In one study

[5], atrial fibrillation was induced during tilt-table tests in one of 73 patients with a positive test (1.4%); in the study by Del Rosso *et al.* [6], three of 119 patients with tilt-induced syncope (2.5%) developed atrial fibrillation after a prolonged asystolic pause.

Coumel *et al.* proposed the concept of "vagal atrial fibrillation." In these patients, paroxysms of atrial fibrillation occur at least 90% of the time during sleep or after dinner, when vagal tone is predominant [7,8]. It is not known whether there is a possible relationship between cases of atrial fibrillation induced by vasovagal syncope and vagal fibrillation in the sense of the Coumel definition. In a recent report, van der Berg *et al.* [9] found that patients with presumed vagal atrial fibrillation were characterized by increased vagal tone (referring to overall long-term activity of the autonomic nervous system) but normal vagal reactivity (short-term reactivity to vagal stimulation).

References

1 Lewis T, Drury AN, Bulger HA. Observations upon flutter and fibrillation, vii: the effects of vagal stimulation. *Heart* 1921; **8**: 141–69.

2 Kneller J, Zou R, Vigmond EJ, Wang Z, Leon LJ, Nattel S. Cholinergic atrial fibrillation in a computer model of two-dimensional sheet of canine atrial cells with realistic ionic properties. *Circ Res* 2002; **90**: E73–E78.

3 Hirose M, Carlson MD, Laurita KR. Cellular mechanism of vagally mediated atrial tachyarrhythmia in isolated arterially perfused canine right atria. *J Cardiovasc Electrophysiol* 2002; **13**: 926–8.

4 Leitch J, Klein G, Yee R, *et al.* Neurally mediated syncope and atrial fibrillation. *N Engl J Med* 1991; **324**: 495–6.

5 García Civera R, Sanjuán R, Ruiz R, *et al.* "Patrones" electrocardiográficos de cardioinhibición durantel las pruebas de basculación. Un estudio controlado con registros de Holter [abstract]. *Rev Esp Cardiol* 2001; **54** (Suppl 2): 133.

6 Del Rosso A, Bartoli P, Bartoletti A, *et al.* Shortened head-up tilt testing potentiated with sublingual nitroglycerin in patients with unexplained syncope. *Am Heart J* 1998; **135**: 564–70.

7 Coumel P, Attuel P, Lavallee J, Flammang D, LeClercq JF, Slama R. The atrial arrhythmia syndrome of vagal origin. *Arch Mal Coeur Vaiss* 1978; **71**: 645–56.

8 Coumel P. Autonomic influences in atrial tachyarrhythmias. *J Cardiovasc Electrophysiol* 1996; **7**: 999–1007.

9 van der Berg MP, Hassink RJ, Baljé-Volkers C, Crijns HJGM. Role of the autonomic nervous system in vagal atrial fibrillation. *Heart* 2003; **89**: 333–4.

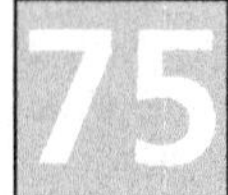

CASE 75

Effort presyncope due to idiopathic right ventricular tachycardia

R. García Civera, R. Ruiz Granell, S. Morell Cabedo, R. Sanjuán Mañez

Case report

A 22-year-old woman, who was a marathon runner, was referred for examination due to presyncopal attacks associated with rapid palpitations during heavy exercise. In the previous few months, the patient had had three episodes of paroxysmal palpitations and presyncopal symptoms (instability, light-headedness, and blurring vision) that forced her to interrupt her sports activity. Once she had stopped the exercise, the palpitations ended suddenly and spontaneously within a few minutes. The physical examination was normal. The electrocardiogram (Fig. 75.1) was also normal, and an echocardiographic examination did not show any valvular or obstructive abnormalities.

An exercise stress test with a modified Mader protocol was carried out. In the 20th minute of exercise, regular tachycardia at 170 beats/min with a wide QRS complex developed (Fig. 75.2), associated with presyncopal symptoms. The QRS during the tachycardia

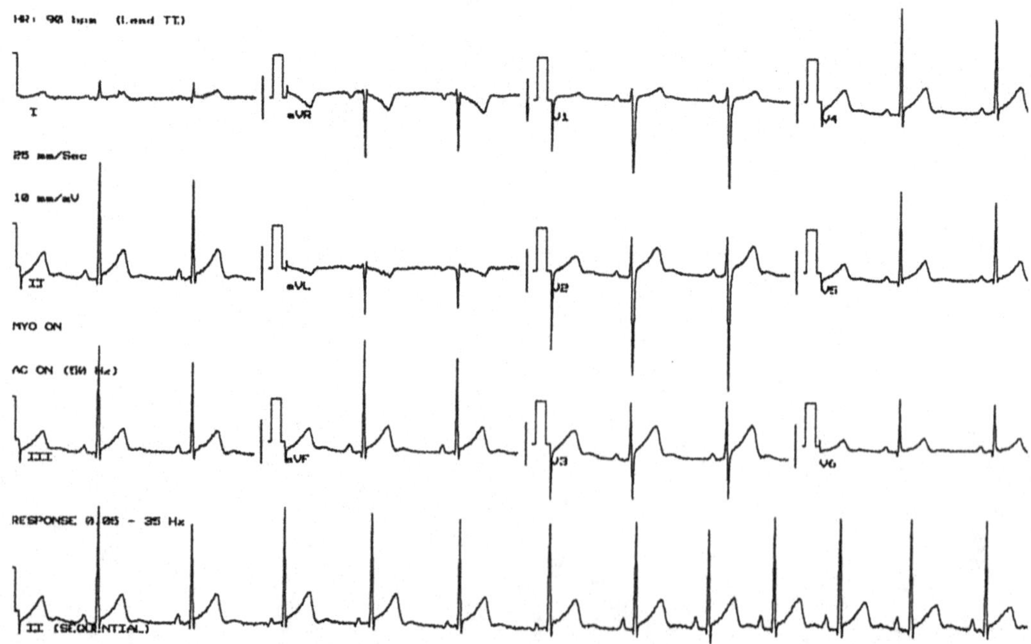

Figure 75.1 The baseline electrocardiogram.

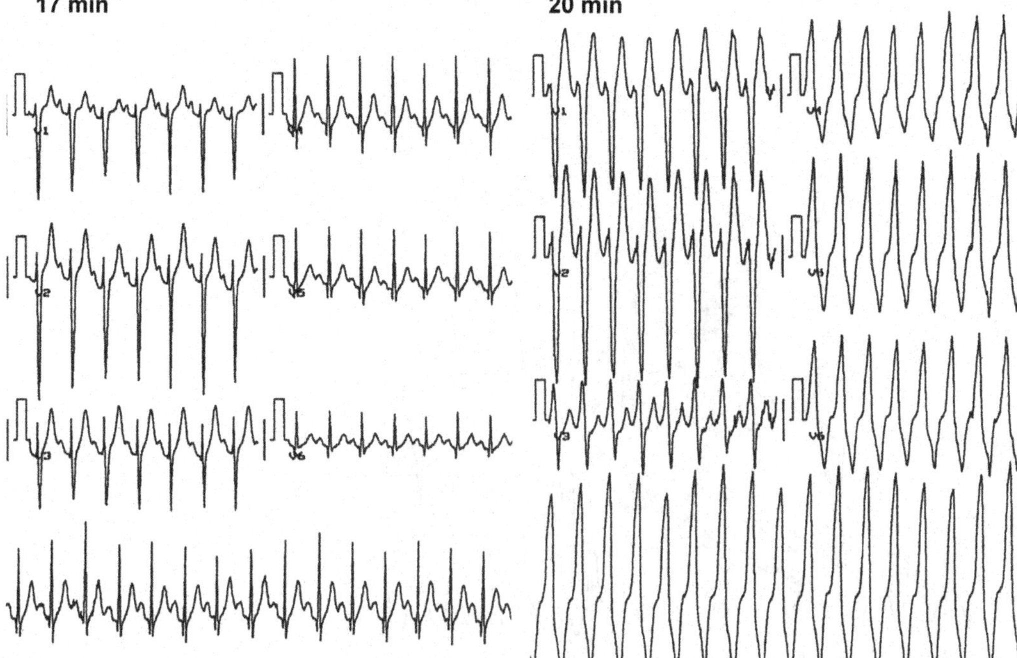

Figure 75.2 Exercise stress test.

had a left bundle-branch block configuration and a right inferior frontal plane axis. The tachycardia ended spontaneously once the exercise was stopped.

An electrophysiological study was conducted, on the basis of a suspicion of idiopathic ventricular tachycardia of the right ventricular outflow tract. At the baseline, programmed heart stimulation did not induce any arrhythmia. After isoproterenol infusion, rapid ventricular stimulation was able to induce short runs of ventricular tachycardia originating in the right outflow tract and a QRS morphology similar to that seen during the exercise test. Precise localization of the origin of the tachycardia was obtained by pace mapping (Fig. 75.3), and radiofrequency ablation was carried out. After ablation, the patient returned to competitive sports activities.

Comment

Syncope during effort can be due to obstructive, arrhythmic, or neurally mediated causes.

Effort syncope of arrhythmic cause can be present in patients with or without structural heart disease. Although a great variety of arrhythmias can be induced during effort, ventricular tachycardia is the most characteristic. In chronic ischemic heart disease, ischemia and the increase in catecholamines induced by the effort can trigger ventricular arrhythmias and syncope [1]. However, in patients with chronic recurrent ventricular tachycardia after myocardial infarction, the induction of the tachycardia by effort is relatively infrequent. Conversely, the ventricular tachycardia of arrhythmogenic right ventricular dysplasia [2] and idiopathic monomorphic ventricular tachycardias [3] are frequently induced by effort. In congenital long QT syndromes, polymorphic ventricular tachycardia (*torsade de pointes*) can be induced by effort. Indeed, in the three better-characterized congenital long QT syndromes (LQT1, LQT2, and LQT3), effort was the trigger of 66% of the events in LQT1 patients, 19% of those in LQT2 patients, and only in 8% of those in LQT3 patients [4]. Effort is also the main trigger of the rare cases of polymorphic catecholamine-dependent idiopathic ventricular tachycardia [5].

Infrequently, effort can induce high-degree atrioventricular (AV) block. When this happens, it is, practically always, in patients with a previous bundle-branch block. Exercise-induced AV block has been shown to be invariably located distal to the AV node

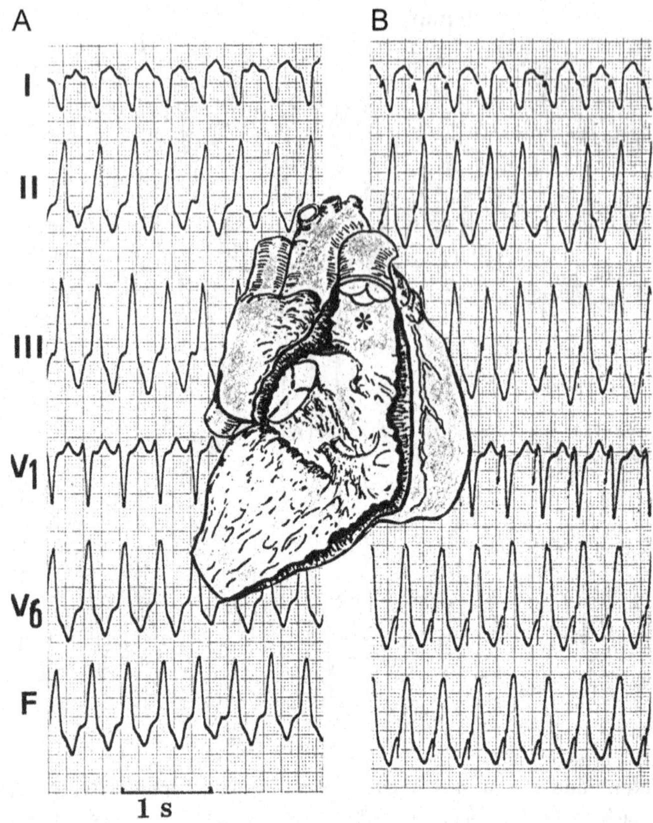

Figure 75.3 **A.** Induced ventricular tachycardia (150 beats/min). **B.** Pace mapping in the right ventricular outflow tract.

and is a prognostic finding for progression to chronic AV block [6–8].

Idiopathic ventricular tachycardia arising from the outflow tract of the right ventricle is frequently related to effort and is often initiated during exercise testing [3]. Induction of the tachycardia by programmed stimulation of the heart is generally possible, but isoproterenol infusion is often necessary [3]. The mechanism of this type of tachycardia is not fully clarified. On the basis of the response to programmed stimulation and the effect of several drugs in terminating the tachycardia, Lerman *et al.* [9] suggested that the mechanism is triggered activity mediated by cyclic adenosine monophosphate (cAMP).

References

1 Coumel P, Leenhardt A, Haddad G. Exercise ECG: prognostic implications of exercise induced arrhythmias. *Pacing Clin Electrophysiol* 1994; **17**: 417–27.

2 Marcus FI, Fontaine GH. Arrhythmogenic right ventricular dysplasia/cardiomyopathy: a review. *Pacing Clin Electrophysiol* 1995; **18**: 1298–314.

3 Mont LL, Seixas T, Brugada P, *et al.* Clinical and electrophysiologic characteristics of exercise related idiopathic ventricular tachycardia. *Am J Cardiol* 1991; **68**: 897–900.

4 Schwartz PJ. The long QT syndrome. In: Camm AJ, ed. *Clinical Approaches to Tachyarrhythmias*, vol. 7. Futura Publishing, Armonk, New York, 1997: 56.

5 Leenhardt A, Lucet V, Denjoy I, Grau F, Ngoc DD, Coumel P. Catecholaminergic polymorphic ventricular tachycardia in children: a 7-year follow-up of 21 patients. *Circulation* 1995; **91**: 1512–9.

6 Woelfel AK, Simpson RJ Jr, Gettes LS, Foster JR. Exercise-induced distal atrioventricular block. *J Am Coll Cardiol* 1983; **2**: 578–81.

7 Barra M, Brignole M, Menozzi C, Sartore B, De Marchi E, Bertulla A. [Intermittent atrioventricular block induced by exertion: description of three cases; in Italian.] *G Ital Cardiol* 1985; **15**: 1051–5.

8 Finci A, Bruno A, Perondi R. Exercise-induced paroxysmal atrioventricular block during nuclear perfusion stress testing: evidence for transient ischemia of the conduction system. *G Ital Cardiol* 1999; **29**: 1313–7.

9 Lerman BB, Belardinelli L, West GA, *et al.* Adenosine sensitive ventricular tachycardia: evidence suggesting cyclic AMP-mediated triggered activity. *Circulation* 1986; **74**: 270–80.

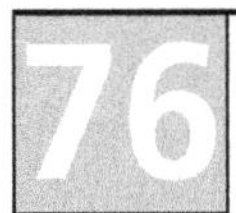

CASE 76

Syncope due to idiopathic left ventricular tachycardia

L. García Riesco, A. Pedrote Martínez, E. Arana, G. Barón Esquivias, F. Errázquin Sáenz de Tejada

Case report

A 25-year-old man without any significant medical history presented at a local emergency room after a syncopal episode. He had previously noted palpitations while playing football. A wide complex tachycardia at 200 beats/min with a right bundle-branch block and left axis deviation morphology in the QRS was documented on a 12-lead electrocardiogram (ECG) (Fig. 76.1).

The tachycardia did not respond to 12 mg of intravenous adenosine, but ended after intravenous administration of 15 mg of verapamil. The physical examination was normal. The cardiac evaluation showed a normal resting ECG and chest radiograph. Transthoracic echocardiography was also normal, with no evidence of structural heart disease.

The tachycardia tracing suggested ventricular tachycardia originating from the left ventricle. An electrophysiological study was subsequently carried out, and a sustained monomorphic ventricular tachycardia with a single morphology was induced from the right ventricular apex by using double and triple ventricular extrastimuli, both in the baseline state and during isoprenaline infusion. The morphology of the tachycardia was identical to that seen at presentation, with a cycle length of 300 ms.

On the basis of the morphology, the tachycardia was thought to originate from the posterior fascicle of the left bundle branch. Pace mapping in this region revealed an area with pace maps identical to the tachycardia. A high-frequency potential, corresponding to the Purkinje system (Fig. 76.2), was identified in this site. Several radiofrequency applications in the region ended the tachycardia. It was later impossible to induce the tachycardia even with isoprenaline. At the time of writing, the patient was still asymptomatic, with no new episodes of tachycardia.

Comment

Idiopathic left ventricular tachycardia generally occurs in young patients with no structural heart disease. This type of ventricular tachycardia often has the morphology of right bundle-branch block with a leftward frontal axis, is frequently provoked by exercise, and may respond to verapamil [1]. It usually originates from the posterior fascicle at the inferior left ventricular apex or midseptal region, although there is another infrequent variety originating in the anterior fascicle. In the latter type, the QRS during the tachycardia shows a right bundle-branch block and right axis deviation [2]. The prognosis in left fascicular tachycardia is generally good, with only rare reports of sudden death [1].

In this case, the clinical presentation (exertional syncope), the response to verapamil, the QRS morphology, and the absence of structural heart disease all suggested the diagnosis of idiopathic ventricular tachycardia originating in the posterior fascicle.

In these cases, high success rates have been reported with radiofrequency catheter ablation. Several different criteria have been used to target successful ablation sites, the most widely accepted being that guided by recordings of Purkinje potentials. However, this finding is not specific for successful ablation [3]. The evidence suggests that the mechanism of this form of ventricular

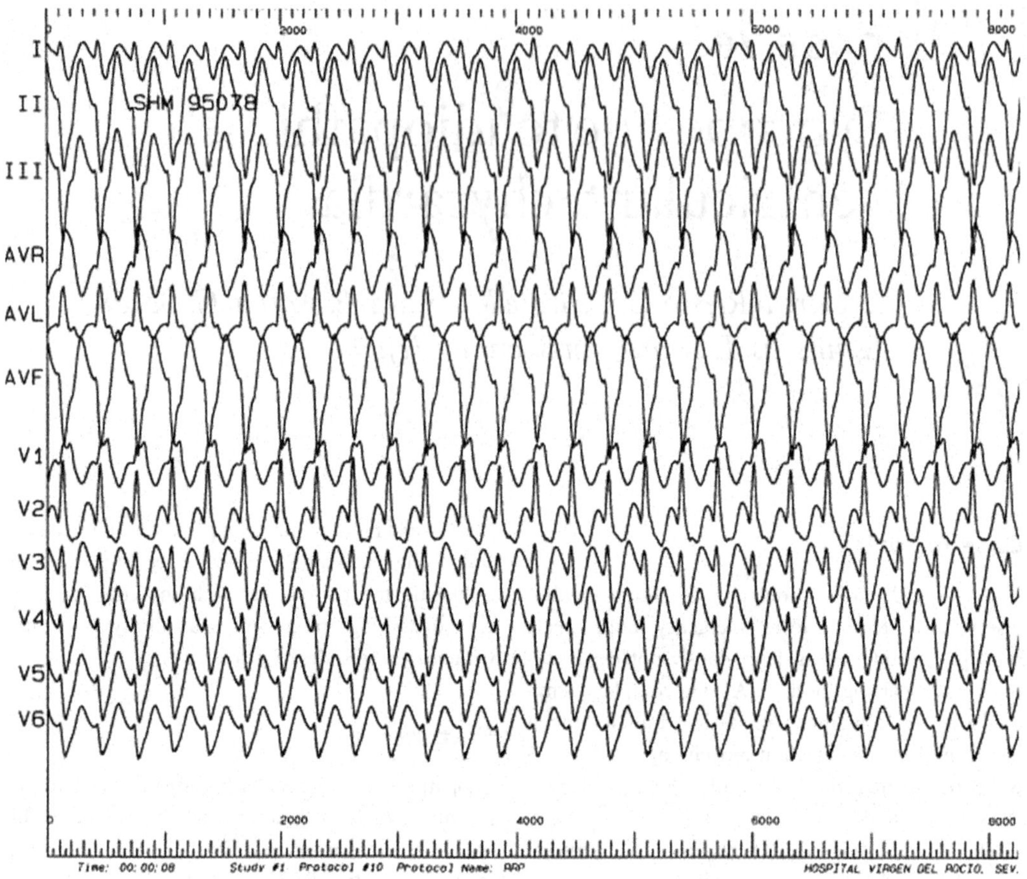

Figure 76.1 Electrocardiography of idiopathic left ventricular tachycardia originating from the left posterior fascicle, with a right bundle-branch block and left axis deviation morphology.

tachycardia is macroreentry with utilization of the Purkinje system. This conclusion was drawn from the characteristic response of the tachycardia to entrainment mapping, with the area of slow conduction of the tachycardia circuit being near the Purkinje network [4]. It has also been demonstrated that the area of slow conduction within the tachycardia circuit is calcium-dependent and that the cycle length of the tachycardia can be extended with verapamil administration [5].

The vast majority of these patients are readily curable with current catheter ablation techniques. The site of successful ablation is the site at which a characteristic high-frequency P-potential is recorded, which appears to identify the exit site of the slow conduction zone. It is therefore advisable to take this type of tachycardia into account in young patients with no structural heart disease who present with ventricular tachycardia, particularly if the tachycardia responds to verapamil.

References

1 Blanck Z. Bundle branch reentrant ventricular tachycardia: cumulative experience in 48 patients. *J Cardiovasc Electrophysiol* 1993; **4**: 253–62.

2 Wen M, Yeh S, Wang C, *et al.* Radiofrequency ablation therapy in idiopathic left ventricular tachycardia with no obvious structural heart disease. *Circulation* 1994; **89**: 1690–6.

3 Nakawaga H, Beckman KJ, McClelland JH, *et al.* Radiofrequency catheter ablation of idiopathic left ventricular tachycardia guided by a Purkinje potential. *Circulation* 1993; **88**: 2607–17.

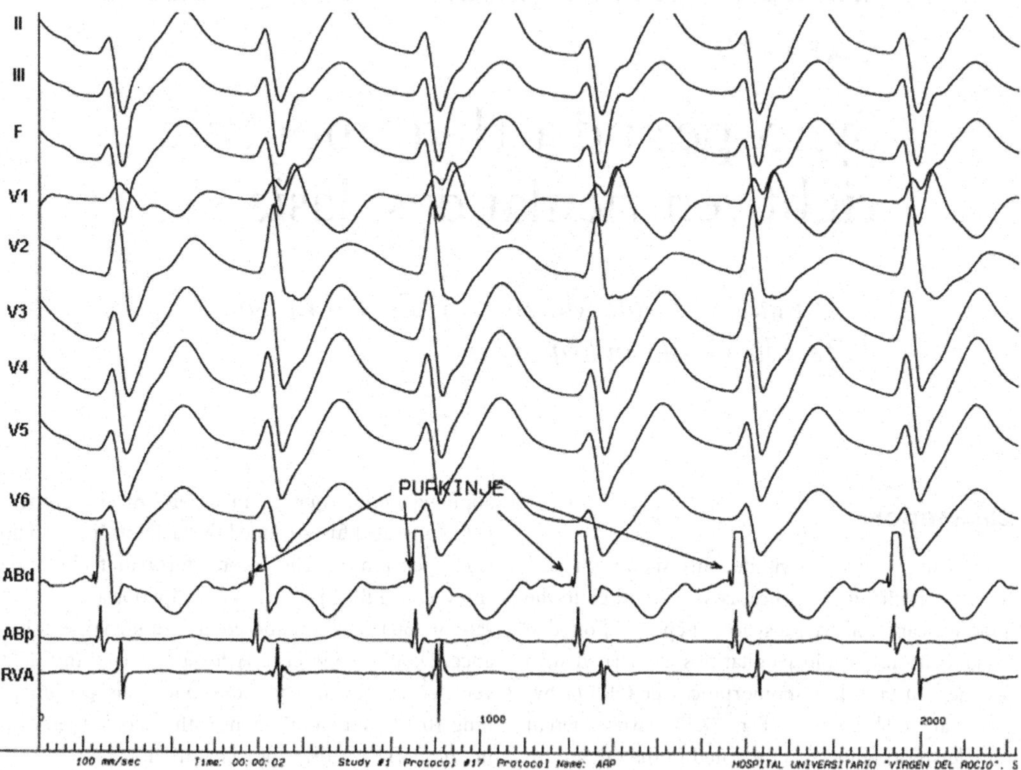

Figure 76.2 Intracardiac electrograms in the zone of the left posterior fascicle, showing the Purkinje potentials that were used as a target for ablating the tachycardia.

4 Maruyama M. Demonstration of the reentrant circuit of verapamil-sensitive idiopathic left ventricular tachycardia: direct evidence for macroreentry as the underlying mechanism. *J Cardiovasc Electrophysiol* 2001; **12**: 968–72.

5 Tsuchiya T. Effects of verapamil and lidocaine on two components of the re-entry circuit of verapamil-sensitive idiopathic left ventricular tachycardia. *J Am Coll Cardiol* 2001; **37**: 1415–21.

CASE 77

Syncope and arrhythmogenic right ventricular dysplasia

E. Arana, A. Pedrote Martínez, F. Errázquin Sáenz de Tejada, G. Barón Esquivias

Case report

A 22-year-old woman without any significant personal or familial medical history was admitted to the intensive-care unit after a syncopal episode preceded by sudden-onset rapid palpitations, associated with complex, sustained, monomorphic wide QRS tachycardia at 260 beats/min (Fig. 77.1). Two different complex morphologies were noted in the QRS, both similar to left bundle-branch block (LBBB), but one with the superior axis in the frontal plane and the other with the inferior axis. Suppression of the arrhythmia required an external direct-current shock of 150 J. Acute causes of ventricular tachycardia were excluded (myocardial ischemia, prolonged QT interval, electrolyte imbalance, etc.). The physical examination was normal. The baseline electrocardiogram showed a sinus rhythm, with the frontal axis at 30°, a PR interval of 160 ms, a QRS duration in lead V_1 of 119 ms, and T wave inversion in the right precordial leads (V_1 to V_4). The QT interval was normal.

Image studies included a normal echocardiogram and cardiac magnetic resonance imaging, which identified pulmonary infundibular hypokinesia with mild dilation and wall thinning in the right ventricle. Right ventricle angiography showed a redundant trabeculation in the septal, apical, and infundibular regions. The left ventricle and coronary arteries were normal.

An electrophysiological study was carried out, and two different forms of ventricular tachycardia were induced. The first type of ventricular tachycardia showed an LBBB pattern and an inferior axis, with a rate of 260 beats/min. The origin of the tachycardia was located in the right ventricular outflow tract, and applying radiofrequency in a zone of entrainment with concealed fusion ended the tachycardia, with no later recurrences. The second form of tachycardia showed an LBBB pattern and a superior axis, with a rate of 230 beats/min and good hemodynamic tolerance. Despite good criteria for ablation at the right ventricular apex (mesodiastolic potentials, pace mapping 10/12, and entrainment with fusion), there was no success in ablating this tachycardia.

Treatment with sotalol was started, and another electrophysiological study was conducted, during which the unablated tachycardia was reproduced (at a lower rate). After the sotalol dosage had been increased, 24-h Holter monitoring showed a mean heart rate of 55 beats/min, with isolated ventricular ectopic beats. The patient continued to be asymptomatic during a 2-year follow-up period.

Comment

Arrhythmogenic right ventricular dysplasia (ARVD) is a myocardial disease characterized by progressive right ventricular dysfunction as a consequence of fibrofatty replacement of the myocardium. Clinical manifestations include ventricular arrhythmias, mainly involving ventricular tachycardia with LBBB morphology, which may lead to sudden death [1].

The etiology, pathogenesis, and real prevalence of ARVD are unknown. In an anatomopathological study, ARVD was found in 20% of patients with sudden death under the age of 35. A familial background has been demonstrated in 30–50% of cases, with an autosomal pattern of inheritance, variable penetrance, and a polymorphic phenotype expression [1].

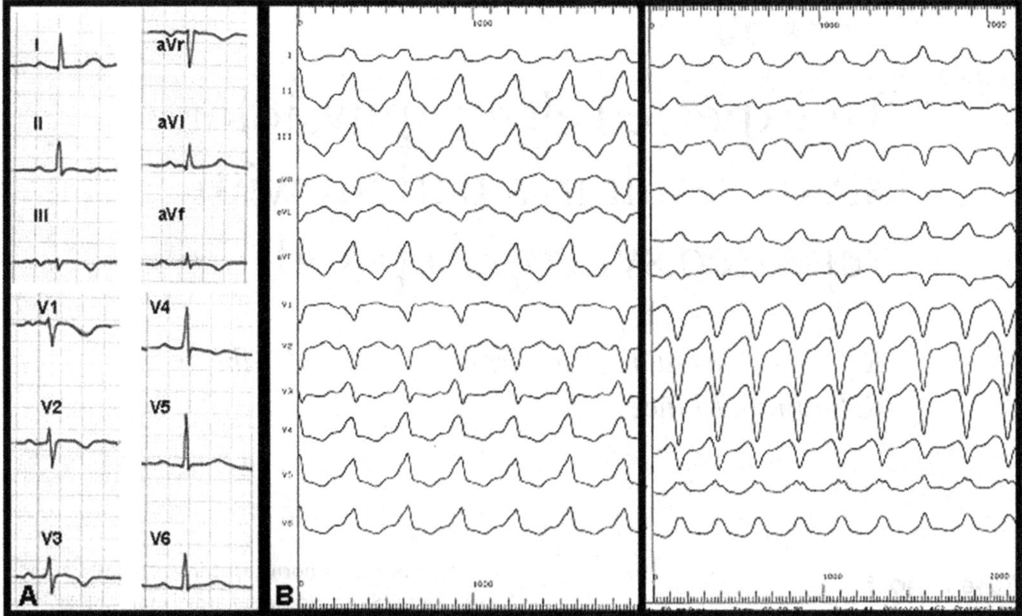

Figure 77.1 A. Electrocardiography in sinus rhythm. **B.** Two tachycardia morphologies are detected.

ARVD is a complex entity. The possible types of presentation include asymptomatic forms, ventricular arrhythmias, and occasionally sudden death [2]. Syncope is common in patients with ARVD and is usually related to ventricular tachycardia, which is often induced by effort.

The differential diagnosis of ARVD includes Uhl's anomaly and cases of idiopathic right ventricular tachycardia. Due to the diagnostic difficulties, the European Society of Cardiology has established standardized diagnostic criteria based on the structural, clinical, histological, and electrocardiographic findings [2]. In the present case, in addition to the findings of the cardiac magnetic resonance, the T wave inversion in the right precordial leads and the induction of more than one ventricular tachycardia strongly suggest the presence of ARVD.

Intracardiac electrophysiological studies are usually carried out in symptomatic patients with suspected ARVD, as well as asymptomatic patients with a high suspicion of "high-risk" ARVD (a familial history of sudden death, unsustained ventricular tachycardia, or depressed ventricular function) [1,3]. The aim in the electrophysiological studies is to evaluate the arrhythmogenic potential, to assess clinical tolerance for induced arrhythmias, and to establish the feasibility of radiofrequency ablation. Catheter ablation is associated with a high rate of initial success (60–90%), but also a high recurrence rate (up to 60% of cases), possibly due to the natural progression of the disease, with the appearance of new arrhythmogenic foci [3].

The implantable cardioverter-defibrillator is indicated in high-risk patients and patients with poorly tolerated ventricular tachycardia that does not respond to pharmacological treatment [4].

References

1 Corrado D, Basso C, Thiene G. Arrhythmogenic right ventricular cardiomyopathy: diagnosis, prognosis, and treatment. *Heart* 2000; **83**: 588–95.

2 Corrado D, Fontaine G, Marcus FI, *et al.* Arrhythmogenic right ventricular dysplasia/cardiomyopathy: need for an international registry. Study Group on Arrhythmogenic Right Ventricular Dysplasia/Cardiomyopathy of the Working Groups on Myocardial and Pericardial Disease and Arrhythmias of the European Society of Cardiology and of the Scientific Council on Cardiomyopathies of the World Heart Federation. *Circulation* 2000; **101**: E101–6.

3 Ellison KE, Friedman PL, Ganz LI, *et al.* Entrainment mapping and radiofrequency catheter ablation of ventricular tachycardia in right ventricular dysplasia. *J Am Coll Cardiol* 1998; **32**: 7424–8.

4 Witcher T, Paul M, Wollmann C, *et al.* Implantable cardioverter/defibrillator therapy in arrhythmogenic right ventricular cardiomyopathy: single-center experience of long-term follow-up and complications in 60 patients. *Circulation* 2004; **109**: 1503–8.

CASE 78

Unexpected electrophysiology study result in a patient with repeated syncopal episodes

R. García Civera, R. Ruiz Granell, S. Morell Cabedo, R. Sanjuán Mañez

Case report

A 72-year-old woman was referred to the electrophysiology laboratory with a history of repeated syncopal attacks during the previous 2 years. The syncopal episodes appeared without triggers or prodromal symptoms. The patient had been evaluated previously, and structural heart disease was ruled out by history, physical evaluation, electrocardiography (ECG), Holter monitoring, and echocardiography. A tilt-table test had also been carried out, with a normal response being obtained.

The ECG recorded in the electrophysiological study (EPS) (Fig. 78.1A) showed a sinus rhythm at a rate of 63 beats/min, a normal PR interval (0.14 s), and a narrow QRS complex with normal morphology. The His bundle recordings in sinus rhythm (Fig. 78.1B) showed a split His bundle deflection (H and H′), with intervals AH, H–H′, and H′V of 110, 60, and 50 ms, respectively. Programmed atrial and ventricular stimulation was not able to induce any significant arrhythmia. After the EPS, the patient had a pacemaker implanted and her syncopal attacks resolved.

Comment

Several studies have shown that the probability of a positive EPS in cases of syncope of unknown cause

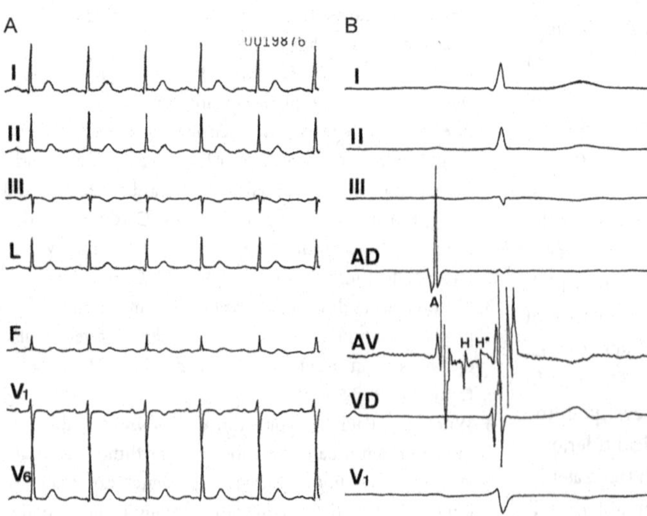

Figure 78.1 Normal electrocardiogram (A) and His bundle recording (B), showing a first-degree intra-His block. I, II, III, L, F, V_1 and V_6 are the electrocardiography leads; AD, bipolar high right atrium; AV, His bundle electrogram; VD, right ventricle.

after the initial clinical evaluation depends on the presence of some of the following criteria [1–4]: structural heart disease; abnormal ECG; significant but nonsyncopal arrhythmias on Holter monitoring; palpitations during the episode; and a family history of sudden death.

The present case does not meet any of the previous criteria, and the possibility of a positive EPS is therefore very low. However, there are always exceptions. In this case, EPS was performed because of the repeated syncopal attacks. A typical intrahisian block was demonstrated in the EPS [5,6], and subsequent pacemaker implantation made the syncopal relapses disappear, suggesting that the cause of the syncope was a high-degree paroxysmal truncal block.

References

1 Brignole M, Alboni P, Benditt DG, *et al.* Task Force on Syncope, European Society of Cardiology. Guidelines on management (diagnosis and treatment) of syncope. *Eur Heart J* 2001; **22**: 1256–306.

2 Krol RB, Morady F, Flacker GC, *et al.* Electrophysiologic testing in patients with unexplained syncope: clinical and noninvasive predictors of outcome. *J Am Coll Cardiol* 1987; **10**: 358–63.

3 Alboni P, Brignole M, Menozzi C, *et al.* Diagnostic value of history in patients with syncope with or without heart disease. *J Am Coll Cardiol* 2001; **37**: 1921–8.

4 Garcia-Civera R, Ruiz-Granell R, Morell-Cabedo S, *et al.* Selective use of diagnostic tests in patients with syncope of unknown cause. *J Am Coll Cardiol* 2003; **41**: 787–90.

5 Garcia-Civera R, Sanjuán R, Ferrero JA, *et al.* Estudio electrofisiológico de los bloqueos tronculares del haz de His. *Rev Esp Cardiol* 1975; **28**: 205–17.

6 Guimond CL, Puech P. Intra-His bundle blocks (102 cases). *Eur J Cardiol* 1976; **4**: 481–93.

CASE 79

Syncope in a patient with right bundle-branch block and alternating anterior and posterior left fascicular block

A. García Alberola

Case report

A 68-year-old woman presented at the emergency department following a syncopal event. She had a history of chronic hypertension (treated with diltiazem and torasemide) and hypercholesterolemia managed with atorvastatin. Type 2 diabetes had been diagnosed 6 months previously, and a hypocaloric diet had been prescribed. Otherwise the patient was healthy, her physical activity was adequate, and she was not taking other drugs.

One year before admission, the patient had suffered an episode of syncope while standing, without prodromal symptoms. She recovered spontaneously within a few seconds and did not ask for medical assistance. A second episode of syncope preceded by dizziness occurred 4 months later while the patient was sitting. Finally, on the day of admission, the patient fainted suddenly while walking, resulting in a mild head injury, with full recovery within a few minutes. A second loss of consciousness occurred some minutes later, and the patient was transferred to the hospital for assessment. In the emergency department, her level of consciousness, orientation, and speech were normal. Her heart rate was 72 beats/min and her blood pressure was 140/80 mmHg. The rest of the physical examination was normal, except for moderate excess weight and a small contusion on her forehead. A standard blood test, chest radiograph, and a brain computed tomography did not produce any relevant findings. The 12-lead electrocardiogram (ECG) showed a sinus rhythm, a PR interval of 160 ms, a QRS duration of 120 ms with a right bundle-branch block (RBBB) morphology, and a left axis deviation, characteristic of left anterior hemiblock (Fig. 79.1).

The patient was admitted to the cardiology department for further evaluation. A check-up ECG 2 days later is shown in Fig. 79.2. The tracing shows a PR interval of 200 ms and an RBBB, but the axis has shifted to the right in the frontal plane. Thus, the first 40–60 ms of the QRS complex has an inferior direction and the rS morphology in lead I with a qR pattern in the inferior leads is highly suggestive of left posterior hemiblock. The existence of RBBB associated with left anterior hemiblock, alternating with left posterior hemiblock, led to a diagnosis of trifascicular block.

In this patient, the recurrent syncope is best explained by a paroxysmal complete atrioventricular (AV) block, and a permanent pacemaker was indicated with no further diagnostic work-up. After pacemaker implantation, the patient did well and was free of syncope or presyncope during a 1-year follow-up period.

Comment

The syndrome of RBBB with intermittent left anterior and posterior fascicular block was described by Rosenbaum *et al.* [1] in a classic textbook, *Los Hemibloqueos*, published in 1967. Electrocardiographically, the condition is characterized by the presence of a fixed RBBB associated with changes in the

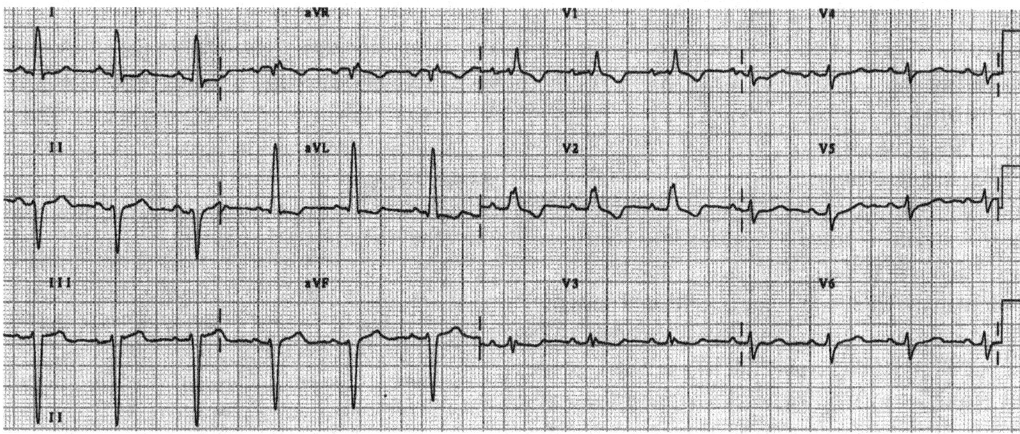

Figure 79.1 The electrocardiogram at admission.

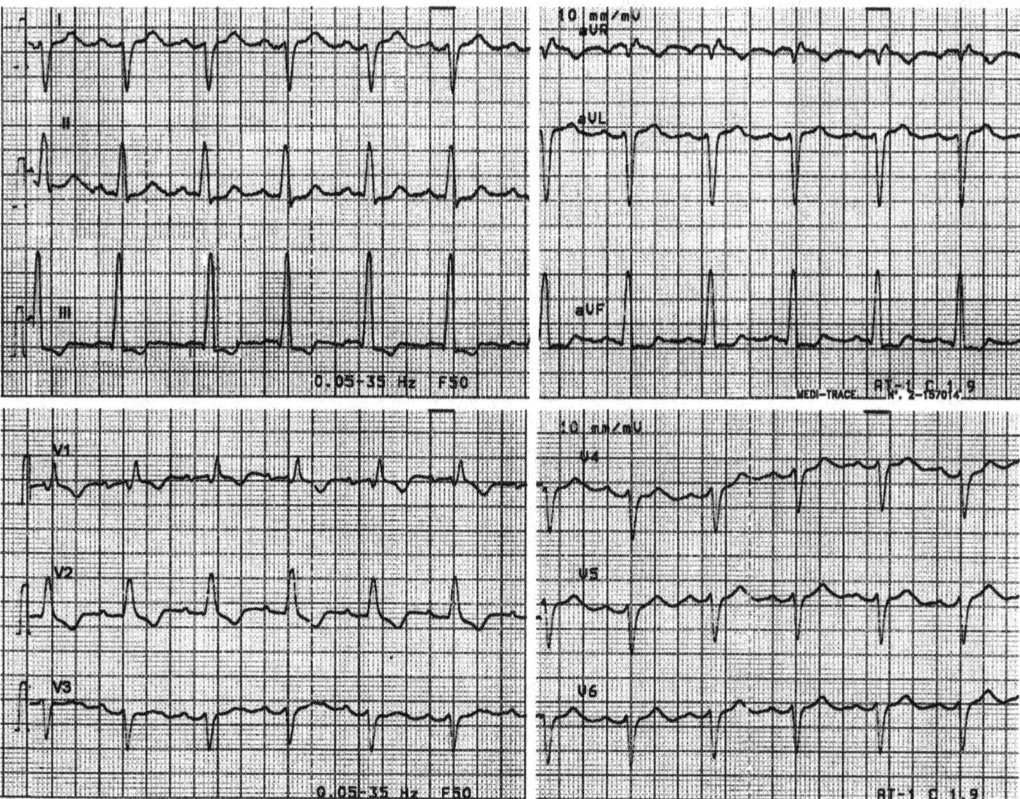

Figure 79.2 Electrocardiogram on the second day of hospitalization.

QRS morphology and frontal axis suggesting left anterior and left posterior fascicular blocks. These changes may be observed in the same ECG tracing, or more frequently in successive ECGs. Generally, the shift from one type of fascicular block to another is associated with changes in the PR interval.

The present case is an example of RBBB with intermittent left anterior and posterior fascicular block.

The most plausible interpretation of the ECG findings is that there is a fixed RBBB and impaired conduction in the two left fascicles. In the first ECG, conduction by the anterior fascicle is delayed in relation to the posterior fascicle, resulting in an ECG morphology of RBBB and anterior hemiblock. In the second ECG, an increase in the conduction time or block of the conduction in the posterior fascicle allows ventricular activation via the anterior fascicle, resulting in a change in the QRS morphology (RBBB and posterior hemiblock) and prolongation of the PR interval.

The electrocardiographic findings in this case are diagnostic of trifascicular block and have the same physiopathological and clinical significance as alternating right and left bundle-branch block—a condition associated with a high risk of AV block [2]. In this case, therefore, there is a high probability of paroxysmal AV block being the cause of the syncope, and the implantation of a pacemaker without further diagnostic tests appears to be an appropriate strategy [3].

References

1 Rosenbaum MB, Elizari MV, Lazzari JO. El síndrome de "bloqueo de rama derecha con hemibloqueo anterior y posterior intermitentes". In: Rosenbaum MB, Elizari MV, Lazzari JO, eds. *Los Hemibloqueos.* Editorial Paidos, Buenos Aires, 1967: 181–7.

2 Josephson ME, Seides SF. *Clinical Cardiac Electrophysiology.* Lea & Febiger, Philadelphia, 1979: 114–5.

3 García Civera R, Ruiz Granell R, Morell S, *et al.* Bloqueos de conducción AV e intraventriculares. In: Merino Lloréns J, ed. *Arritmología Clínica.* Momento Médico, Madrid, 2003: 51–65.

CASE 80

Vasovagal syncope in a patient with bundle-branch block

R. García Civera, R. Ruiz Granell, S. Morell Cabedo

Case report

In September 2002, a 73-year-old male presented after suffering a single syncopal episode. The patient had a history of chronic lung disease and benign prostate hypertrophy. The syncopal episode occurred in a restaurant. After a copious meal and abundant alcohol intake, the patient began to feel nausea and cold perspiration, and when he stood up to go to the toilet, he lost consciousness and fell to the floor. The loss of consciousness lasted only 1 min, followed by spontaneous recuperation without neurological sequelae.

The physical examination was normal. The electrocardiogram (ECG) (Fig. 80.1) showed a sinus rhythm at 90 beats/min and a PR interval of 0.16 s. The QRS duration was 0.13 s, with morphology compatible with right bundle-branch block and left anterior–superior fascicular block. Carotid sinus massage and orthostatic stress tests were normal. A two-dimensional echocardiogram and Doppler studies documented normal cardiac chambers and preserved ventricular function (with a left ventricular ejection fraction of 62%).

The diagnosis was typical vasovagal syncope, and no further tests were scheduled. The patient was instructed about general measures for avoiding vasovagal fainting, and clinical follow-up was recommended because of the intraventricular conduction defect. The patient remained asymptomatic until January 2004, when he

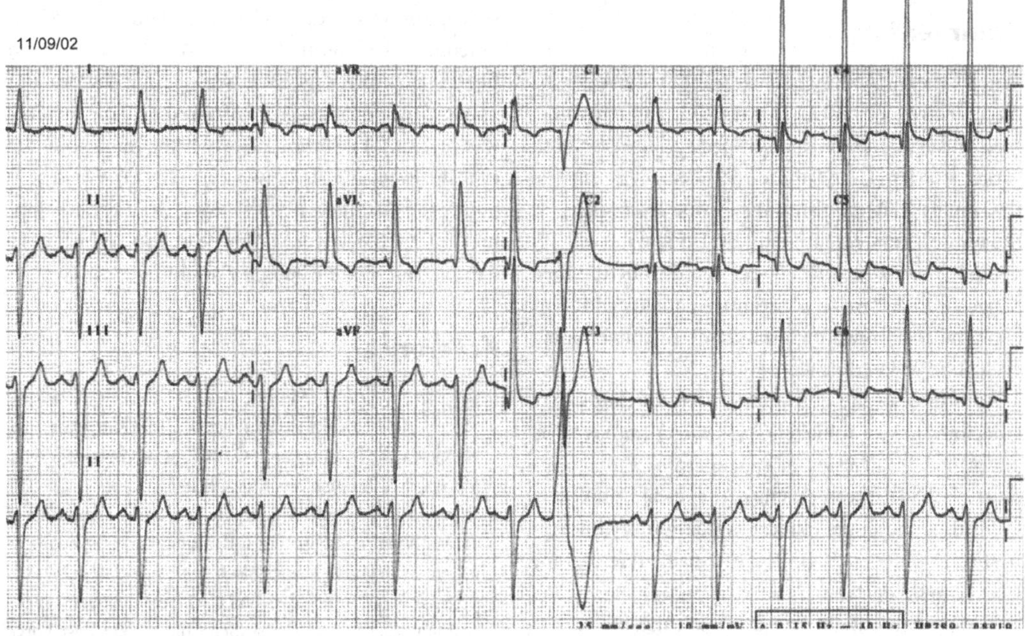

Figure 80.1 The initial electrocardiogram.

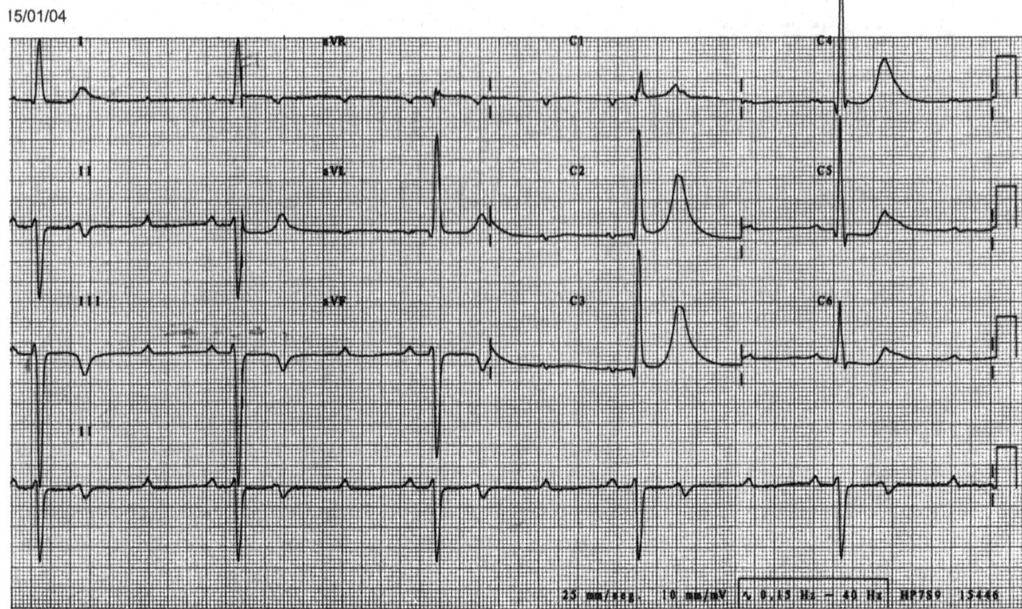

Figure 80.2 The electrocardiogram after 15 months of follow-up.

consulted again due to fatigue and a slow pulse. The ECG (Fig. 80.2) at this time showed a 3 : 1 atrioventricular (AV) block with a QRS of similar morphology to that on the previous ECGs. Subsequently, the patient underwent implantation of a DDD pacemaker.

Comment

When a patient with syncope is found to have a bundle-branch block (BBB) on the ECG, an arrhythmic mechanism for the syncope is suspected. However, both earlier studies [1] and more recent ones [2] suggest that multiple mechanisms of syncope are possible in these cases. In a recent study by Donateo *et al.* [2], neurally mediated syncope was found to be the final diagnosis in 40% of 55 consecutive patients with syncope and BBB in whom a standardized conventional evaluation was performed.

According to the European Society of Cardiology guidelines [3], an initial clinical evaluation has to be performed in all cases of syncope and a diagnosis must be made if well-established clinical criteria are fulfilled. If the initial clinical evaluation is nondiagnostic, patients with BBB are usually referred for electrophysiological studies.

The present patient had a bifascicular block, but the circumstances and warning symptoms clearly suggested a neuromediated cause of syncope. On the other hand, the syncopal episode was the first, and good ventricular function was demonstrated on echocardiography. Consequently, no further examinations were scheduled and general prevention measures were recommended. After 15 months of follow-up, the patient developed a high-grade AV block without syncope or presyncope. What is the significance of this outcome? Was the first diagnosis incorrect? Should further examinations have been performed? In our opinion, the initial diagnosis of neuromediated syncope was correct. The clinical history is the most powerful tool in the diagnosis of syncope, and in this case it points to neuromediated syncope. The later development of AV block would only be a sequela during the natural course of the bifascicular block.

References

1 Sanjuan R, Muñoz J, Morell S, García Civera R, Llavador J. Síncope y trastornos de conducción intraventricular. In: García Civera R, Sanjuán R, Cosín J, López Merino V, eds. *Síncope*. MCR, Barcelona, 1989: 271–7.

2 Donateo P, Brignole M, Alboni P, *et al.* A standardized conventional evaluation of the mechanism of syncope in patients with bundle branch block. *Europace* 2002; **4**: 357–60.

3 Brignole M, Alboni P, Benditt D, *et al.* Guidelines on management (diagnosis and treatment) of syncope. Task Force on Syncope, European Society of Cardiology. *Eur Heart J* 2001; **22**: 1256–306.

CASE 81

Intermittent atrioventricular block suggested by an electrophysiological study

A. Guisado, A. Aguilera, F. Errázquin Sáenz de Tejada, A. Pedrote Martínez

Case report

An 80-year-old man was admitted to hospital due to four episodes of syncope without previous symptoms during the previous 4 months. There were no findings on the physical examination. The electrocardiogram (ECG) (Fig. 81.1) showed a sinus rhythm with masquerading bundle-branch block (right bundle-branch block plus left anterior fascicular block, which appears similar to a left bundle-branch block in the frontal leads) and a normal PR interval (180 ms). Echocardiography showed no evidence of structural disease, and 24-h Holter monitoring and the tilt test were also normal.

An electrophysiological study (EPS) was carried out. The sinus node recovery time and corrected sinus

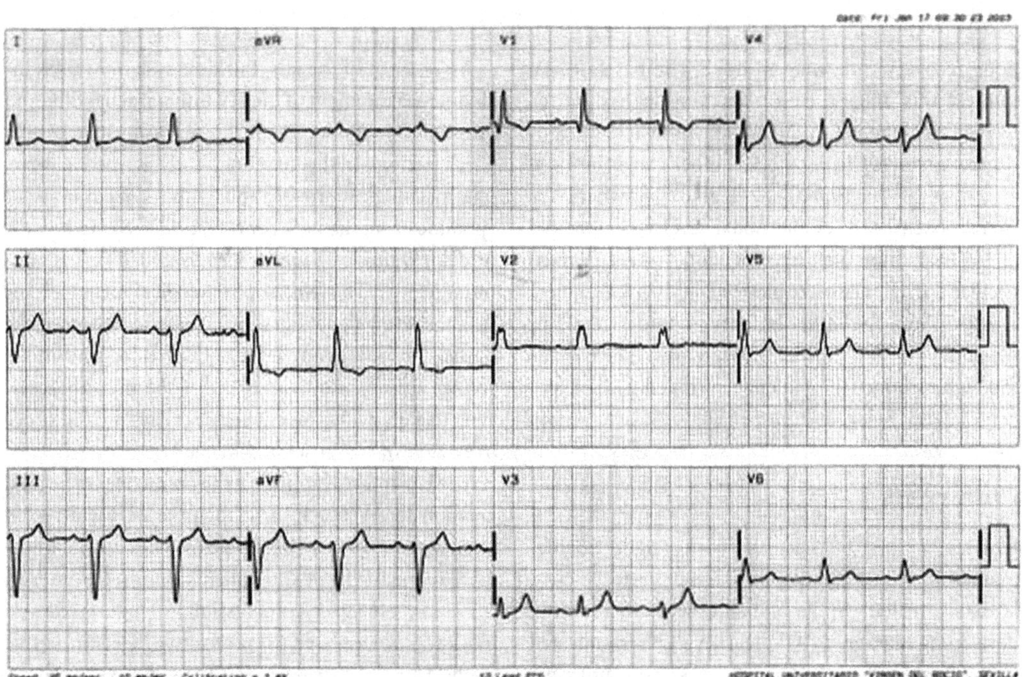

Figure 81.1 The baseline electrocardiogram, showing a bifascicular bundle-branch block.

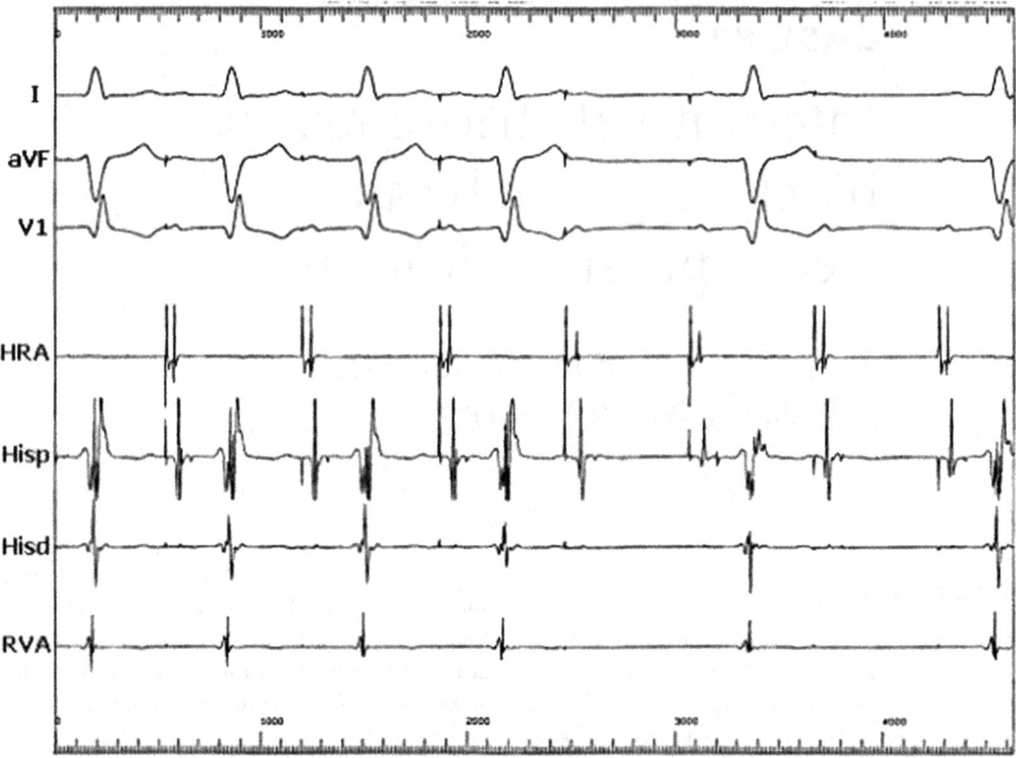

Figure 81.2 Infra-His second-degree atrioventricular block during incremental atrial pacing.

node recovery time were normal. The baseline HV interval was 108 ms (infra-His first-degree block). During incremental atrial pacing, infra-His second-degree atrioventricular (AV) block was induced at a rate of 100 beats/min (Fig. 81.2), whereas a Wenckebach block at the nodal level was obtained at 160 beats/min. Neither ventricular nor supraventricular arrhythmias were induced.

After these findings, the patient underwent implantation of a permanent pacemaker. During the follow-up period, the patient developed a persistent complete AV block.

Comment

Patients with a bifascicular block (right bundle-branch block plus left anterior or left posterior fascicular block, or left bundle-branch block) are at risk of developing high-grade AV block. An EPS is indicated in these cases when the cause of syncope is not clear after a noninvasive clinical evaluation [1].

Assessment of the His–Purkinje system in EPSs includes measurement of the HV interval at baseline and His–Purkinje conduction with stress using incremental atrial pacing. If the baseline study is inconclusive, pharmacological provocation, with a slow infusion of ajmaline (1 mg/kg i.v.), procainamide (10 mg/kg i.v.), or disopyramide (2 mg/kg i.v.), is added unless contraindicated. The electrophysiological protocol for diagnosing syncope also should include measurement of the sinus node recovery time, corrected sinus node recovery time, and assessment of the inducibility of ventricular and supraventricular arrhythmia in order to exclude other causes of syncope [1].

The HV interval appears to be predictive of the progression to AV block. Scheinman *et al.* [2] detected this progression in 12% of patients with an HV interval > 70 ms and in 24% of patients with an HV interval > 100 ms. However, progression to high-grade AV block was not assessed using sensitive detectors in this study. Later, Bergfeldt *et al.* [3] used a bradycardia-detecting pacemaker to detect progression; in their study, the sensitivity and positive predictive value for an HV interval > 70 ms were 47% and 88%, respectively.

The development of intra-His or infra-His block in incremental atrial pacing is highly predictive of a future AV block. In some studies, it has been found that progression to complete AV block occurs in 78% of patients with this finding [4]. However, it is observed only in 6–9% of patients with syncope and bundle-branch block undergoing EPSs. This low sensitivity is probably due to the fact that supra-His block may occur before intra-His or infra-His block and mask this finding.

A pharmacological stress test with class IA antiarrhythmic drugs is the next step in the study. The occurrence of high-degree AV block during spontaneous rhythm or the presence of an intra-His or infra-His block during incremental atrial pacing or after short sequences of ventricular pacing suggests a high risk of AV block. However, the prognostic value of a pharmacologically prolonged HV interval without induction of an AV block is uncertain.

An EPS is considered to predict progression to AV block when any of the following criteria are found: baseline HV interval of > 70 ms, second-degree or third-degree His–Purkinje block demonstrated during incremental atrial pacing, or high-degree His–Purkinje block elicited by intravenous administration of class IA antiarrhythmic drugs.

The sensitivity of EPSs can be low, however. Recently, Brignole *et al.* [5] used an implantable loop recorder to follow 52 patients with any type of bundle-branch block with QRS > 100 ms, no documentation of second-degree or third-degree AV block, and a negative EPS. Fourteen of these patients had syncope or presyncope with documented sudden complete AV block, and three patients developed nonsyncopal persistent complete AV blocks. In this study, the negative predictive value of EPS was thus only 67%.

In conclusion, a positive electrophysiological test appears to be highly predictive of progression to a high-degree AV block in patients with syncope and a bifascicular block, whereas a negative study has a low predictive value.

References

1 Brignole M, Alboni P, Benditt D, *et al.* Guidelines on management (diagnosis and treatment) of syncope. Task Force on Syncope, European Society of Cardiology. *Eur Heart J* 2001; **22**: 1256–306.

2 Scheinman MM, Peters RW, Suave MJ, *et al.* Value of the H-Q interval in patients with bundle branch block and the role of prophylactic permanent pacing. *Am J Cardiol* 1982; **50**: 1316–22.

3 Bergfeldt L, Edvardsson N, Rosenqvist M, Vallin H, Edhag O. Atrioventricular block progression in patients with bifascicular block assessed by repeated electrocardiography and a bradycardia-detecting pacemaker. *Am J Cardiol* 1994; **74**: 1129–32.

4 Petrac D, Radic B, Birtic K, Gjurovic J. Prospective evaluation of infrahisal second-degree AV block induced by atrial pacing in the presence of chronic bundle branch block and syncope. *Pacing Clin Electrophysiol* 1996; **19**: 784–92.

5 Brignole M, Menozzi C, Moya A, *et al.* Mechanism of syncope in patients with bundle branch block and negative electrophysiological test. International Study on Syncope of Uncertain Etiology (ISSUE) Investigators. *Circulation* 2001; **104**: 2045–50.

CASE 82

Syncope in a patient with bundle-branch block and negative electrophysiological study

S. Morell Cabedo, R. Sanjuán Mañez, R. Ruiz Granell, R. García Civera

Case report

A 73-year-old man was referred to the electrophysiology laboratory for evaluation of syncopal attacks. He had had several syncopal episodes during the previous year. Loss of consciousness occurred abruptly, without warning symptoms and without any specific triggers.

The physical examination, orthostatic tests, and an echocardiogram were all normal. The baseline electrocardiogram (ECG) showed a sinus rhythm at 56 beats/min, a PR interval of 150 ms, and a QRS duration of 120 ms, with features of right bundle-branch block and anterosuperior left hemiblock. Carotid sinus massage and a 24-h Holter recording were carried out, with negative results.

During the electrophysiological study (EPS), the baseline AH interval was 110 ms and the HV interval was 40 ms. Sinus node function was normal (with a corrected sinus node recovery time of 394 ms). A Wenckebach-type nodal atrioventricular (AV) block was obtained with atrial stimulation at 150 beats/min. Programmed atrial and ventricular stimulation (two cycles, two sites, and up to three extrastimuli in the right ventricle) did not induce any significant arrhythmia. After intravenous administration of procainamide (10 mg/kg over 5 min), the HV interval duration was 58 ms and no AV block was observed.

After the negative EPS testing, a tilt-table test with a nitroglycerin challenge and an adenosine triphosphate (ATP) test were carried out, without abnormal findings.

With the patient under local anesthesia, a Reveal Plus implantable loop recorder (ILR) (Medtronic, Inc., Minneapolis, Minnesota, USA) was implanted subcutaneously in the left parasternal region. During the follow-up, an ILR-documented syncopal event occurred 3 months after implantation, and the electrograms stored in the ILR showed a paroxysmal AV block causing syncope (Fig. 82.1). A ventricular pacemaker was implanted, and the patient did not suffer any further syncopal episodes.

Comment

Patients with bifascicular block are at high risk of developing high-degree AV block. However, other causes of syncope should be excluded. In an unselected population of 55 patients with bundle-branch block (BBB), cardiac syncope was observed in 25 patients (AV block in 20 patients, sick sinus syndrome in two, sustained ventricular tachycardia in one, and aortic stenosis in two); neuromediated syncope was found in 22 patients (40%; carotid sinus syndrome in five, tilt-induced syncope in 15, and adenosine-sensitive syncope in two). The syncope remained unexplained in eight patients (15%) [1].

In the present case, an ILR monitor was implanted after a complete evaluation including EPS testing, and a paroxysmal AV block was documented as the cause of syncope.

In the International Study of Syncope of Uncertain Etiology (ISSUE), an ILR was implanted in 52 patients with BBB and negative EPS [2]. During a follow-up period of 3–15 months, syncope recurred in 22 patients (42%), and the event was documented in 19

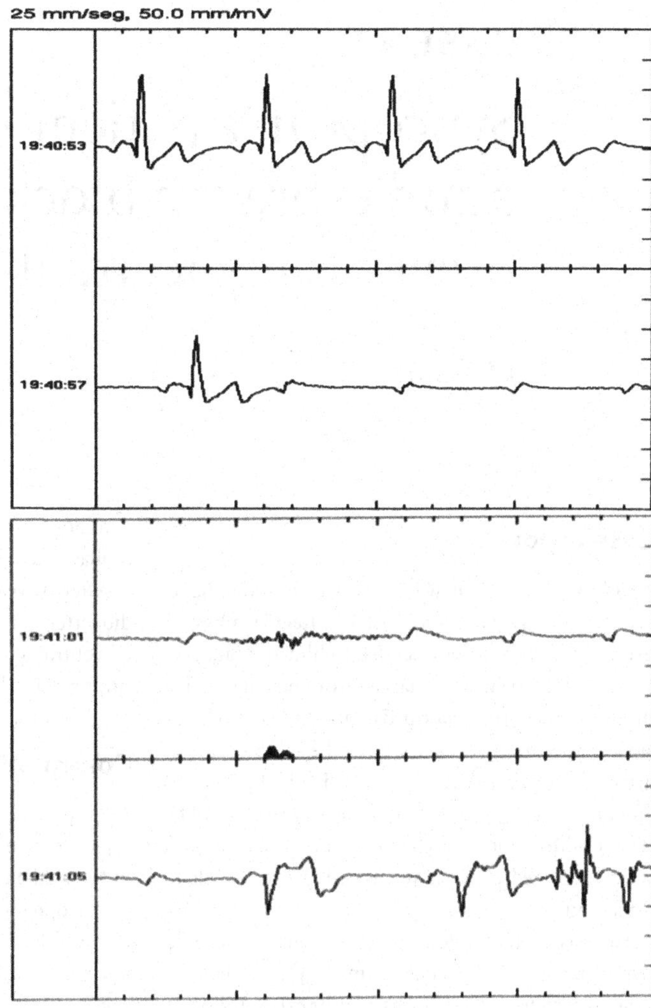

Figure 82.1 The implantable loop recorder tracing during syncope.

patients after a median of 48 days. The most frequent finding, in 17 patients, was prolonged asystolic pauses, mainly due to AV block. The remaining two patients with syncope and ILR activation had a normal sinus rhythm and sinus tachycardia during the event. In addition, three other patients developed asymptomatic persistent third-degree AV block, and two patients had presyncope due to AV block with asystole. No clinical variable at the baseline was capable of predicting the development of an AV block. No patients had injury due to recurrent syncope. The conclusions of the ISSUE study were: firstly, the sensitivity of the EPS for detecting paroxysmal AV block is low; secondly, in patients with BBB and negative EPS, most episodes of recurrent syncope have a homogeneous mechanism that is characterized by prolonged asystolic pauses, mainly attributable to paroxysmal AV block; thirdly, an ILR-guided strategy appears to be reasonable in these patients; and fourthly, owing to the high rate of AV blocks observed, the only acceptable alternative strategy is to implant a pacemaker in all patients with BBB and unexplained syncope.

References

1 Donateo P, Alboni P, Brignole M, *et al.* The mechanism of syncope in patients with bundle branch block [abstract]. *Europace* 2000; Suppl 2: A43.

2 Brignole M, Menozzi C, Moya A, *et al.* Mechanism of syncope in patients with bundle branch block and negative electrophysiological test. *Circulation* 2001; **104**: 2045–50.

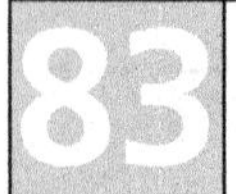

CASE 83

Syncope in a patient with bundle-branch block and previous myocardial infarction

J.J. Blanc

Case report

A 70-year-old patient was still in very good shape, exercising every day for at least 1 h. Regular physical exercise had been recommended to him 10 years previously, when he was discharged from hospital with a diagnosis of inferior myocardial infarction with occlusion of the right coronary artery (the other coronary arteries were considered normal). He had remained completely asymptomatic for almost 10 years until he was admitted due to a characteristic syncopal spell, which occurred while he was running a few yards to catch a bus.

He was receiving long-term treatment for mild hypertension (metoprolol 100 mg/day), but had no other risk factors or cardiovascular or extracardiovascular disease. History-taking and physical examination showed no abnormalities. Electrocardiography revealed a long PR interval (235 ms) and a right bundle-branch block with wide Q waves in the inferior leads. Echocardiography showed an akinetic inferior area, but a preserved left ventricular ejection fraction (LVEF) and no other abnormalities.

In accordance with the current guidelines, an electrophysiological study (EPS) was carried out in this patient with coronary disease and conduction abnormalities. EPS demonstrated a long AH interval, a normal HV interval (50 ms), and a normal response to atrial pacing, while right ventricular apical pacing at a driven cycle of 600 ms with three extrastimuli (280 ms, 250 ms, and 220 ms) resulted in the induction of rapid, sustained monomorphic ventricular tachycardia (cycle length 280 ms) (Fig. 83.1). The patient lost consciousness, and sinus rhythm was restored by a biphasic external direct-current shock.

After 1 year of follow-up, the implantable cardioverter-defibrillator recordings showed one episode of ventricular tachycardia, which was converted to sinus rhythm by a burst of rapid ventricular pacing.

Comment

In a patient with bundle-branch block, previous myocardial infarction, and syncope of unknown cause in the initial clinical evaluation, an arrhythmic cause of syncope must be suspected and an EPS is indicated. In the EPS, infrahisian conduction was found to be normal at the baseline and during atrial pacing, while ventricular tachycardia was induced by programmed ventricular stimulation.

The sensitivity and specificity of inducing sustained ventricular tachycardia in patients with syncope, in the absence of documented spontaneous episodes, are still a matter of debate [1]. However, in patients with coronary heart disease—particularly those with earlier myocardial infarction and altered left ventricular function—the induction of ventricular tachycardia is considered to be diagnostic and has been classified as a class 1 indication for the diagnosis of syncope [2].

Although this patient had a preserved LVEF and the tachycardia was induced with a relatively aggressive protocol, the authors recommended placement of an implantable cardioverter-defibrillator. The occurrence of syncope during sudden exercise was an additional argument in this active man (as there are no hard data to support the view that syncope

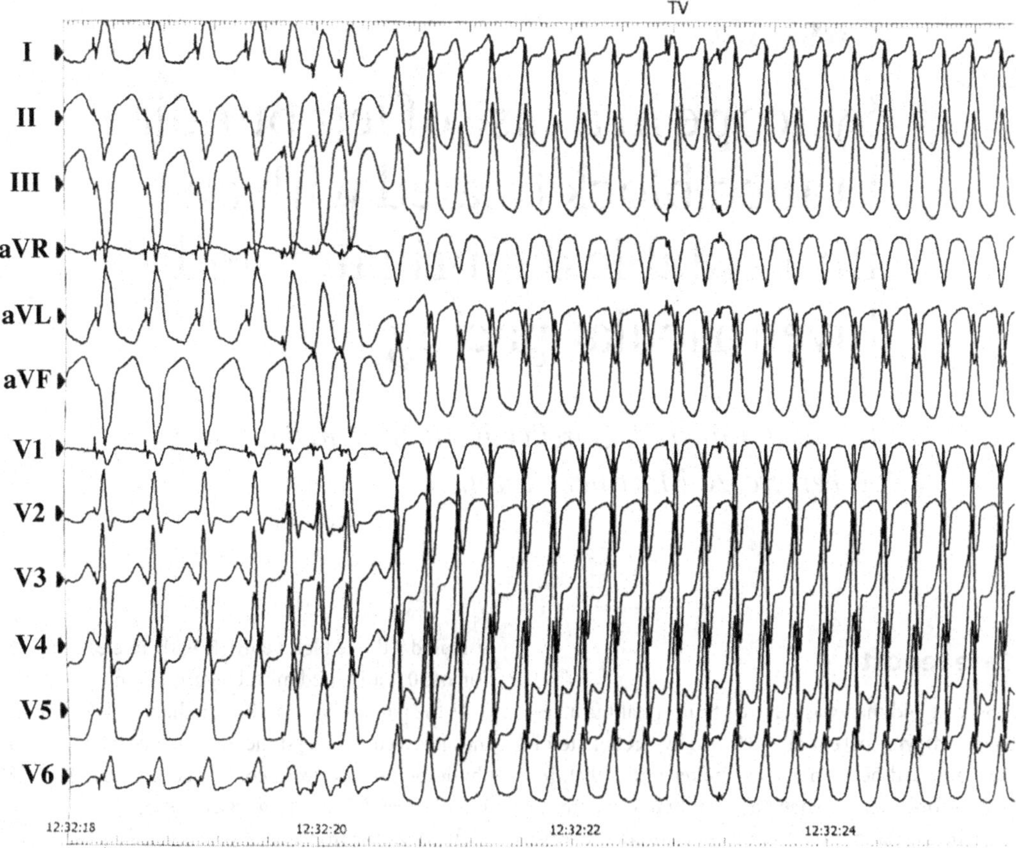

Figure 83.1 Induction of sustained monomorphic ventricular tachycardia.

during exercise is often a consequence of ventricular tachycardia).

References

1 Bigger JT, Reiffel JA, Livelli FD, *et al.* Sensitivity, specificity and reproducibility of programed ventricular stimulation. *Circulation* 1986; **73** (Suppl II): 73–8.

2 Brignole M, Alboni P, Benditt DG, *et al.* Guidelines on management (diagnosis and treatment) of syncope: update 2004. Task Force on Syncope, European Society of Cardiology. *Europace* 2004; **6**: 467–537.

CASE 84

Syncope in a case of left bundle-branch block treated with an implantable defibrillator and biventricular pacing

R. Ruiz Granell, R. García Civera, S. Morell Cabedo, A. Ferrero, A. Martínez Brotons

Case report

A 64-year-old man was referred to hospital for investigation of syncopal episodes. He had hypercholesterolemia and had been an active smoker until 1994, ten years before referral, when he had suffered an anterior myocardial infarction with an uneventful acute course. Selective coronary angiography showed a 99% proximal stenosis in the anterior descending branch of the coronary artery, which was successfully dilated with angioplasty. The left ventricular ejection fraction was 56%. The patient remained asymptomatic during the follow-up. In 1999, the development of a complete left bundle-branch block (LBBB) was noted on the electrocardiogram (ECG). Since then, symptoms of heart failure had developed and progressed, causing severe limitation of his functional capacity—New York Heart Association (NYHA) class III. The patient had received treatment with furosemide, spironolactone, angiotensin-converting enzyme (ACE) inhibitors, carvedilol, simvastatin, and aspirin, with improvement of his functional status to NYHA class II.

In 2003–4, the patient had had five syncopal episodes without warning symptoms, and with mild head trauma during the last one. The ECG showed a complete LBBB. Carotid sinus massage did not elicit abnormal responses, a Holter recording did not show any significant arrhythmia, and the echocardiogram disclosed a dilated left ventricle with an ejection fraction of 30% and mild mitral regurgitation.

As the patient had an LBBB, ischemic heart disease, and left ventricle systolic dysfunction, an electrophysiological study was conducted. The baseline HV interval was 85 ms (Fig. 84.1). Programmed electrical stimulation from the right ventricular apex induced monomorphic sustained ventricular tachycardia (Figs. 84.2, 84.3), which was poorly tolerated by the patient and had to be electrically cardioverted with a 100-J direct-current shock.

Implantation of a defibrillator was indicated, but as the patient had an advanced intraventricular conduction defect, with a high probability of developing a high-grade atrioventricular (AV) block and hence a need for permanent pacing, in addition to the systolic dysfunction and LBBB, it was decided to implant a biventricular device, with right atrial and right ventricular endocardial leads and a left ventricular epicardial lead implanted through the coronary sinus in a lateral vein.

Since implantation, the patient has experienced appropriate activation of the defibrillator caused by ventricular tachycardia, which was successfully suppressed by antitachycardia pacing. He has had no further recurrences of syncope, his functional status has improved to functional class I, the echocardiographic size of the left ventricle has declined, and the ejection fraction has improved to 40%.

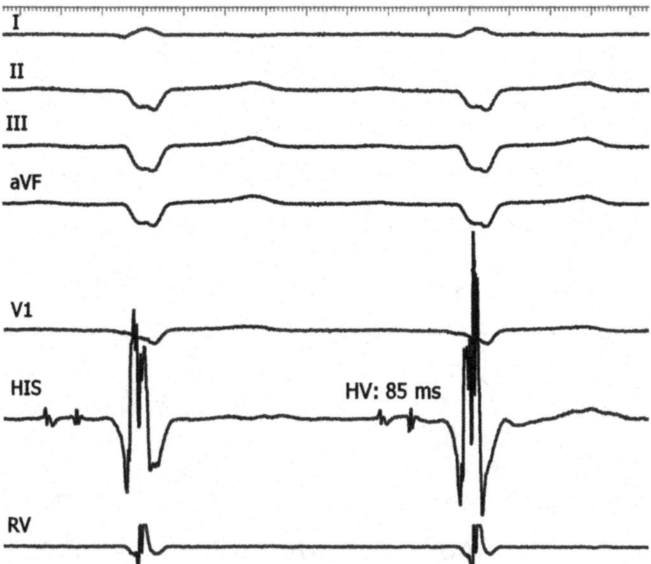

Figure 84.1 Baseline recordings obtained during the electrophysiological study, showing an HV interval of 85 ms.

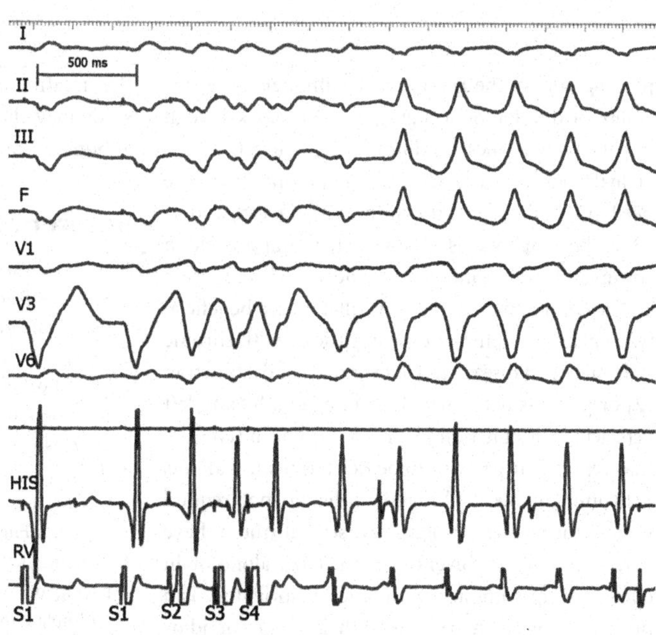

Figure 84.2 Introducing three ventricular extrastimuli into the right ventricular apex induces sustained monomorphic ventricular tachycardia.

Comment

The differential diagnosis of causes of syncope is especially important in patients with structural heart disease, since malignant causes are highly prevalent in this group. In these patients, extensive and complete evaluation is warranted. The diagnostic protocol has to include tests that can exclude or confirm high-risk causes. In patients with heart disease and a negative initial evaluation, electrophysiological studies appear to be the most appropriate approach [1]. Some findings can be confusing or open to misinterpretation, preventing completion of the diagnostic work-up. This can be the case with bundle-branch blocks or

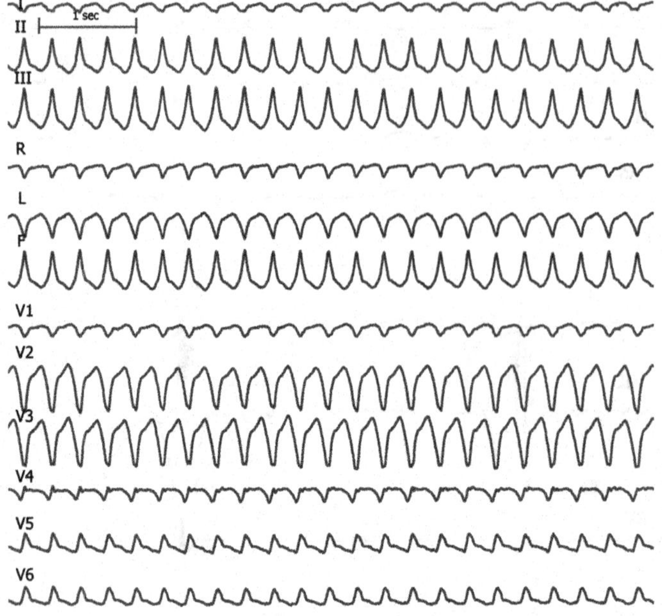

Figure 84.3 The 12-lead electrocardiogram shows the ventricular tachycardia induced during the electrophysiological study.

prolongation of the HV interval. Although the probability of developing a high-grade AV block is high in patients with these findings, malignant ventricular arrhythmias can also cause syncope and therefore need to be ruled out through in-depth investigations. After the diagnosis is established, the approach to treatment has to be integral and individualized.

Automatic implantable defibrillators are beneficial when placed prophylactically in patients with chronic ischemic heart disease and left ventricular dysfunction [2] or patients with dilated cardiomyopathy and left ventricular dysfunction [3]. It has also been reported that ventricular pacing can be deleterious in patients with implantable defibrillators who do not require permanent pacing [4]. Recently, several studies have demonstrated that biventricular pacing, alone or in combination with an automatic defibrillator, can prolong survival in patients with ischemic or idiopathic dilated cardiomyopathy, heart failure, and LBBB [5,6].

In the case presented here, it could be argued that the patient met the criteria for implantation of a biventricular defibrillator without the need for further investigations, and indeed even before developing syncope. However, it appears to be more reasonable to confirm the diagnosis initially and then to establish the treatment. Moreover, the electrophysiological study may elicit a treatable form of arrhythmia, such as bundle-branch reentry ventricular tachycardia.

References

1 García-Civera R, Ruiz-Granell R, Morell-Cabedo S, *et al.* Selective use of diagnostic tests in patients with syncope of unknown cause. *J Am Coll Cardiol* 2003; **41**: 787–90.

2 Moss AJ, Zareba W, Hall WJ, *et al.* Prophylactic implantation of a defibrillator in patients with myocardial infarction and reduced ejection fraction. *N Engl J Med* 2002; **346**: 877–83.

3 Bardy GH, Lee KL, Mark DB, *et al.* Amiodarone or an implantable cardioverter-defibrillator for congestive heart failure. *N Engl J Med* 2005; **352**: 225–37.

4 Wilkoff BL, Cook JR, Epstein AE, *et al.* Dual-chamber pacing or ventricular backup pacing in patients with an implantable defibrillator: the Dual Chamber and VVI Implantable Defibrillator (DAVID) Trial. *J Am Med Assoc* 2002; **288**: 3115–23.

5 Cleland JG, Daubert JC, Erdmann E, *et al.* The effect of cardiac resynchronization on morbidity and mortality in heart failure. *N Engl J Med* 2005; **352**: 1539–49.

6 Bristow MR, Saxon LA, Boehmer J, *et al.* Cardiac resynchronization therapy with or without an implantable defibrillator in advanced chronic heart failure. *N Engl J Med* 2004; **350**: 2140–50.

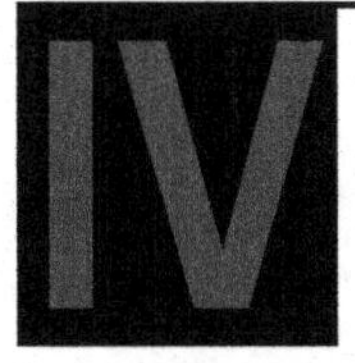

PART IV

Syncope and cardiovascular disease

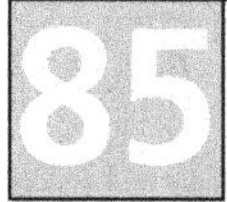

CASE 85

Acute coronary syndrome presenting as syncope

R. García Civera, R. Ruiz Granell, S. Morell Cabedo, R. Sanjuán Mañez

Case report

A 67-year-old woman was admitted to the emergency department after a syncopal attack occurred without warning at home. The patient had a history of diabetes, hypercholesterolemia, and depression (treated with tricyclic antidepressants and benzodiazepines). After recovering from the syncopal episode, the patient had a sensation of oppression in the chest and nausea. At admission, she was alert and oriented, with a blood pressure of 170/100 mmHg, and the physical examination was normal.

The 12-lead electrocardiogram (ECG) (Fig. 85.1) showed a sinus rhythm at 67 beats/min, a PR interval of 0.16 s, a QRS duration of 0.10 s, and a QT interval of 0.39 s (corrected QT 0.41 s). The QRS showed q waves in leads II, III, and aVF, and discrete ST elevation in leads II, III, aVF and in leads V_2 and V_3. Laboratory tests showed normal glucose and electrolyte levels and elevated troponin I (4.6 ng/mL) and creatine kinase myocardial-bound (CKMB) mass (32 ng/mL). A diagnosis of acute coronary syndrome was made, treatment with aspirin, clopidogrel, and nitrites was initiated, and the patient was transferred to the intensive coronary unit (ICU).

In the first hours in the ICU, the patient developed several syncopal episodes related to polymorphic ventricular tachycardia (Fig. 85.2). Control of the

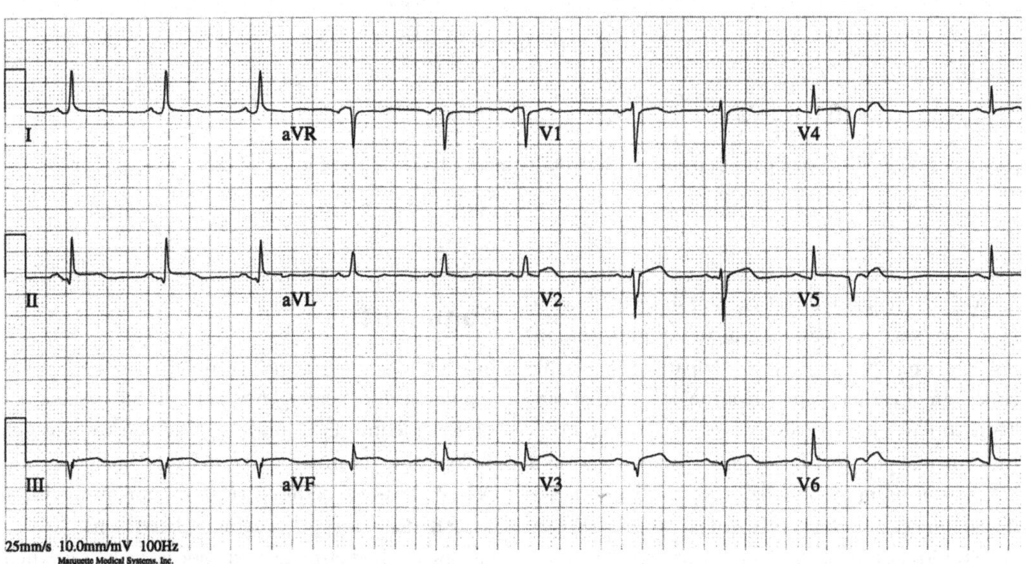

Figure 85.1 The electrocardiogram at admission.

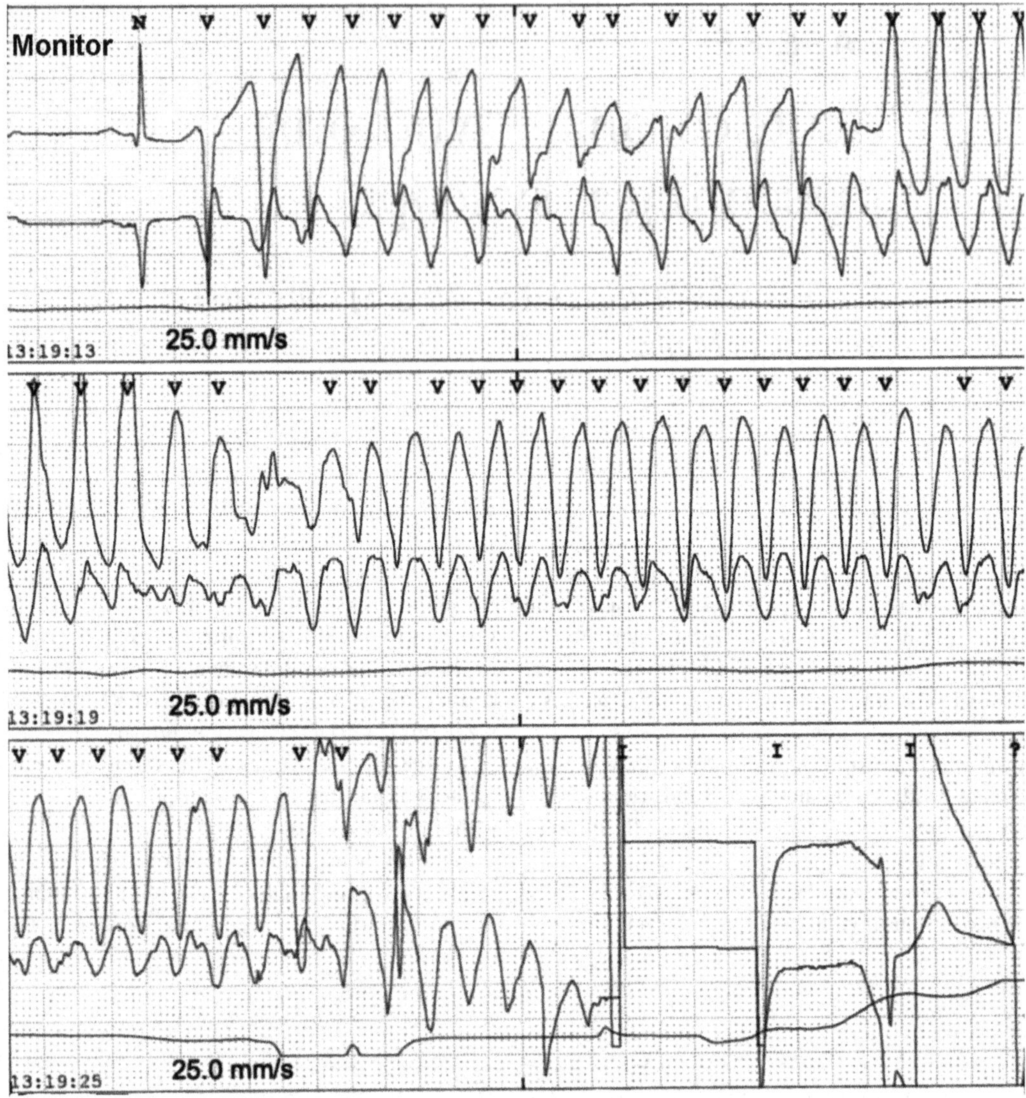

Figure 85.2 Syncopal polymorphic ventricular tachycardia, terminated with a direct-current shock.

arrhythmias required direct-current shocks, lidocaine infusion, and magnesium sulfate administration. Six days after admission, with the patient in a stable condition, a cardiac catheterization was carried out. The coronary angiography showed 90% occlusion in the proximal portion of the right coronary artery and 80% occlusion in the middle portion of the anterior descending coronary artery. Coronary bypass surgery was performed.

Comment

In this case, an acute coronary syndrome was diagnosed in the emergency ward on the basis of the clinical picture, ECG findings, and the response of biological myocardial markers. Up to this point, the exact mechanism of the syncope was not known, but a general diagnosis of ischemia-related syncope was possible. Ischemia-related syncope is diagnosed when symptoms are present in addition to ECG evidence of acute ischemia with or without myocardial infarction, regardless of the mechanism involved [1,2]. In these cases, the mechanism of the syncope can be acute cardiac dysfunction [3], cardiac arrhythmia [4], or the Bezold–Jarisch reflex (bradycardia–hypotension syndrome) [5], but the management is primarily that of the ischemia.

After the patient was admitted to the ICU, the cause of the syncope became evident: a repetitive polymorphic ventricular tachycardia with the appearance of *torsade de pointes,* but with a normal QT interval. Acute ischemia is the most probable mechanism for the arrhythmia, although it is possible that the chronic medication with tricyclic antidepressants and benzodiazepines could have played a role, despite the normal QT interval.

References

1 Brignole M, Alboni P, Benditt DG, *et al.* Task Force on Syncope, European Society of Cardiology. Guidelines on management (diagnosis and treatment) of syncope. *Eur Heart J* 2001; **22**: 1256–306.

2 Dixon MS, Thomas P, Sheridan DI. Syncope as the presentation of unstable angina. *Int J Cardiol* 1988; **19**: 125–29.

3 Hart TT, Kern MG. Coronary spasm presenting as syncope during ventricular demand pacing. *Am Heart J* 1986; **112**: 405–7.

4 Pantridge JF, Adgey AJ. Prehospital coronary care: the mobile coronary care unit. *Am J Cardiol* 1969; **24**: 666–73.

5 Chadda KD, Lichtein E, Gupta PK, Choy R. Bradycardia–hypotension syndrome in acute myocardial infarction: reappraisal of the overdrive effects of atropine. *Am J Med* 1975; **59**: 158–64.

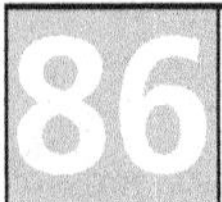

CASE 86

Syncope as an isolated manifestation of left main coronary artery occlusion

A. Sánchez González, J.A. Fournier Andray, S.M. Ballesteros Pradas, L.S. Díaz de la Llera, M. Villa Gil-Ortega

Case report

A 48-year-old man who was a taxi-driver and smoked 20 cigarettes a day, with no other coronary risk factors or previous ischemic history, was admitted to hospital due to an episode of loss of consciousness. The episode started with general discomfort and dizziness while he was driving, followed by loss of consciousness when he got out of the car. The patient spontaneously recovered consciousness after a period of time not well established, and remained asymptomatic. He came to the hospital driving his own car. The clinical, electrocardiographic, and echocardiographic examinations showed no notable abnormalities. The arterial blood pressure was 110/87 mmHg and the pulse was regular at 95 beats/min. The serum cardiac enzymes were within the normal limits. An initial diagnosis of possible vasovagal syncope was then established.

A treadmill test was carried out on the second day after admission. During the first stage of the Bruce protocol, when he reached a heart rate of 107 beats/min, he showed silent ischemia, with a 3-mm ST-segment depression in the inferior and anterior leads. The exercise was then stopped, and the tracing slowly returned to normal. In the subsequent catheterization study, the left ventriculogram showed no contraction abnormalities and the ejection fraction was 54%. The right coronary artery was angiographically normal, with collateral circulation visualized in the entire left coronary tree as far as the level of the left main trunk (Fig. 86.1A). The left main coronary artery was totally occluded before its bifurcation (Fig. 86.1B). The patient underwent uneventful coronary surgery, with grafting of an internal mammary artery to the left anterior descending artery and a saphenous vein to the first marginal branch of the circumflex artery. The patient had no further syncopal episodes during a 5-year follow-up period.

Comment

Total occlusion of the left main coronary artery is a rare angiographic diagnosis. Its prevalence is estimated at between 0.06% and 0.6% of coronary angiography studies [1]. Most cases occur in patients with depressed left ventricular function or malignant ventricular arrhythmias, during or immediately after an extensive anterior myocardial infarction [2]. The prognosis for these patients is very poor, and the reported cases of survival represent a natural selection of patients who reach the catheterization laboratory alive [3–5]. In some patients with gradual occlusion of the left main coronary artery, the development of collateral circulation could avoid a myocardial infarction, presenting progressive angina [4] or congestive cardiac failure [1]. Other forms of presentation, such as silent ischemia [5,6] or syncope [6], are exceptional. Although fibrinolytic treatment [7] and heart transplantation [3] have been reported in case reports, urgent percutaneous or surgical revascularization is the required treatment.

Benign vasovagal syncope is the most frequent

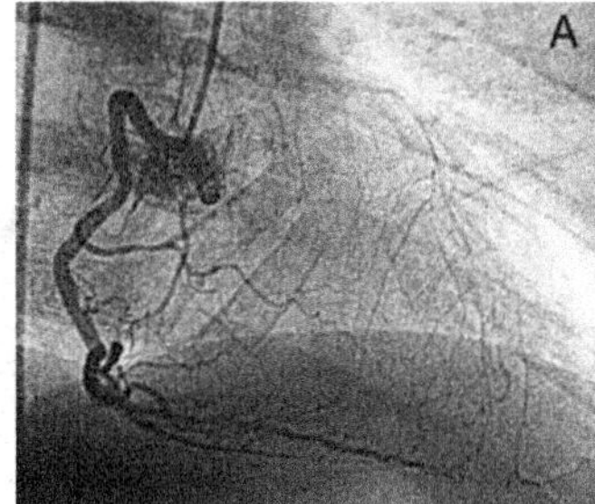

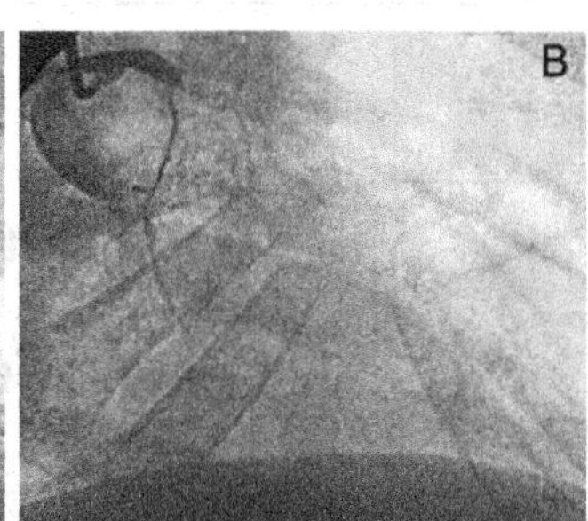

Figure 86.1 Coronary angiography. **A.** The left coronary tree as far as the level of the left main trunk. **B.** The left main coronary artery is totally occluded before its bifurcation.

cause of syncope in the general population. The European guidelines on the management of syncope do not recommend routine exercise testing in the general population, but only in patients with exercise-related syncope [8]. Nevertheless, in selected patients at high risk for coronary artery disease who present with syncope, a search for a coronary cause can be useful. The mechanisms involved can include:

- Triggering of a reflex cardiac response, producing cardioinhibitory and vasodepressor syncope.
- Transitory hypotension due to cardiac dysfunction, reduced contractility, and low cardiac output.
- Induction of a self-limited major ventricular arrhythmia.

References

1 Zimmern SH, Rogers WJ, Bream PR, *et al.* Total occlusion of left main coronary artery: the Coronary Artery Surgery Study (CASS) experience. *Am J Cardiol* 1982; **49**: 2003–10.

2 Cohen MC, Ferguson DW. Survival after myocardial infarction caused by acute left main coronary artery occlusion: case report and review of the literature. *Cathet Cardiovasc Diagn* 1989; **16**: 230–8.

3 Abecia AC, Alegría E, Fidalgo ML, Cabañero J, Herreros J, Martínez Caro D. [Acute nonlethal complete occlusion of the left main coronary artery; in Spanish.] *Rev Esp Cardiol* 1993; **46**: 119–21.

4 Vliegen HW, Cats VM. Nineteen years survival after occlusion of the left main coronary artery by virtue of an anomalous septal branch. *Cathet Cardiovasc Diagn* 1993; **29**: 283–4.

5 DePace NL, Kimbiris C, Iskandrian AS, Bemis CE, Segal BL. Total occlusion of the left main coronary artery without angina pectoris. *Arch Intern Med* 1983; **143**: 1064–5.

6 Sánchez González A, Fournier Andray JA, Pérez Fernandez-Cortacero JA, Ruiz Borrell M, Revello A. [Occlusion of left main coronary artery with silent ischemia and syncope; in Spanish.] *Rev Esp Cardiol* 1997; **50**: 363–5.

7 De Feyter PJ, Serruys PW. Thrombolysis of acute total occlusion of the left main coronary artery in evolving myocardial infarction. *Am J Cardiol* 1984; **53**: 1727–8.

8 Brignole M, Alboni P, Benditt DG, *et al.* Task Force on Syncope, European Society of Cardiology. Guidelines on management (diagnosis and treatment) of syncope. *Eur Heart J* 2001; **22**: 1256–306.

CASE 87

Syncope in a patient with myocardial infarction

P. Castellant, J.J. Blanc

Case report

A 56-year-old man, who was a smoker and was receiving treatment for hypercholesterolemia, had never complained of chest pain, dizziness, or palpitations when suddenly, and without any previous exertion, he fell and lost consciousness for a few seconds. He recovered immediately without any symptoms, but 10 min later he started to have epigastric pain, with nausea and fatigue. His family practitioner arrived quickly and measured his arterial pressure at 100/60 mmHg and his heart rate as regular but rather slow (50 beats/min). Figure 87.1 shows the electrocardiogram, with an ST-segment elevation in the inferior leads. A diagnosis of acute inferior myocardial infarction was made, and the patient was immediately admitted to the catheterization laboratory.

The coronary angiogram shows occlusion of the proximal right coronary artery, which was immediately opened using angioplasty. During the procedure, the patient had a syncopal episode, and the tracing shows a long ventricular asystolic pause without atrial activity while the coronary artery was occluded by the balloon (Fig. 87.2). Normal sinus rhythm resumed after a few seconds, and the follow-up was uneventful.

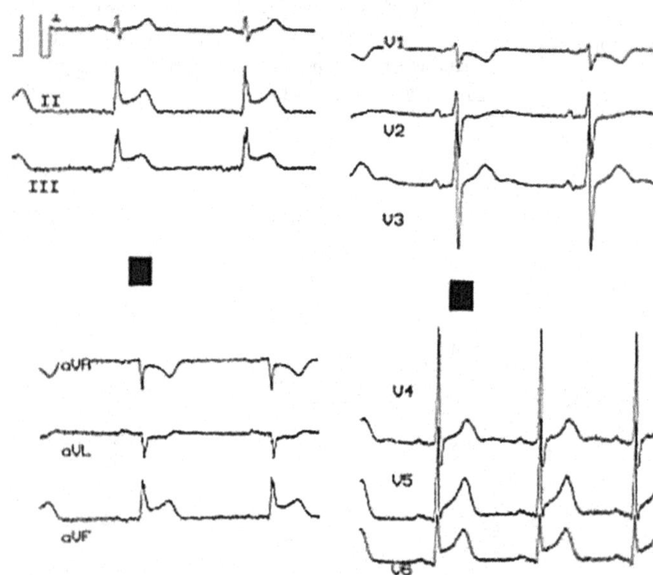

Figure 87.1 The electrocardiogram at admission.

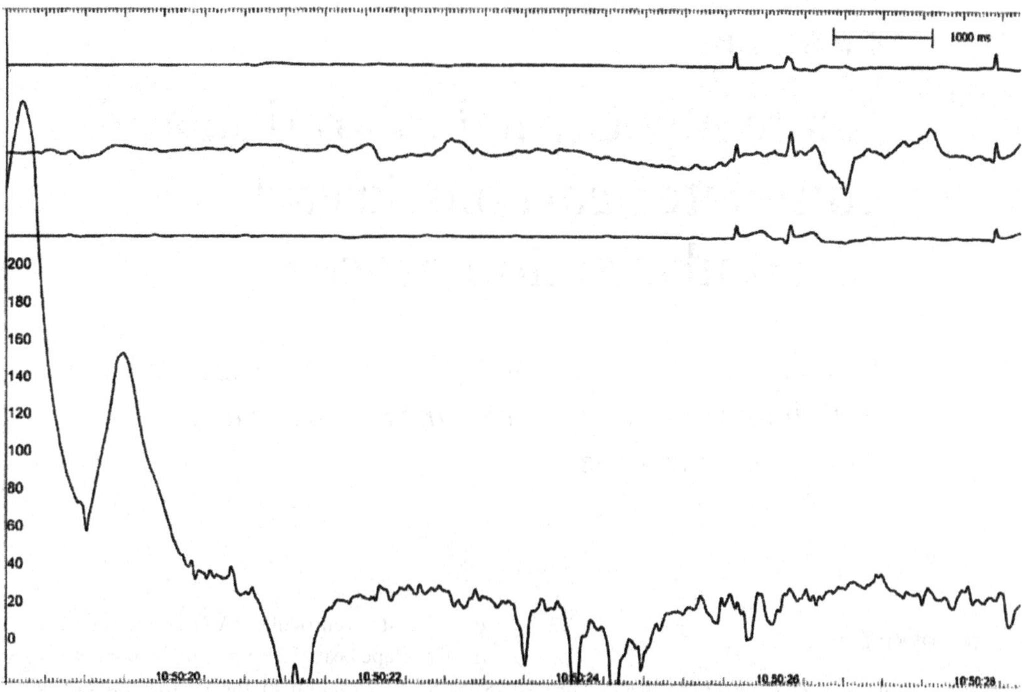

Figure 87.2 A long ventricular asystolic pause and syncope during right coronary artery angioplasty.

Comment

It is well known—although the data are not precisely quantified—that the first manifestation of myocardial infarction can be syncope, and this is particularly frequent with infarcts in inferior locations. These syncopes can be classified globally as "ischemic syncope," although the exact mechanism remains undetermined. However, there are many reasons for assuming that, in most cases, the syncope is the consequence of a reflex and not of acute atrioventricular block or ventricular tachycardia [1]. This mechanism could also explain the long atrial standstill in the present case while the right artery was occluded during angioplasty [2,3].

References

1 Mark AL. The Bezold–Jarisch reflex revisited: clinical implications of inhibitory reflexes originating in the heart. *J Am Coll Cardiol* 1983; **1**: 90–102.

2 Wei JY, Markis JE, Malagold M, Braunwald E. Cardiovascular reflexes stimulated by reperfusion of ischemic myocardium in acute myocardial infarction. *Circulation* 1983; **67**: 796–801.

3 Koren G, Weiss AT, Ben-David Y, Hasin Y, Luria MH, Gotsman MS. Bradycardia and hypotension following reperfusion with streptokinase (Bezold–Jarisch reflex): a sign of coronary thrombolysis and myocardial salvage. *Am Heart J* 1986: **112**: 468–71.

CASE 88

Acute myocardial infarction and complete heart block: early revascularization procedure

S. Gómez Moreno, G. Barón Esquivias, L.S. Díaz de la Llera, A. Pedrote Martínez, F. Errázquin Sáenz de Tejada, A. Martínez Martínez

Case report

A 48-year-old man presented to the emergency department due to experiencing precordial oppression for the previous 90 min. He had a history of hypertension, which was well controlled with diuretics, and smoked 20 cigarettes a day. While the patient was being evaluated in the emergency room, he had a loss of consciousness lasting a few seconds, and the electrocardiogram, which was immediately recorded, showed a complete atrioventricular (AV) block with a ventricular escape beat at 50 beats/min and an abnormal ST-segment elevation in the II, III, and aVF leads (Fig. 88.1). At this point, his blood pressure was 100/50 mmHg. Pacing was initiated with an external pacing system, and the patient was referred urgently for hemodynamic and angiographic evaluation.

In the hemodynamic laboratory, a transvenous electrocatheter was inserted and connected to an external pacemaker. The coronary angiography showed that

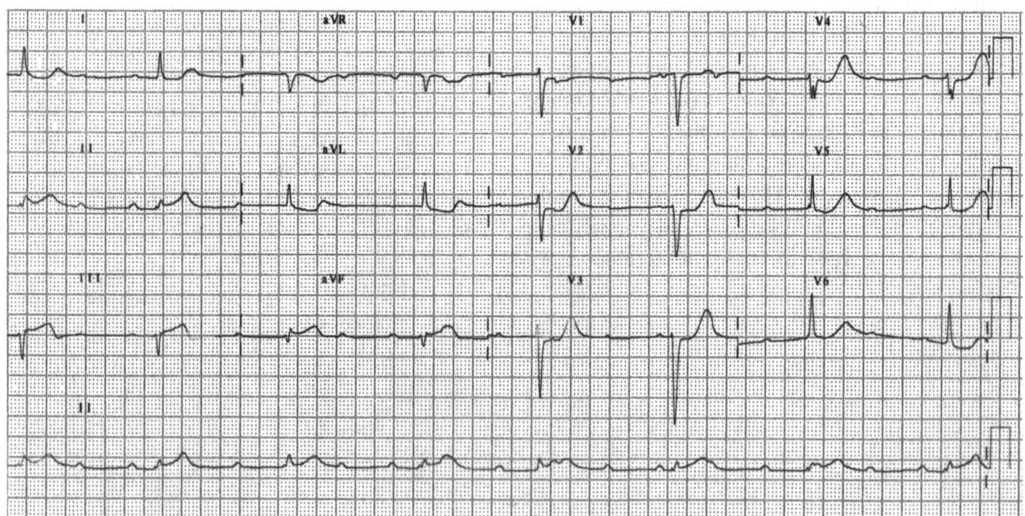

Figure 88.1 The12-lead electrocardiogram shows a complete atrioventricular block with a ventricular escape beat of 50 beats/min and abnormal ST-segment elevation in the II, III, and aVF leads.

the right coronary artery was occluded in the proximal segment. An angioplasty was carried out, and a stent was placed in the right coronary artery, producing anterograde Thrombolysis in Myocardial Infarction (TIMI) grade III flow. At this moment, the monitor showed an accelerated idioventricular rhythm as a sign of reperfusion, followed by sinus rhythm with 1 : 1 AV conduction.

The temporary electrocatheter was removed 24 h later when the patient was asymptomatic and maintaining a sinus rhythm at 60–70 beats/min, with a PR interval of 160 ms and a narrow QRS. The patient was seen at the outpatient cardiology clinic 3 months later and was still asymptomatic. The electrocardiogram only showed Q waves and negative T waves in the inferior leads.

Comment

Complete AV block is a frequent complication of inferior wall acute myocardial infarction (AMI), which is associated with a high incidence of in-hospital morbidity and mortality [1,2]. The appearance of an AV block in the setting of acute inferior infarction is associated with proximal right coronary artery obstruction and frequently with right ventricular involvement [3]. Other factors, such as parasympathetic reflexes or ischemic release of metabolites such as adenosine or extracellular potassium, can also play a role in the development of AV block [4,5].

The present case illustrates the effect of early reperfusion in the resolution of an AV block. In addition, early reperfusion can reduce the infarct size and avoid other complications. A few studies have suggested that reperfusion can rapidly resolve AV blocks presenting in inferior AMI [6–8]. For example, in the study by Kimura *et al.* [8], reperfusion was carried out in 19 consecutive patients with inferior AMI of less than 6 h duration and complete AV blocks resistant to atropine treatment. In 16 of the 19 patients, the AV block resolved immediately (within 3 min) after reperfusion, and in two other patients within an hour of the reperfusion.

References

1 Berger PB, Ryan T. Inferior myocardial infarction high-risk subgroups. *Circulation* 1989; **81**: 401–11.
2 Goldberg RJ, Zevallos JC, Yarzebski J, *et al.* Prognosis of acute myocardial infarction complicated by complete heart block (the Worcester Heart Attack Study). *Am J Cardiol* 1992; **69**: 1135–41.
3 Braat S, de Zwaan C, Brugada P, *et al.* Right ventricular involvement with acute myocardial infarction identifies high risk of developing atrioventricular nodal conduction disturbances. *Am Heart J* 1984; **107**: 1183–7.
4 Feigl D, Ashkenazy J, Kishon Y. Early and late atrioventricular block in acute inferior myocardial infarction. *J Am Coll Cardiol* 1984; **4**: 35–8.
5 Strasberg B, Bassevich R, Mager A, Kusniec J, Sagie A, Sclarovsky S. Effects of aminophylline on atrioventricular conduction in patients with late atrioventricular block during inferior wall acute myocardial infarction. *Am J Cardiol* 1991; **67**: 527–8.
6 Clemmensen P, Bates ER, Califf RM, *et al.* Complete atrioventricular block complicating inferior wall acute myocardial infarction treated with reperfusion therapy. *Am J Cardiol* 1991; **67**: 225–30.
7 McNeill AJ, Roberts MJ, Purvis JA, *et al.* Thrombolytic therapy administered to patients with complete heart block complicating acute myocardial infarction. *Coron Artery Dis* 1992; **3**: 223–9.
8 Kimura K, Kosuge M, Ishikawa T, *et al.* Comparison of the results of early reperfusion in patients with inferior wall acute myocardial infarction with and without complete atrioventricular block. *Am J Cardiol* 1999; **84**: 731–3.

CASE 89

Syncope in chronic ischemic heart disease: ventricular tachycardia induced during an electrophysiological study

A. Moya i Mitjans, C. Alonso

Case report

A 78-year-old patient was admitted to hospital due to a syncopal episode. In 1991, he had had an acute myocardial infarction that was not well localized due to the presence of a left bundle-branch block. At that time, an angiographic study had been conducted which showed three-vessel disease that was considered unsuitable for revascularization, with a left ventricular ejection fraction of 35%. The patient was still in New York Heart Association (NYHA) class II and was receiving treatment with enalapril and atenolol.

The current syncopal episode was sudden and was not preceded by typical prodromal signs or palpitations. After recovery, he reported anginal pain, and no other symptoms were present. When the patient arrived at the emergency department, he was conscious, had no angina, and there were no signs of heart failure. Electrocardiography (ECG) was carried out, which showed a sinus rhythm at 60 beats/min, with a left bundle-branch block. A blood sample was taken for analysis, and no abnormalities were found in cardiac enzymes.

The patient was admitted to the hospital. A gammagraphic stress test was carried out, which showed inferoposterior necrosis, but no evidence of reversible ischemia was demonstrated. An echocardiogram showed global depression of left ventricular function, with a left ventricular ejection fraction of 40%. On 24-h ECG monitoring, the patient remained in sinus rhythm, with no supraventricular or ventricular arrhythmias.

At this point, an electrophysiological study (EPS) was indicated in order to assess conduction system properties as well as the possible inducibility of arrhythmias. The EPS showed a normal AH interval (116 ms), a prolonged HV interval (70 ms), and a normal corrected sinus node recovery time (325 ms). No supraventricular arrhythmias were induced, and with programmed ventricular stimulation, with two extrastimuli from the right ventricular apex (S1–S1 600 ms, S1–S2 240 ms, S2–S3 240 ms), a monomorphic sustained ventricular tachycardia, with a cycle length of 280 ms, was induced (Fig. 89.1). The tachycardia was not well tolerated by the patient. A burst was sent to interrupt the arrhythmia, but in fact it was accelerated (Fig. 89.2), with presyncopal symptoms, and the patient was successfully cardioverted.

An implantable cardioverter-defibrillator (ICD) was indicated. As the patient had a left bundle-branch block and a long HV interval, a dual-chamber defibrillator, Prizm 2 DR (Guidant Corporation, Indianapolis, Indiana, USA), was implanted.

The patient has remained asymptomatic during the follow-up. In May 2002, it was noted that the patient had had an episode of asymptomatic ventricular tachycardia, which was recognized by the device and correctly treated with antitachycardia pacing (Fig. 89.3).

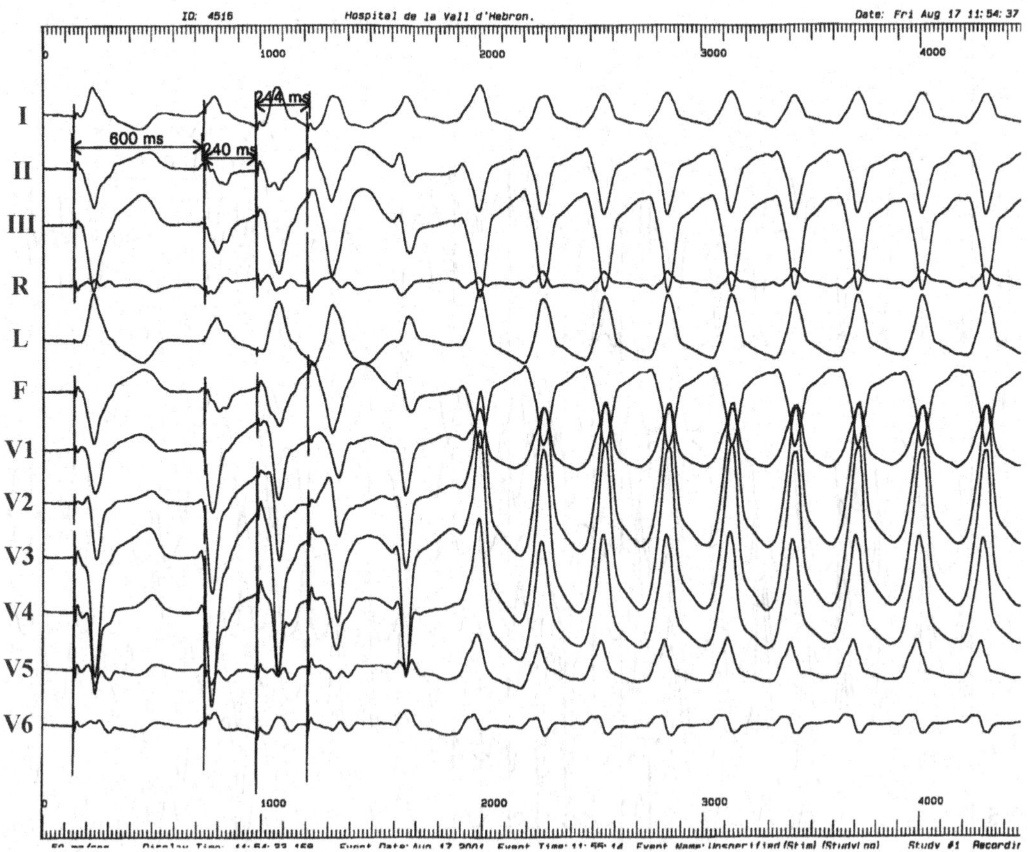

Figure 89.1 Induction of sustained monomorphic ventricular tachycardia with programmed ventricular stimulation from the right ventricular apex, with S1 600 ms, S2 240 ms, S3 240 ms. The induced arrhythmia had a cycle length of 280 ms and a morphology of right bundle-branch block and left superior axis deviation.

Comment

Ten years after a previous myocardial infarction, this patient with chronic ischemic heart disease had a syncopal episode. According to the guidelines, patients with unexplained syncope and structural heart disease or an abnormal ECG have to be admitted to hospital, as these patients have a higher probability of having an arrhythmic cause of syncope [1] and a poorer prognosis in terms of survival [2,3]. In these patients, a complete cardiac evaluation should be carried out, including an assessment of ventricular function, as well as ruling out the possibility that the syncope was due to an acute ischemic episode. In the present patient, this possibility was reasonably ruled out, as he had normal cardiac enzymes and an absence of reversible ischemia in the stress test.

It has been shown that, in patients with ischemic heart disease and a very low left ventricular ejection fraction, implantation of an automatic ICD improves survival, even in asymptomatic patients [4]. However, in patients with ischemic heart disease and syncope, it has been suggested that the inducibility of ventricular arrhythmias on EPS identifies a group of patients who are at higher risk of having ventricular arrhythmias during the follow-up [5–7].

It can be argued that, in these patients, although an ICD can be useful to prevent sudden death, it cannot be adequate for syncope treatment, as the ICD does not prevent the development of the ventricular tachycardia and syncopal symptoms can develop while a shock is being delivered. However, it has been shown that, if antitachycardia pacing is programmed for fast ventricular tachycardias, many

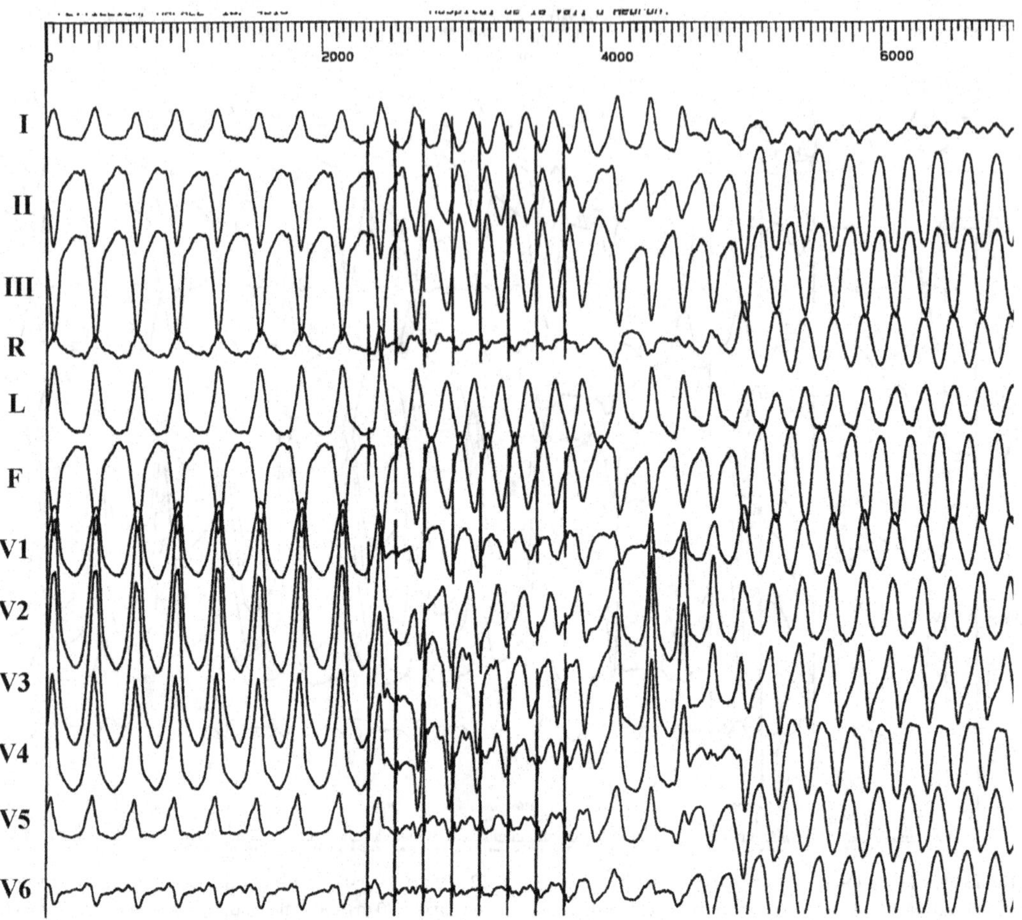

Figure 89.2 Acceleration of sustained ventricular tachycardia with a burst of pacing, leading to ventricular flutter, which required immediate cardiac defibrillation.

of these arrhythmias can be terminated quickly and without pain, preventing syncope in many of these patients [8].

This case is a good illustration of the way in which antitachycardia pacing terminates fast ventricular tachycardia within a few seconds, preventing syncope and palpitations.

References

1 Brignole M, Alboni P, Benditt D, *et al.* Task Force on Syncope, European Society of Cardiology. Guidelines on management (diagnosis and treatment) of syncope. *Eur Heart J* 2001; **22:** 1256–306.

2 Kapoor WN, Hanusa B. Is syncope a risk factor for poor outcomes? Comparison of patients with and without syncope. *Am J Med* 1996; **100:** 646–55.

3 Colivicchi F, Ammirati F, Melina D, Guido V, Imperoli G, Santini M. Development and prospective validation of a risk stratification system for patients with syncope in the emergency department: the OESIL risk score. *Eur Heart J* 2003; **24:** 811–9.

4 Moss AJ, Zareba W, Hall WJ, *et al.* Prophylactic implantation of a defibrillator in patients with myocardial infarction and reduced ejection fraction. *N Engl J Med* 2002; **346:** 877–83.

5 Militianu A, Salacata A, Seibert K. Implantable cardioverter utilization among device recipients presenting exclusively with syncope or near-syncope. *J Cardiovasc Electrophysiol* 1997; **8:** 1087–97.

6 Mittal S, Iwai S, Stein KM, Markowitz SM, Slotwiner DJ, Lerman BB. Long-term outcome of patients with unexplained syncope treated with an electrophysiologic-guided approach in the implantable cardioverter-defibrillator era. *J Am Coll Cardiol* 1999; **34:** 1082–9.

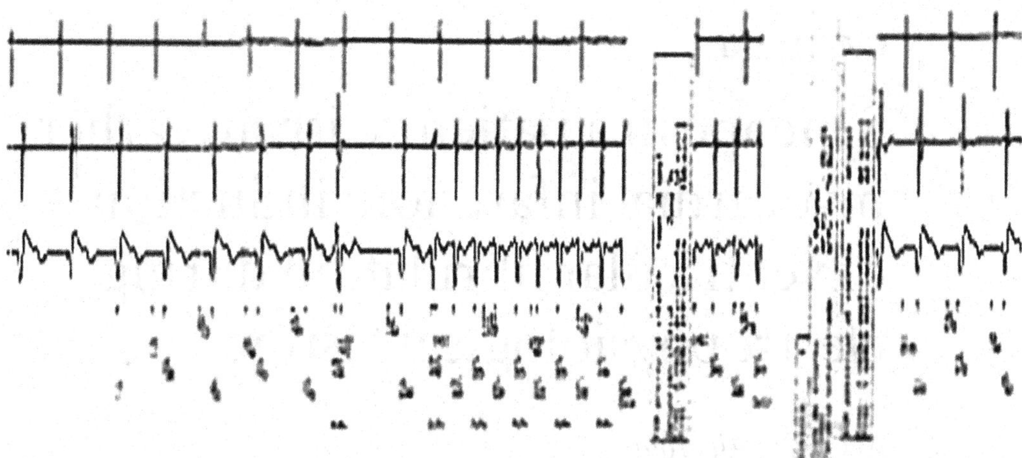

Figure 89.3 Recordings from the implantable cardioverter-defibrillator. At the top is the intracavitary recording of the atrial electrogram, in the middle the ventricular electrogram, and at the bottom the morphology electrogram. At the beginning of the tracing, the patient is in sinus rhythm. After a premature ventricular beat, there is a pause, followed by a ventricular tachycardia, confirmed by the change in morphology of the electrogram as well as by atrioventricular dissociation. Once the arrhythmia has been recognized by the device, a burst of antitachycardia pacing is delivered, and the tachycardia stops, with a return to sinus rhythm.

7 Andrews NP, Fogel RI, Pelargonio G, Evans JJ, Prystowsky EN. Implantable defibrillator event rates in patients with unexplained syncope and inducible sustained ventricular tachyarrhythmias: a comparison with patients known to have sustained ventricular tachycardia. *J Am Coll Cardiol* 1999; **34:** 2023–30.

8 Wathen MS, Sweeney MO, DeGroot PJ, *et al.* Shock reduction using antitachycardia pacing for spontaneous rapid ventricular tachycardia in patients with coronary artery disease. *Circulation* 2001; **104:** 796–801.

CASE 90

Syncope in a patient with an earlier myocardial infarction: induction of ventricular fibrillation during electrophysiological testing

A. García Alberola

Case report

A 62-year-old man presented with recurrent syncope. He had a history of chronic obstructive pulmonary disease, with stable moderate dyspnea on exertion (New York Heart Association class II). He had developed adult-onset diabetes and hypercholesterolemia 4 years earlier, and was receiving treatment with glibenclamide and atorvastatin. In 1998, the patient had been admitted to another hospital with an inferior acute myocardial infarction, which was managed with thrombolytic therapy. The postinfarction period was uneventful, and chronic beta-blocker treatment was prescribed. He had not experienced any episodes of chest pain or palpitations after discharge.

The day before admission, the patient had experienced a sudden-onset loss of consciousness while he was walking at a normal pace. There were no prodromal symptoms, and the episode resolved spontaneously after a few minutes. On the day of admission, a second episode of syncope had occurred while the patient was sitting. According to the patient, he had not noticed any chest pain or palpitations before or after either of the syncope episodes. Nor was there any confusion after the episode, tongue biting, or incontinence. The patient presented at the emergency unit 1 h after the last syncope. The physical examination was unremarkable and the electrocardiogram (ECG) showed sinus rhythm, a small q wave in leads II, III, and aVF, a tall R wave in lead V_2, and a normal repolarization pattern (Fig. 90.1). The myocardial enzymes were within normal values. Echocardiography showed a postero-inferior hypokinetic area, with a global left ventricular ejection fraction (LVEF) of 45%. Continuous ECG monitoring for 48 h showed a stable sinus rhythm, with a normal heart rate and infrequent isolated premature ventricular contractions.

A tilt test potentiated with sublingual nitroglycerin resulted in progressive and symptomatic hypotension after the administration of the drug. The patient became pale and experienced dizziness for 40–60 s, finally developing light-headedness and near-syncope when his systolic blood pressure fell below 60 mmHg and the tilt test was stopped (Fig. 90.2). The symptoms elicited by the tilt test had not been present before the spontaneous episodes, according to the patient. Coronary angiography showed chronic occlusion in the mid-right coronary artery and an absence of lesions in the rest of the coronary vessels. On the fifth day after admission, an electrophysiological study (EPS) was carried out. The rhythm and baseline intervals were normal (HV interval 42 ms), as was the assessment of sinus function and atrioventricular conduction. During programmed ventricular stimulation, a sustained ventricular fibrillation (VF) was induced and converted uneventfully to sinus rhythm after 17 s with an external 200-J direct-current shock. Arrhythmia was induced with two extrastimuli delivered from the apex of the right ventricle, at a baseline cycle length of 500 ms and with coupling intervals of 250/200 ms (Fig. 90.3).

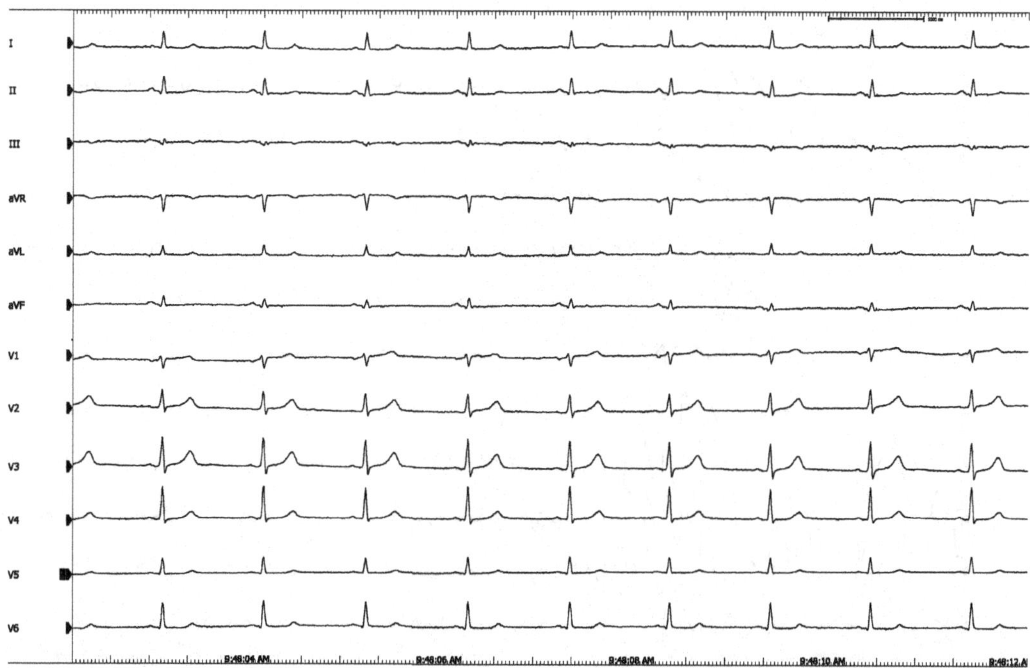

Figure 90.1 The electrocardiogram at admission.

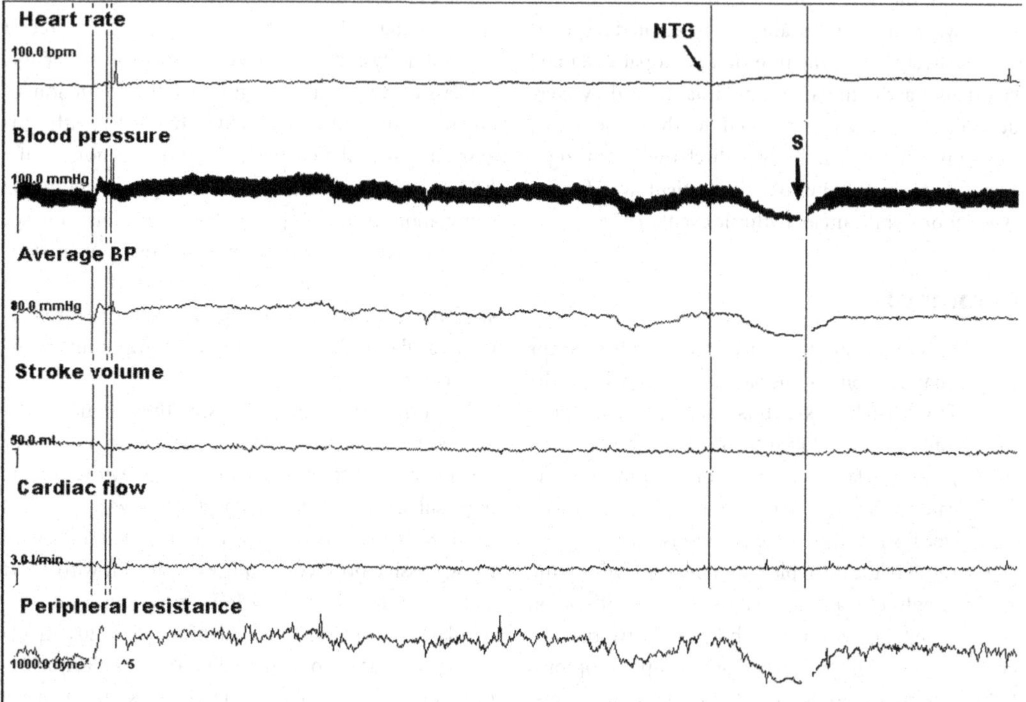

Figure 90.2 The tilt-table test. BP, blood pressure; NTG, nitroglycerin; S, syncope.

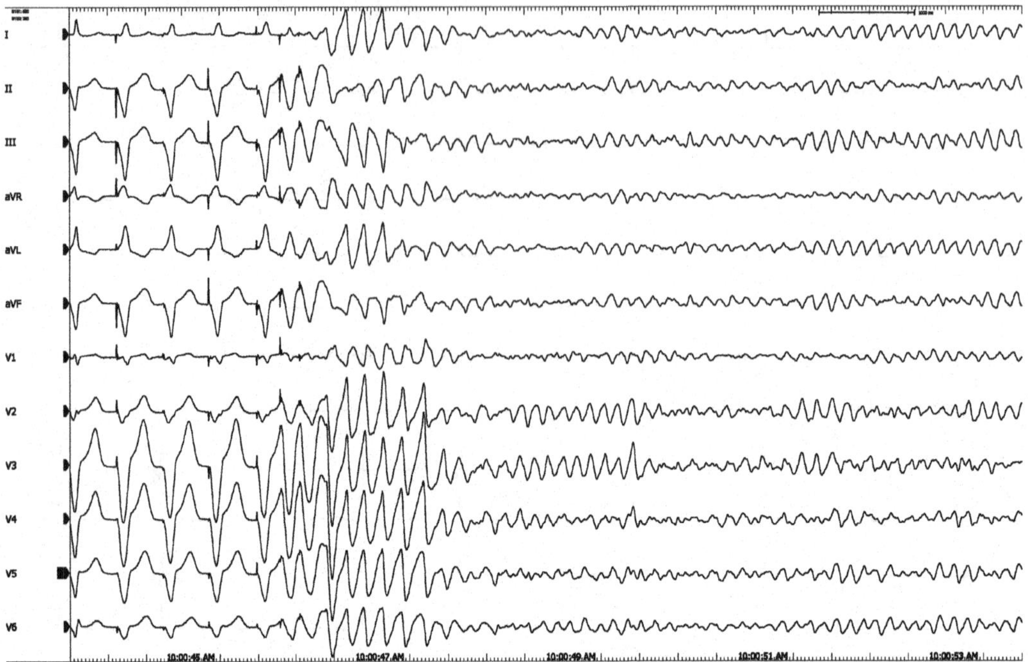

Figure 90.3 Induction of ventricular fibrillation during electrophysiological testing.

Due to the patient's history of an earlier myocardial infarction, the lack of similarity between the spontaneous syncopal episodes, and the tilt-elicited response and relatively easy induction of a syncopal sustained ventricular arrhythmia, an implantable cardioverter-defibrillator was recommended to the patient and was implanted before he was discharged. During a 1-month follow-up period, the patient was free of syncope or significant arrhythmic events.

Comment

Three important questions need to be addressed for proper management of this patient: firstly, what is the value of the tilt-table test in this case? Secondly, what is the significance of induced VF during the EPS? And thirdly, is prophylactic implantation of a cardioverter-defibrillator indicated? Unfortunately, there are no unequivocal answers to these questions.

The result of the tilt-table test in this case is doubtful. After nitroglycerin administration, the patient's blood pressure fell progressively, while his heart rate increased slightly. The patient had presyncopal symptoms (which were not present during the spontaneous attacks), and finally the test was stopped without a clear vasovagal reaction being observed. This behavior in the tilt test is compatible with an orthostatic intolerance pattern [1], which suggests a certain degree of autonomic dysfunction but not true vasovagal syncope.

Classically, it was thought that the induction of polymorphic ventricular tachycardia or VF with programmed stimulation of the heart was a nonspecific finding, mainly related to the aggressiveness of the stimulation protocol [2–5]. However, this concept probably needs modification depending on the clinical setting. For example, in patients with Brugada syndrome, the induction of polymorphic ventricular tachycardia or VF appears to be an important prognostic finding [6].

Recently, two studies addressed the significance of the induction of VF in patients with coronary artery disease with syncope of unknown cause, with conflicting results. Mittal *et al.* [7] reported follow-up findings for 118 of these patients who underwent EPS with an aggressive protocol (triple extrastimuli with short coupling intervals, two cycle lengths, two right ventricular sites, and isoproterenol infusion). In 20 patients (16%), VF was the only inducible arrhythmia; fibrillation was not inducible in 45 patients (the control group). During a follow-up period of 25.3 months, six patients with inducible VF and 10 of those in the control group died. There were therefore no significant differences in relation to overall survival for patients with or without inducible VF. In contrast, Link *et al.* [8] found that VF and ventricular flutter (regular monomorphic ventricular tachycardia with a cycle length of ≤ 230 ms), induced in EPSs, have prognostic significance for the occurrence of arrhythmia in patients presenting with syncope. In this study of 274 consecutive patients who underwent EPS, VF was induced in 32 patients (8%) and ventricular flutter in 24 (9%). During a 37-month follow-up period, ventricular arrhythmias occurred in three patients (13%) with inducible VF and seven (30%) with inducible ventricular flutter, but only in four (3%) of 144 patients with noninducible conditions ($P < 0.001$ for induced VF and flutter versus noninducible patients). In this study, the risk of ventricular arrhythmias during the follow-up in inducible patients was similar, regardless of whether the conditions were inducible by double or triple extrastimuli. Both of these studies have important limitations; both were retrospective, and the numbers of patients with inducible VF were small in both. In the study by Mittal *et al.* [7], the aggressiveness of the protocol might have been responsible for a high rate of VF induction, suggesting that this end point is nonspecific. In the study by Link *et al.* [8], the combination of patients with VF and flutter makes it difficult to assess the significance of VF induction alone.

An important point that is not fully addressed in the above studies is the influence of ventricular function on the patients' subsequent course. In the study by Link *et al.* [8], the risk of ventricular arrhythmia after 3 years in patients with inducible VF and an LVEF > 35% was only 6.7%. In the International Study on Syncope of Uncertain Etiology (ISSUE) [9], an implantable loop recorder was used during the follow-up of 35 patients with previous myocardial infarction or cardiomyopathy and negative EPS. In this group, ventricular function was moderately depressed (mean LVEF of 47 ± 17%). During the follow-up, episodes of recurrent syncope were never due to ventricular arrhythmias, which were documented in only one patient and caused presyncope. Interestingly, the induction of polymorphic ventricular tachycardia or VF during the EPS (which was regarded as a negative result) was of no value for predicting syncopal events or ventricular tachyarrhythmia.

Given the uncertainty of the significance of VF induction, the authors' approach of implanting a defibrillator seems reasonable. Nevertheless, as this patient had relatively well-preserved ventricular function, a "wait and see" strategy with placement of an implantable loop recorder might also be acceptable.

References

1 Brignole M, Menozzi C, del Rosso A, *et al.* New classification of haemodynamics of vasovagal syncope: beyond the VASIS classification. Analysis of the presyncopal phase on the tilt test without and with nitroglycerine challenge. *Europace* 2000; **2**: 66–7.

2 Wellens HJJ, Brugada P, Stevenson WG. Programmed electrical stimulation of the heart in patients with life-threatening ventricular arrhythmias: what is the significance of induced arrhythmias and what is the correct stimulation protocol? *Circulation* 1985; **72**: 1–7.

3 Denniss AR, Richards DAB, Cody DV, *et al.* Prognostic significance of ventricular tachycardia and fibrillation induced at programmed stimulation and delayed potentials detected on the signal-averaged electrocardiograms of survivors of acute myocardial infarction. *Circulation* 1986; **74**: 731–45.

4 Bourke JP, Richards DAB, Ross DL, McGuire MA, Uther JB. Does the induction of ventricular flutter or fibrillation at electrophysiological testing after myocardial infarction have any prognostic significance? *Am J Cardiol* 1995; **75**: 431–5.

5 DiCarlo LA Jr, Morady F, Schwartz AB, *et al.* Clinical significance of ventricular fibrillation-flutter induced by ventricular programmed stimulation. *Am Heart J* 1985; **109**: 959–63.

6 Brugada J, Brugada R, Brugada P. Determinants of sudden cardiac death in individuals with the electrocardiographic pattern of Brugada syndrome and no previous cardiac arrest. *Circulation* 2003; **108**: 3092–6.

7 Mittal S, Hao SC, Iwati S, *et al.* Significance of inducible ventricular fibrillation in patients with coronary artery disease and unexplained syncope. *J Am Coll Cardiol* 2001; **38**: 371–6.

8 Link MS, Saeed M, Gupta N, Homoud MK, Wang PJ, Estes M. Inducible ventricular flutter and fibrillation predict the arrhythmia occurrence in coronary artery disease patients presenting with syncope of unknown origin. *J Cardiovasc Electrophysiol* 2002; **13**: 1103–8.

9 Menozzi C, Brignole M, Garcia-Civera R, *et al.* Mechanism of syncope in patients with heart disease and negative electrophysiologic test. International Study on Syncope of Uncertain Etiology (ISSUE) investigators. *Circulation* 2002; **105**: 2741–5.

CASE 91

Syncope in a patient with dilated cardiomyopathy, a negative electrophysiological study, and poor left ventricular function

A. Pedrote Martínez, L. García Riesco, G. Barón Esquivias, F. López Pardo, F. Errázquin Sáenz de Tejada

Case report

A 45-year-old man was brought to the emergency room after suffering two syncopal episodes in 1 h. The first syncope did not present prodromal symptoms, and neurological recovery was complete without sequelae. The second occurred when he was in the supine position and was preceded by blurred vision and accompanied by convulsions. On arrival in the emergency room, the patient was asymptomatic. He had no risk factors for cardiovascular disease. He reported having experienced exertional dyspnea in the previous few months. The physical examination revealed a normal state of consciousness; his blood pressure was 130/70 mmHg and his heart rate was 90 beats/min. There was a systolic cardiac murmur in the apex, the lungs were normal, and there were no signs of heart failure. Serum electrolytes and glucose levels were also normal. The chest radiograph showed cardiomegaly, and the resting electrocardiogram showed a left bundle-branch block (with a QRS duration of 145 ms) with left axis deviation. Transthoracic echocardiography showed a dilated left ventricle (65 mm) and an ejection fraction of 0.30. Color Doppler analysis showed that there was a slight mitral regurgitation. A 24-h Holter recording showed polymorphic ventricular premature beats and asymptomatic episodes of monomorphic nonsustained ventricular tachycardia. The R–R interval variability was within normal limits, and the QT interval was also normal. A normal coronary system was seen on angiography.

Using three 6-Fr catheters (located in the high right atrium, the right ventricle, and the His zone), an electrophysiological study (EPS) was performed with up to three extrastimuli at two sites in the right ventricle, apex, and output tract, using two cycle lengths (400 and 500 ms), without isoprenaline. The conduction intervals were normal (HV 55 ms), and no sustained arrhythmia was induced. Despite the negative results of the electrophysiologically programmed stimulation, the patient had syncope in the setting of a nonischemic dilated cardiomyopathy (NIDCM). An implantable cardioverter-defibrillator (ICD) was placed in the left subpectoral region. The ICD was programmed with two zones (VT zone between 370 ms and 330 ms and ventricular fibrillation zone for cycle lengths < 330 ms).

Two months after ICD implantation an episode of sustained monomorphic ventricular tachycardia with a cycle length of 260 ms occurred, which was interrupted by a 29-J ICD discharge (Fig. 91.1).

Comment

During the past 10 years, observational studies of patients with left ventricular dysfunction who present with syncope have found that there is a high risk of mortality from all causes and a greater incidence of

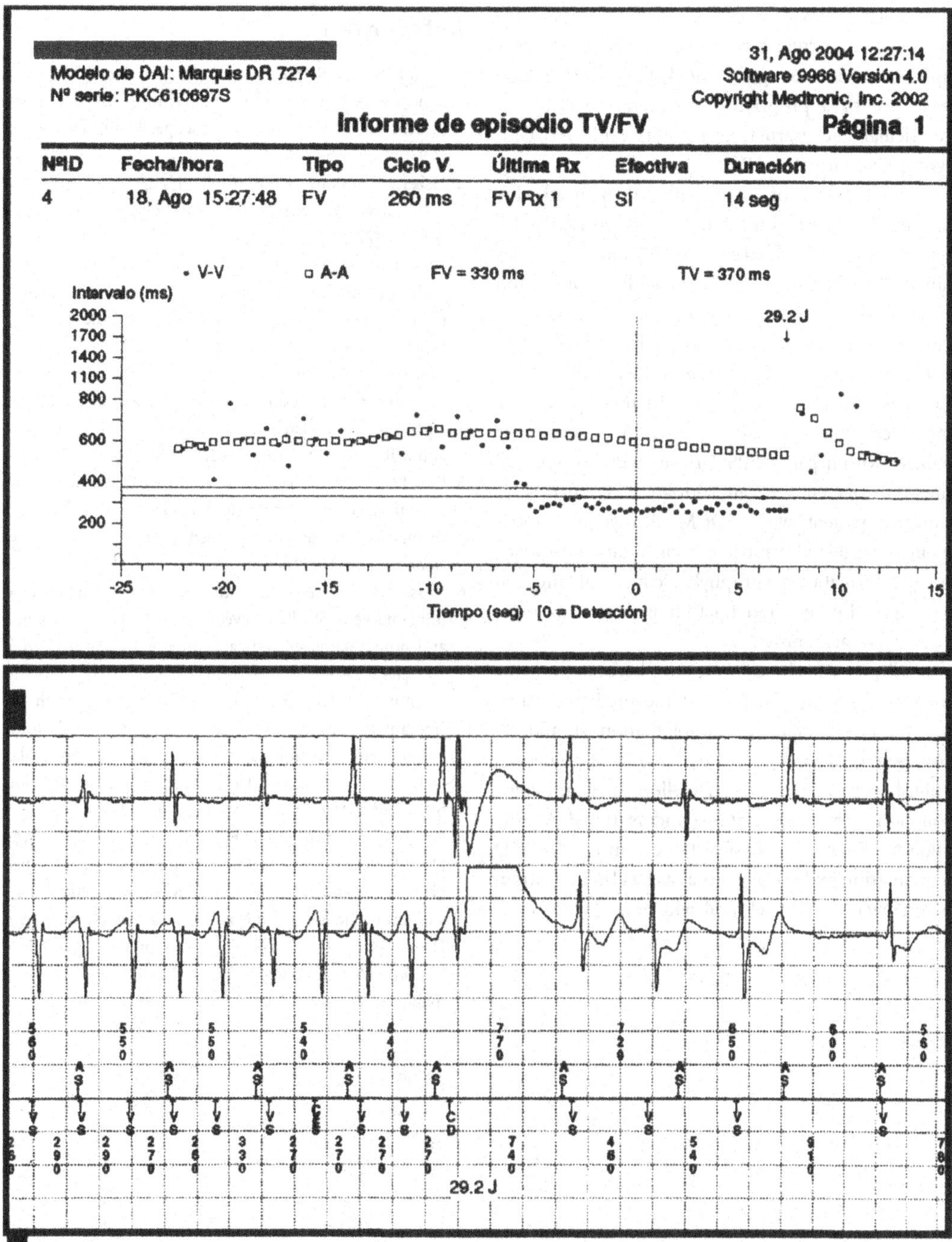

Figure 91.1 Implantable cardioverter-defibrillator telemetry showing an episode of ventricular tachycardia, followed by a defibrillation shock of 29 J and reversion to sinus rhythm.

sudden cardiac death in these patients [1]. The etiology of syncope in patients with NIDCM and left ventricular dysfunction includes a high incidence of ventricular arrhythmias, while other causes (bradyarrhythmias, supraventricular tachycardia, and noncardiac etiologies) are less prevalent [1].

The predictive value of EPS in NIDCM is poor [2], and patients with syncope who do not have inducible ventricular tachycardia during EPS may experience sustained ventricular arrhythmias during the follow-up. In addition, Knight *et al.* [3] reported a high incidence of appropriate ICD therapy (50%) for ventricular tachycardia in patients with NIDCM, syncope, and negative EPS.

Medical treatment to prevent sudden death due to ventricular arrhythmias in patients with NIDCM, syncope, and a depressed ejection fraction (< 0.35) has not been effective [4]. Patients with NIDCM and syncope without documented ventricular tachycardia have been excluded from large clinical trials with ICDs, and the data are limited to uncontrolled observational clinical studies [3,5,6]. In these series, the incidence of ICD shocks is nearly 50%, including patients with negative EPS. Grimm *et al.* [7] reported that the incidence of appropriate ICD therapy is similar in patients with NIDCM with syncope, documented sustained ventricular tachycardia or ventricular fibrillation, or prophylactic ICD implantation for a very low ejection fraction with nonsustained ventricular tachycardia.

Until primary clinical trial data become available for this group of patients and the predictive value of EPS is clarified, ICD implantation should be considered. At present, the updated 2002 guidelines published by the American College of Cardiology, American Heart Association, and National Association for Sport and Physical Education classify ICD implantation in these patients as a class IIb indication, with a low rank (C) of clinical evidence [8].

References

1 Middlekauff HR, Stevenson WG, Stevenson LW, *et al.* Syncope in advanced heart failure: high risk of sudden death regardless of origin of syncope. *J Am Coll Cardiol* 1993; **21**: 110–6.

2 Hsia H, Marchlinski F. Electrophysiology studies in patients with dilated cardiomyopathies. *Cardiac Electrophysiol Rev* 2002; **6**: 472–81.

3 Knight BP, Goyal R, Pelosi F, *et al.* Outcome of patients with nonischemic dilated cardiomyopathy and unexplained syncope treated with an implantable defibrillator. *J Am Coll Cardiol* 1999; **33**: 1964–70.

4 Fonarow G, Feliciano Z, Boyle N, *et al.* Improved survival in patients with nonischemic advanced heart failure and syncope treated with an implantable cardioverter-defibrillator. *Am J Cardiol* 2001; **85**: 981–5.

5 Saeed M, Saba S, Swygman C, *et al.* High risk of ventricular arrhythmia in long-term follow-up of patients with dilated cardiomyopathy and unexplained syncope [abstract]. *Circulation* 2000; **102**: 1809.

6 Russo AM, Verdino R, Schorr C, *et al.* Occurrence of implantable defibrillator events in patients with syncope and nonischemic dilated cardiomyopathy. *Am J Cardiol* 2001; **88**: 1444–6.

7 Grimm W, Hoffmann JJ, Muller HH, Maisch B. Implantable defibrillator event rates in patients with idiopathic dilated cardiomyopathy, nonsustained ventricular tachycardia on Holter and left ventricular ejection fraction below 30%. *J Am Coll Cardiol* 2002; **39**: 780–7.

8 Gregoratos G, Abrams J, Epstein AE, *et al.* ACC/AHA/NASPE 2002 guideline update for implantation of cardiac pacemakers and antiarrhythmia devices: summary article: a report of the American College of Cardiology/American Heart Association Task Force on practice guidelines (ACC/AHA/NASPE Committee to Update the 1998 Pacemaker Guidelines). *Circulation* 2002; **106**: 2145–61.

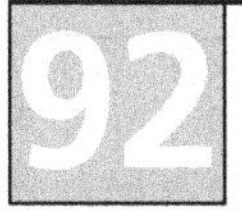

CASE 92

Syncope in a patient with obstructive hypertrophic cardiomyopathy and left bundle-branch block

J. García Sacristán, R. Ceres, J. Fedriani

Case report

A 55-year-old patient was referred for cardiac evaluation due to recurrent syncopal episodes. Four years before, he had been diagnosed with obstructive hypertrophic cardiomyopathy (HCM) after a heart murmur had been detected during a medical check-up for renewal of his driving license. Two years later, when the patient was asymptomatic, a new left bundle-branch block was noted on the electrocardiogram (ECG). Three months before the current consultation, he had started to experience syncopal episodes without warning signs or precipitating events.

At auscultation, a systolic ejection murmur with maximum intensity at the left sternal edge was noted. The ECG showed a normal sinus rhythm at 66 beats/min, a normal PR interval, and a complete left bundle-branch block. Doppler ultrasonography showed hypertrophy of the septum (21 mm) with systolic anterior movement of the anterior leaflet of the mitral valve and subaortic obstruction (with a maximum instantaneous gradient of 122 mmHg). Several Holter recordings were not diagnostic, and a head-up tilt-table test with nitroglycerin challenge was negative.

An electrophysiological study (EPS) was carried out. In sinus rhythm with a cycle length of 900 ms, the AH interval was 120 ms and the HV interval 65 ms (Fig. 92.1). Sinus node function was normal. No atrial arrhythmias were induced. During programmed ventricular stimulation with a basic cycle length of 600 ms, the introduction of three ventricular extrastimuli (coupled to 280, 220 and 220 ms) induced ventricular fibrillation (Fig. 92.1) which was reverted with a direct-current (DC) shock. After the DC shock, a transient infrahisian complete atrioventricular block was observed (Fig. 92.2). After sinus rhythm had resumed, ventricular stimulation at a cycle length of 400 ms and with up to three extrastimuli was not able to induce any arrhythmia. A procainamide test was negative.

As the results of the EPS were considered nondiagnostic, an implantable loop recorder (ILR) (Reveal Plus, Medtronic, Minneapolis, Minnesota, USA) was placed. Six months after the implantation, the patient had a new syncopal episode with automatic activation of the device, and a paroxysmal atrioventricular block with a long asystolic pause was documented as the cause of the syncope (Fig. 92.3). Subsequently, the patient received a DDD pacemaker and has remained asymptomatic during a 2-year follow-up period.

Comment

Syncope is not uncommon in patients with HCM, and the evaluation of these patients is complex and frequently frustrating. The complex pathophysiology of HCM means that hemodynamic, arrhythmic, neuromediated, and ischemic causes can play a role

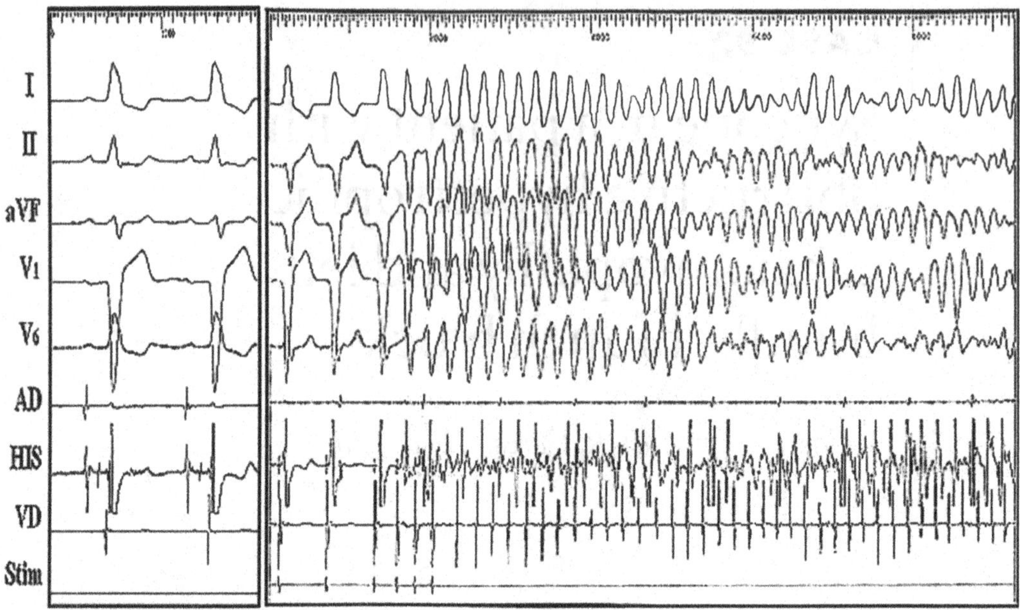

Figure 92.1 Baseline conduction intervals (*right*) and induction of ventricular fibrillation (*left*) during the electrophysiological study.

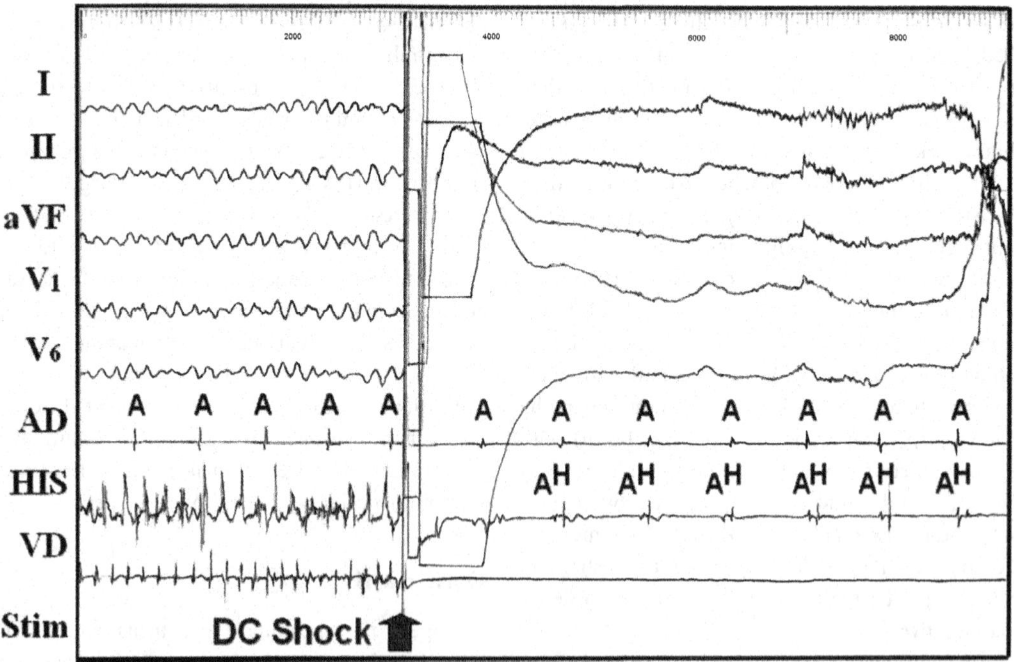

Figure 92.2 Interruption of ventricular fibrillation by a direct-current (DC) shock was followed by a transient complete infrahisian atrioventricular block.

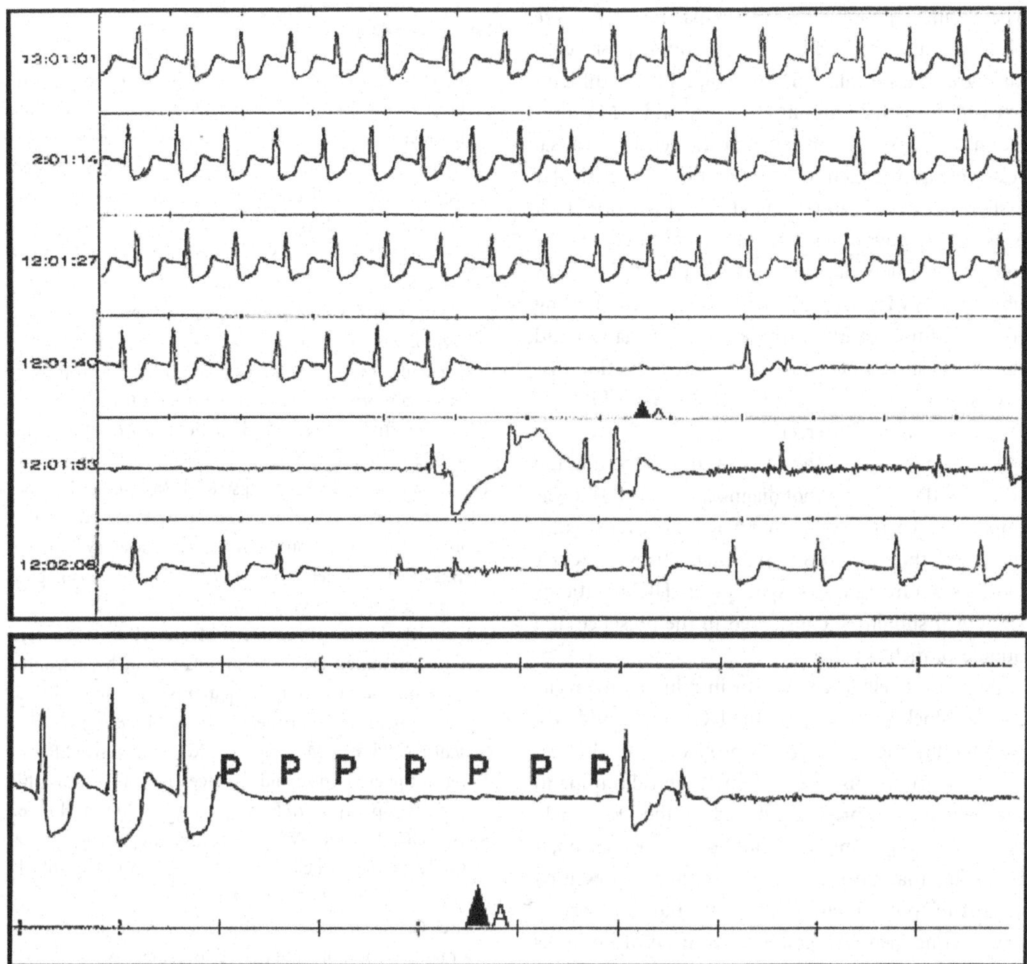

Figure 92.3 The implantable loop recorder tracing during the syncopal episode. The lower panel shows an enlarged view of the start of asystole; blocked P waves can be seen. The triangle marks the moment at which automatic activation of the device took place.

in the production of syncope [1]. In the study by Nienaber *et al.* [2], only three of the clinical, morphological, electrophysiological, and hemodynamic variables present in patients with HCM were predictive of syncope:

- Age under 30.
- A reduced left ventricular end-diastolic volume index (< 60 mL/m^2).
- Presence of nonsustained ventricular tachycardia on Holter monitoring.

The authors suggest that the more common mechanism of syncope in HCM patients is a low-input–low-output failure induced by a sudden increase in heart rate in the presence of a low filling volume.

Because of the possible connection with sudden death, arrhythmic causes are the principal concern, and EPSs are frequently carried out. Unfortunately, the results of EPS in relation to ventricular arrhythmias are difficult to evaluate. Sustained monomorphic ventricular tachycardias are rarely induced, while the induction of polymorphic ventricular tachycardias/ventricular fibrillation is common. In a study by Fananapazir *et al.* [3], sustained monomorphic ventricular tachycardia was induced in 10% of the patients and polymorphic ventricular tachycardia in 33%. The authors found a significant correlation between the induction of sustained ventricular arrhythmias and the occurrence of cardiac arrest and syncope [4].

The results reported by Fananapazir *et al.* were obtained in a referred high-risk population with an aggressive stimulation protocol, and it is difficult to extrapolate these findings to a general HCM population. Other studies have failed to identify a causal relationship between the induction of ventricular arrhythmias at EPS and the incidence of syncope [1,5]. Most electrophysiologists therefore consider that the induction of polymorphic ventricular tachycardia or fibrillation in HCM patients is a nonspecific finding [6]. Other uses of EPS include the investigation and treatment of patients with suspected conduction disease, supraventricular tachycardia, Wolff–Parkinson–White syndrome, flutter, etc.

In the present case, the authors considered that the results of the EPS were not diagnostic, and an ILR was implanted. This demonstrated that an atrioventricular block was the cause of the syncope. Atrioventricular block is a rare cause of syncope in HCM patients [7], but it should be considered in the presence of a bundle-branch block.

Retrospectively, the transient infrahisian atrioventricular block observed after the DC shock could be a valuable finding. The authors probably thought that the block was a consequence of mechanical trauma to the right bundle branch induced by the DC shock. Although this possibility cannot be entirely rejected, it is possible that the atrioventricular block represented a "fatigue" phenomenon in the His–Purkinje system due to concealed retrograde penetration of impulses during ventricular fibrillation. Similar cases of bundle-branch block or transient atrioventricular block have been described after termination of ventricular tachycardia spontaneously [8], with DC shock [9], or with thumpversion [10].

References

1 Betocchi S, Manganelli. Syncope in hypertrophic cardiomyopathy: what are the potential mechanisms and therapeutic implications? In: Raviele A, ed. *Cardiac Arrhythmias 2001: Proceedings of the 7th International Workshop on Cardiac Arrhythmias, Venice, 7–10 October 2001.* Springer, Milan, 2002: 50–6.

2 Nienaber CHA, Hiller S, Spielman RP, Geiger M, Kuck KHK. Syncope in hypertrophic cardiomyopathy: multivariate analysis of prognostic determinants. *J Am Coll Cardiol* 1999; **15**: 984–55.

3 Fananapazir L, Tracy CM, Leon MB, *et al.* Electrophysiological abnormalities in hypertrophic cardiomyopathy: a consecutive analysis of 155 patients. *Circulation* 1989; **80**: 1259–68.

4 Fananapazir L, Chang AC, Epstein SE, McAreavey D. Prognostic determinants in hypertrophic cardiomyopathy: prospective evaluation of a therapeutic strategy based on clinical, Holter, hemodynamic, and electrophysiological findings. *Circulation* 1992; **86**: 730–40.

5 Kuck KH, Kunze KP, Schlueter M, Nienaber CA, Costard A. Programmed electrical stimulation in hypertrophic cardiomyopathy: results in patients with and without cardiac arrest and syncope. *Eur Heart J* 1988; **9**: 177–85.

6 Behr ER, Elliot P, McKenna WJ. Role of invasive EP testing in the evaluation and management of hypertrophic cardiomyopathy. *Card Electrophysiol Rev* 2002; **6**: 482–6.

7 Kair GC, Bamrath VS. Syncope in hypertrophic cardiomyopathy: association with atrioventricular block. *Am Heart J* 1985; **110**: 1081–3.

8 Fisch C. Bundle branch block after ventricular tachycardia: a manifestation of "fatigue" or "overdrive suppression." *J Am Coll Cardiol* 1984; **3**: 1562–4.

9 Babuty D, Charniot JC, Fauchier JP. Complete infrahisian block after endocavitary shock delivered by an automatic implantable cardiac defibrillator. *J Electrocardiol* 1996; **29**: 249–53.

10 Barold SS. Atrioventricular block following thumpversion of ventricular tachycardia. *Pacing Clin Electrophysiol* 2000; **23**:1703–4.

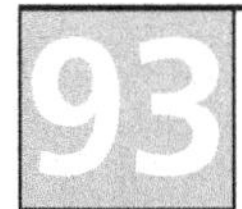

CASE 93

Atrial flutter with 1 : 1 atrioventricular conduction in a patient with hypertrophic cardiomyopathy

R. García Civera, R. Ruiz Granell, S. Morell Cabedo, R. Sanjuán Mañez

Case report

A 58-year-old man was admitted to hospital due to a syncopal episode followed by palpitations. A year before the admission, the patient had been diagnosed with hypertrophic cardiomyopathy without obstruction (Fig. 93.1), and treatment with oral amiodarone was initiated owing to the presence of nonsustained ventricular tachycardia on the Holter recording.

After recovering consciousness, the patient felt intense weakness and fast palpitations and went to the emergency room, where the electrocardiogram (ECG) shown in Fig. 93.2 was recorded. The ECG shows regular tachycardia with a wide QRS complex at 200 beats/min. The QRS during tachycardia has a configuration resembling a right bundle-branch block and a duration of 160 ms. Applying the ECG differential-diagnostic criteria (Brugada's algorithm [1]) suggested a supraventricular origin of the tachycardia and, in addition, atrial flutter waves appeared to be observed in lead aVF. Shortly after the recording of this ECG, a spontaneous change in the ECG was observed (Fig. 93.3). The flutter waves were then clearly identifiable in leads II, III, and aVF and the atrioventricular (AV) conduction ratio was 3 : 2. Electrical cardioversion of the atrial flutter was carried out, and the patient underwent an electrophysiological study (EPS).

During the EPS, a typical (counterclockwise) atrial flutter was induced and ablation of the cavo-tricuspid

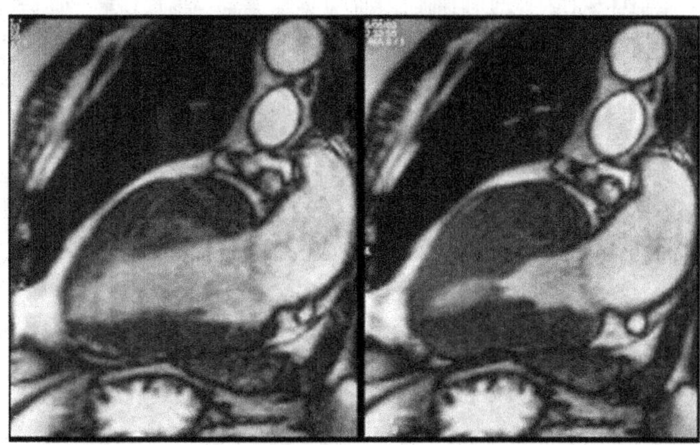

Figure 93.1 Magnetic resonance images, showing hypertrophic cardiomyopathy.

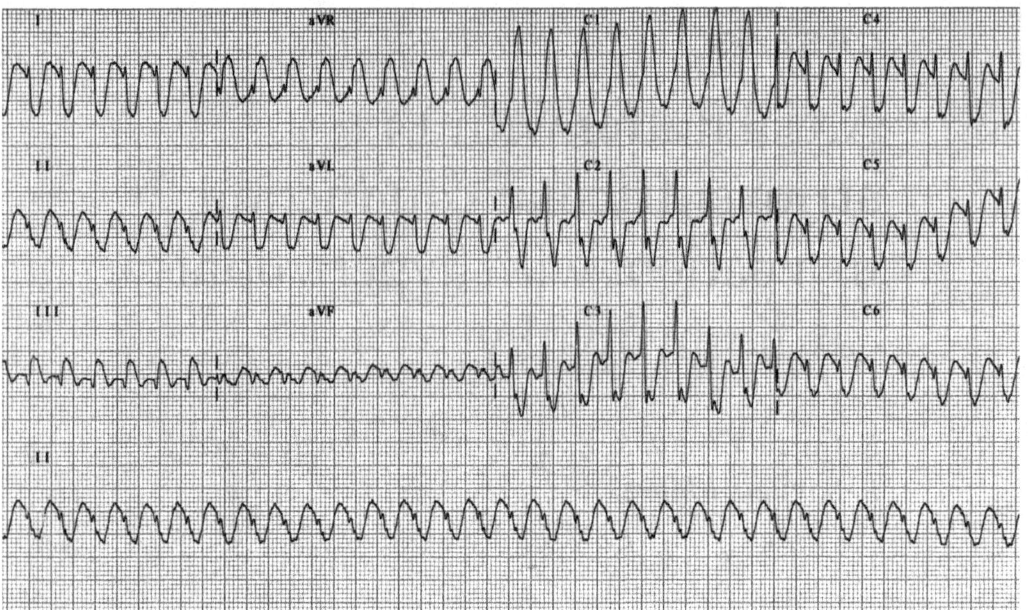

Figure 93.2 The initial electrocardiogram.

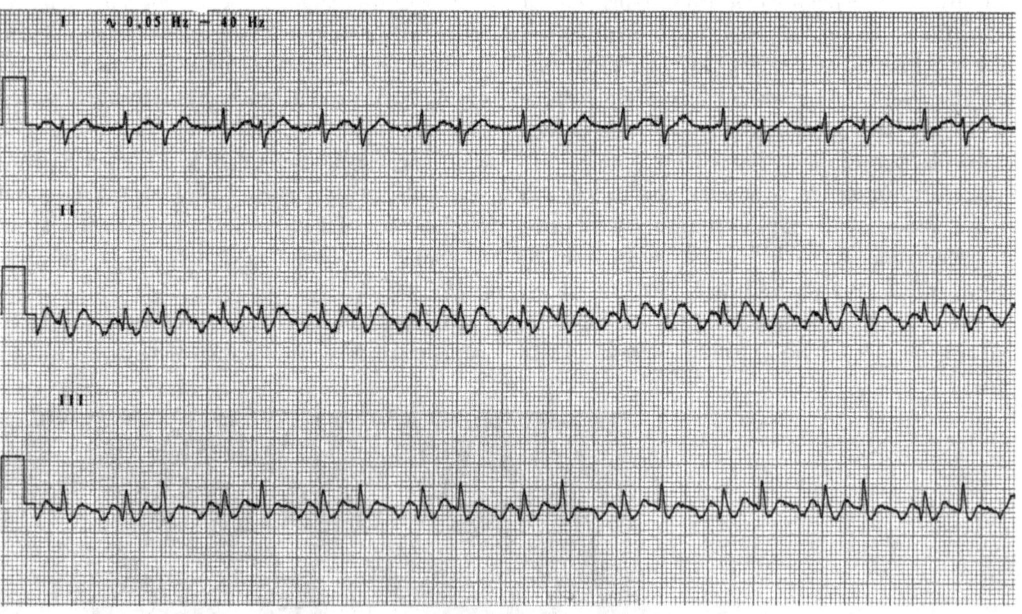

Figure 93.3 Spontaneous change in the electrocardiogram.

isthmus was carried out. The patient has remained asymptomatic during the follow-up period.

Comment

In the absence of fast conducting accessory pathways, 1 : 1 AV conduction during atrial flutter is unusual. In this case, the relatively slow rate of the atrial flutter waves (200 beats/min), probably due to chronic treatment with amiodarone, would have facilitated the 1 : 1 AV conduction.

Diastolic dysfunction is common in patients with hypertrophic cardiomyopathy. In these patients, fast atrial rates with 1 : 1 AV conduction can lead to acute hemodynamic deterioration. It has been demonstrated that supraventricular tachycardia (as induced by rapid atrial pacing) can produce hypotension and presyncope in 25% of patients with hypertrophic cardiomyopathy, and this hemodynamic effect is more frequent in patients with a history of syncope [2]. Moreover, López Gil *et al.* [3] reported that rapid atrial pacing induced ventricular fibrillation in three patients with hypertrophic cardiomyopathy. In some cases, therefore, rapid atrial rates may lead to hemodynamic collapse by critically impairing left ventricular filling or may trigger ventricular arrhythmias, causing syncope.

References

1 Brugada P, Brugada J, Mont L, Smeets J, Andries EW. A new approach to the differential diagnosis of a regular tachycardia with a wide QRS complex. *Circulation* 1991; **83**: 1649–59.

2 Nakatani M, Yokota Y, Yokoyama M. Acute hemodynamic deterioration during rapid atrial pacing in patients with HCM. *Clin Cardiol* 1996; **19**: 385–92.

3 López Gil M, Arribas F, Cosío FG. Ventricular fibrillation induced by rapid atrial rates in patients with hypertrophic cardiomyopathy. *Europace* 2000; **2**: 327–32.

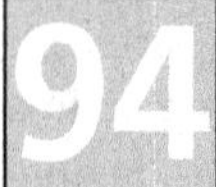

CASE 94

Syncope in hypertrophic cardiomyopathy, atrial fibrillation, and rapid ventricular response

S. Gómez Moreno, G. Barón Esquivias, E. Lage Gallé, A. Pedrote Martínez, F. Errázquin Sáenz de Tejada, A. Martínez Martínez

Case report

A 66-year-old man with hypertrophic cardiomyopathy (HCM) came to hospital because of a syncopal episode preceded by irregular palpitations. He had been diagnosed with HCM at the age of 56. He had a history of paroxysmal atrial fibrillation (AF) with three episodes recorded in the previous year, but had never suffered from syncope or presyncope. An hour before admission, while walking, he began to note palpitations, followed by dizziness and syncope. He recovered consciousness within a minute, but the palpitations persisted.

The physical examination was normal, with the exception of an irregular pulse at approximately 150 beats/min. His arterial blood pressure was 110/80 mmHg. The electrocardiogram showed AF with a rapid ventricular response (Fig. 94.1). Several different blood tests, including tests for triiodothyronine (T_3), thyroxine (T_4), and thyroid-stimulating hormone, were normal.

In an attempt to achieve control of the ventricular rate, the patient was given an intravenous bolus of 300 mg amiodarone followed by a maintenance infusion of 1200 mg/24 h. AF persisted, but after approximately 2 h of intravenous amiodarone administration

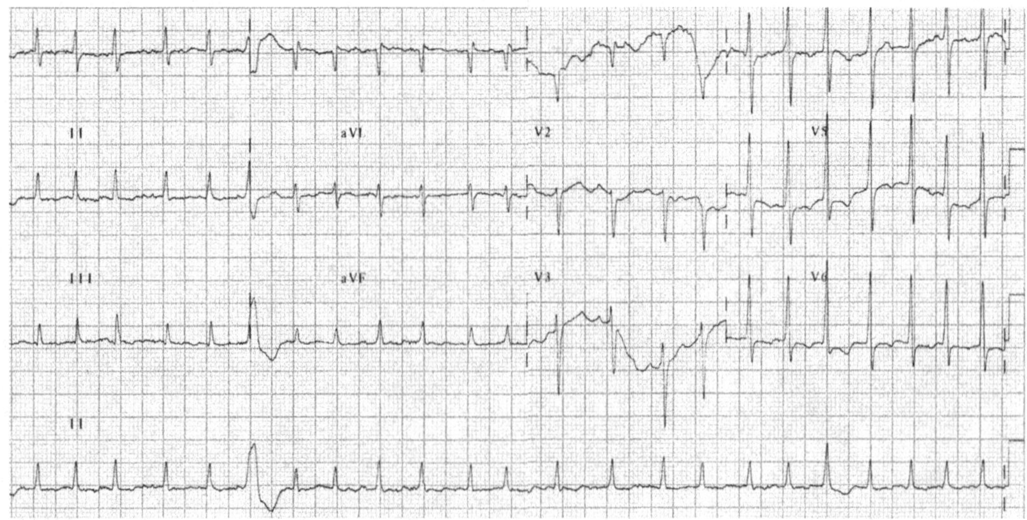

Figure 94.1 The electrocardiogram at admission.

and after intravenous therapy with digoxin, the ventricular rate was controlled.

The patient was discharged and treated with oral amiodarone, digoxin, and oral anticoagulation.

Comment

This case report illustrates the important clinical consequences of AF in patients with HCM. The sudden onset of this arrhythmia, accompanied by a rapid ventricular response, resulted in hemodynamic deterioration which, in this case, led to syncope, although it could have been pulmonary edema.

AF is a particularly important form of arrhythmia in HCM, reportedly occurring in up to 20% of patients with this disease [1]. From a pathophysiological point of view, this type of cardiomyopathy is characterized by diastolic dysfunction, which is exacerbated by the appearance of atrial tachyarrhythmias with a high ventricular response, especially AF, due to the loss of atrial contraction, which is the most powerful compensatory mechanism when protodiastolic filling is compromised. However, chronic AF appears to be reasonably well tolerated as long as the ventricular rate is controlled [2].

The high incidence of stroke in patients with HCM who develop AF justifies efforts to achieve and maintain sinus rhythm, in addition to the use of anticoagulant medication [3].

There have been no systematic studies on the treatment of AF in patients with HCM, but several antiarrhythmic drugs have been used, such as disopyramide, propafenone, and amiodarone. Some authors recommend the administration of amiodarone to prevent AF episodes and to control the ventricular rate [4]. Beta-blockers and calcium antagonists are also appropriate methods of controlling heart rate during AF.

Finally, it is always important to consider the need for oral anticoagulation treatment (international normalized ratio 2–3) as recommended for other high-risk patients for prevention of thromboembolism (recommendation class I, level of evidence B) [3].

References

1 Maron BJ, Casey SA, Poliac LC, *et al.* Clinical course of hypertrophic cardiomyopathy in a regional United States cohort. *J Am Med Assoc* 1999; **281**: 650–5.

2 Robinson KC, Frenneaux MP, Stockins B, *et al.* Atrial fibrillation in hypertrophic cardiomyopathy: a longitudinal study. *J Am Coll Cardiol* 1990; **15**: 1279–85.

3 Fuster V, Rydén LE, Asinger RW, *et al.* ACC/AHA/ESC guidelines for the management of patients with atrial fibrillation: executive summary. A report of the American College of Cardiology/American Heart Association Task Force on Practice Guidelines and the European Society of Cardiology Committee for Practice Guidelines and Policy Conferences (Committee to Develop Guidelines for the Management of Patients With Atrial Fibrillation) developed in collaboration with the North American Society of Pacing and Electrophysiology. *Circulation* 2001; **104**: 2118–50; *Eur Heart J* 2001; **22**: 1852–923; *J Am Coll Cardiol* 2001; **38**: 1231–66.

4 McKenna WJ, England D, Doi YL, Deanfield JE, Oakley C, Goodwin JF. Arrhythmia in hypertrophic cardiomyopathy, 1: influence on prognosis. *Br Heart J* 1981; **46**: 168–72.

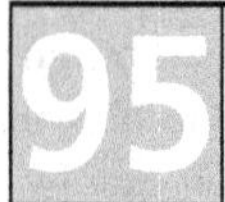

CASE 95

Syncopal ventricular tachycardia in a case of midseptal hypertrophic cardiomyopathy with apical aneurysm

R. Ruiz Granell, S. Morell Cabedo, R. Sanjuán Mañez, R. García Civera

Case report

A 69-year-old man came to the emergency room because of a syncopal episode that had been preceded by fast palpitations and an oppressive sensation in the chest. He recovered from the syncope quickly and without consequences, but palpitations persisted and he came to the hospital. Five years previously, he had consulted a physician due to mild dyspnea, and echocardiography had revealed hypertrophic cardiomyopathy (HCM). The patient was treated with verapamil and had remained asymptomatic until the current episode.

In the emergency room, the patient was conscious and oriented, his blood pressure was 90/60 mmHg, and a regular pulse at 200 beats/min was noted. The electrocardiogram (ECG) (Fig. 95.1) showed regular tachycardia with a wide QRS complex, with a morphology resembling a right bundle-branch block with a superior frontal axis and doubtful atrioventricular (AV) dissociation. Attempts to stop the tachycardia with carotid sinus massage were unsuccessful and, with the patient under mild sedation, a synchronized direct-current (DC) shock was administered, which restored sinus rhythm.

The ECG in sinus rhythm (Fig. 95.2) showed a normal PR interval, a right axis deviation in the frontal plane, profound Q waves in V_2 and V_3, and ST elevation with inverted T waves from V_2 to V_5. Analytical tests, including serial troponin I levels, were normal. The patient was then admitted to hospital for further evaluation.

A transthoracic echocardiogram (Fig. 95.3) showed a dilated left atrium (45 mm), asymmetric septal hypertrophy, and the presence of an apical aneurysm. Cardiac catheterization was carried out, and demonstrated normal coronary arteries, midseptal hypertrophy without obstruction, and severe hypokinesis of the anteroapical left ventricle (Fig. 95.4).

A diagnosis of midseptal HCM with anteroapical aneurysm was made, and an electrophysiological study (EPS) was conducted. Ventricular tachycardia (VT) similar to the clinical form was induced with programmed ventricular stimulation (basic cycle length of 500 ms and two extrastimuli). The tachycardia was poorly tolerated and was ended with DC cardioversion. An automatic cardioverter-defibrillator was finally implanted.

Comment

In patients with HCM, the detection of clinical sustained monomorphic VT is exceptional. In these patients, programmed ventricular stimulation induces sustained ventricular arrhythmias in 36% of cases, but the majority of these arrhythmias are polymorphic VT or ventricular fibrillation [1]. In 1989, Alfonso *et al.* [2] found only two patients with clinical sustained

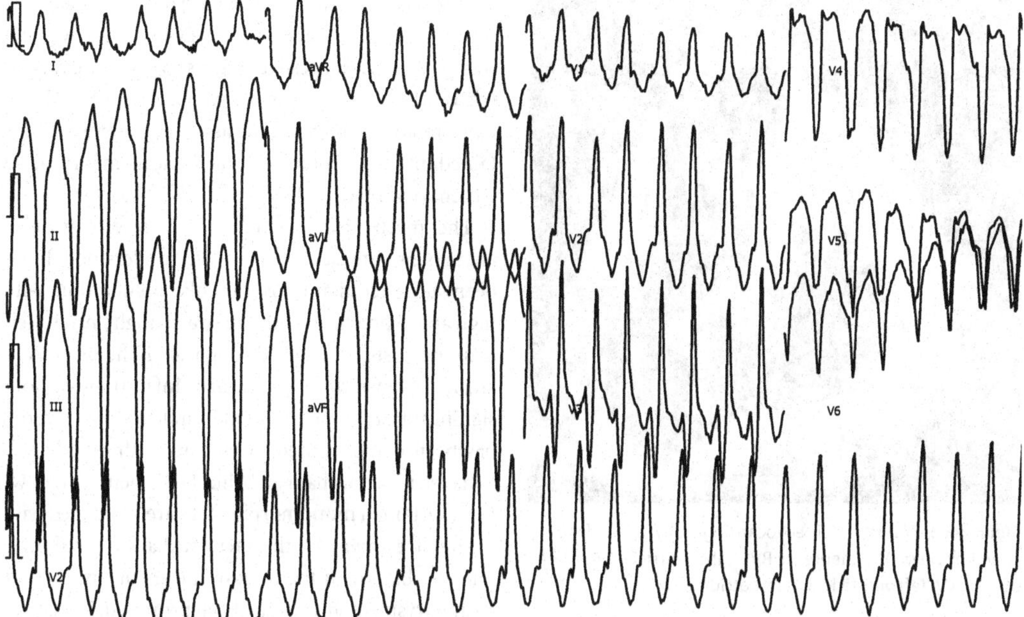

Figure 95.1 The electrocardiogram at admission.

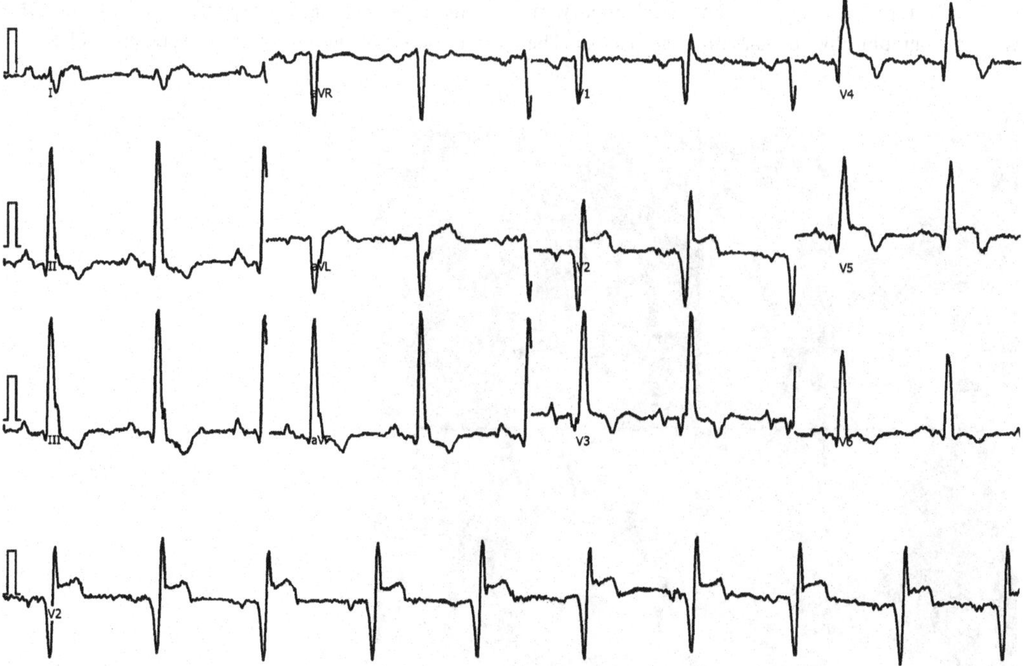

Figure 95.2 The baseline electrocardiogram.

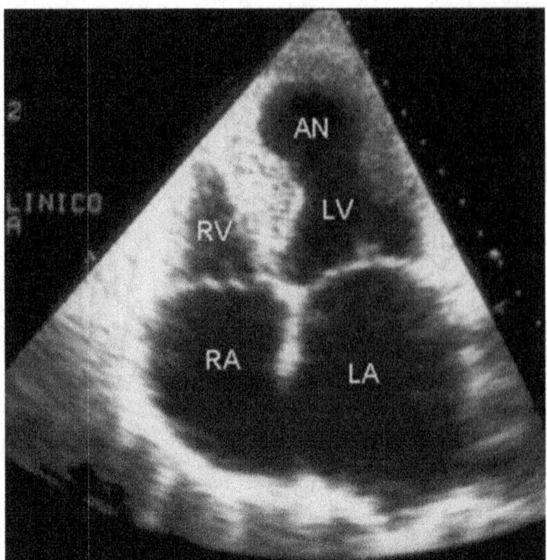

Figure 95.3 Transthoracic echocardiography: apical four-chamber view. AN, aneurysm; RV, right ventricle; RA, right atrium; LV, left ventricle; LA, left atrium.

monomorphic VT among 51 consecutive patients with HCM. Both patients had echocardiographic and ventriculographic evidence of an apical aneurysm, with angiographically normal coronary arteries. The authors also reported the presence of ST-segment elevation in the precordial leads, an ECG pattern which it was previously suggested could serve as a marker of left ventricular aneurysm in patients with HCM [3]. Later reports confirmed the association between sustained monomorphic VT and apical aneurysm in patients with HCM [4–9].

The mechanism leading to the development of aneurysms in these cases is not well understood. It has been suggested that midventricular obliteration, with high apical pressures and wall stress, might lead to cellular necrosis, possibly through an ischemic mechanism. Transmural myocardial infarction without significant stenosis of the extramural coronary arteries has been demonstrated in patients with HCM [10]. Whatever the mechanism behind the aneurysm, however, sustained monomorphic VTs are associated with it, and treatment of the tachycardia with radiofrequency ablation at the neck of the aneurysm [7,8] or by aneurysmectomy [8] has been proposed.

References

1 Fananapazir L, Chang AC, Epstein SE, McAreavey D. Prognostic determinants in hypertrophic cardiomyopathy: prospective evaluation of a therapeutic strategy based on

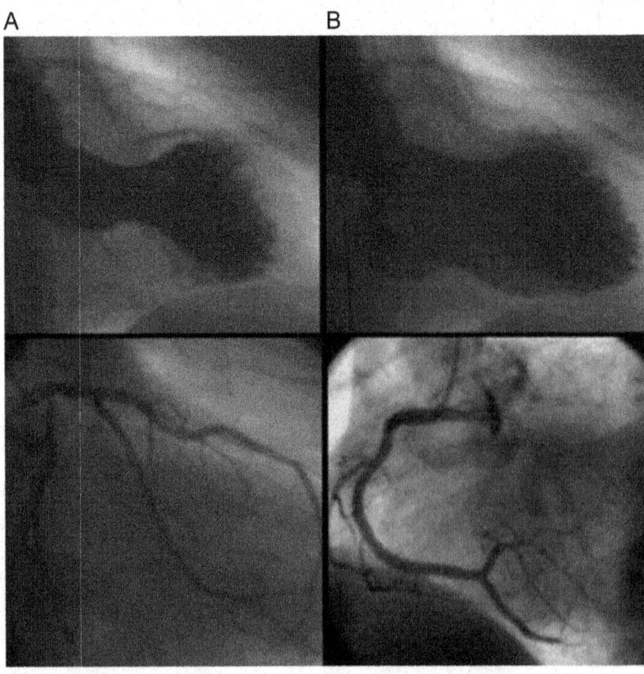

Figure 95.4 Left ventriculography (A, B) and left and right coronary angiography (C, D).

clinical, Holter, hemodynamic, and electrophysiological findings. *Circulation* 1992; **86**: 730–40.

2 Alfonso F, Frenneaux MP, McKenna WJ. Clinical sustained ventricular tachycardia in hypertrophic cardiomyopathy: association with left ventricular apical aneurysm. *Br Heart J* 1989; **61**: 178–81.

3 Gordon EP, Henderson MA, Rakowski H, Wigle ED. Midventricular obstruction with apical infarction and aneurysm formation [abstract]. *Circulation* 1984; **70** (Suppl 2): 145.

4 Wilson P, Marks A, Rastegar H, Manolis AS, Estes NA. Apical hypertrophic cardiomyopathy presenting with sustained monomorphic ventricular tachycardia and electrocardiographic changes simulating coronary artery disease and left ventricular aneurysm. *Clin Cardiol* 1990; **13**: 885–7.

5 Gonzalez Torrecilla E, Fernandez-Yáñez J, García E, Pérez David E, García Fernández MA, Delcán JL. El "síndrome" de obstrucción medioventricular con aneurisma apical en la miocardiopatia hipertrófica: presentación de un caso. *Rev Esp Cardiol* 1997; **50**: 586–9.

6 López-Míngez JR, Marchán Herrera A, Cimboria Ortiga A, *et al.* Taquicardias ventriculares sostenidas en un paciente con miocardiopatia hipertrófica medioventricular y aneurisma apical. *Rev Esp Cardiol* 1997; **50**: 593–6.

7 Rodriguez LM, Smeets JL, Timmermans C, Blommaert D, van Dantzing MEB, Wellens HJ. Radiofrequency catheter ablation of sustained monomorphic ventricular tachycardia in hypertrophic cardiomyopathy. *J Cardiovasc Electrophysiol* 1997; **8**: 803–6.

8 Mantica M, Della Bella P, Arena V. Hypertrophic cardiomyopathy with apical aneurysm: a case of catheter and surgical therapy of sustained monomorphic ventricular tachycardia. *Heart* 1997; **77**: 481–3.

9 Kono K, Higashi T, Hara K, *et al.* [Mid-ventricular obstructive hypertrophic cardiomyopathy associated with an apical aneurysm and sustained ventricular tachycardia: a case report; in Japanese.] *J Cardiol* 2001; **38**: 343–9.

10 Maron BJ, Epstein SE, Roberts WC. Hypertrophic cardiomyopathy and transmural myocardial infarction without significant arteriosclerosis of the extramural coronary arteries. *Am J Cardiol* 1979; **43**: 1086–102.

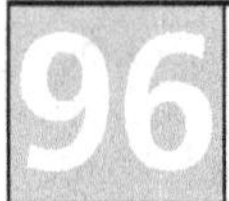

CASE 96
Carcinoid syndrome

S. Gómez Moreno, G. Barón Esquivias, F. López Pardo, M.J. Rodríguez Puras, A. Martínez Martínez

Case report

A 59-year-old woman was admitted to hospital after a single syncopal episode. She had a long history of hypertension that had been treated with enalapril, and 6 months previously had been hospitalized in the gastroenterology department due to dyspnea and an abnormal increase in abdominal girth. During this first hospitalization, two hepatic metastases were identified on magnetic resonance imaging, but the primary tumor was not found. Chemotherapy for an unknown tumor was therefore initiated.

The syncopal episode was brief, with no apparent precipitating events. After recovering, the patient noted a worsening in her usual dyspnea. The physical examination revealed raised jugular venous pressure, hepatomegaly, and discrete bimalleolar edemas. Her blood pressure was 80/60 mmHg, and a loud 2/6 systolic murmur, accentuated by inspiration, was heard over the fifth right intercostal space.

The electrocardiogram and chest radiogram were normal. Transthoracic echocardiography showed normal left chambers, but dilated right chambers. The right ventricle had a telediastolic diameter of 51–56 mm, with marked trabeculation and normal contractility. The right atrium was also dilated (50 mm). The annulus of the tricuspid valve was dilated, with thick leaflets and cordal structures (Fig. 96.1). The leaflets were immobile, and the tricuspid regurgitation was severe (Fig. 96.2). There was pulmonary stenosis, with a gradient of 34 mmHg and mild regurgitation. The pulmonary valve also showed thick leaflets (Fig. 96.3). In conclusion, she had tricuspid and pulmonary valvulopathy, with alterations that suggested carcinoid heart disease.

During hospitalization, the patient had diarrhea, flushing, presyncope, and episodes of thoracic pain that

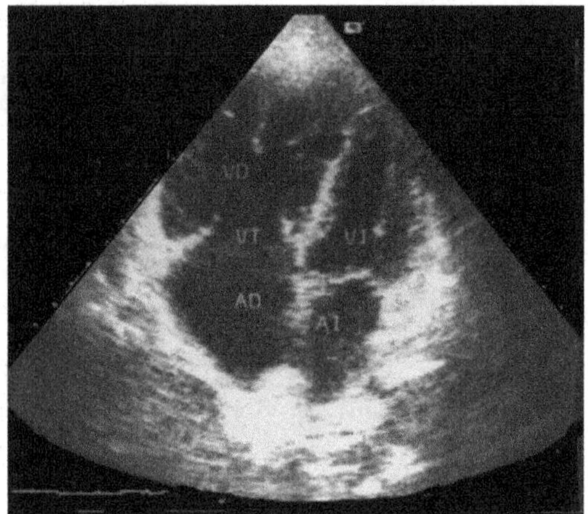

Figure 96.1 Transthoracic echocardiogram, showing dilated right chambers and a tricuspid valve (VT) with a dilated annulus and thick leaflets. VD, right ventricle; VI, left ventricle; AD, right atrium; AI, left atrium.

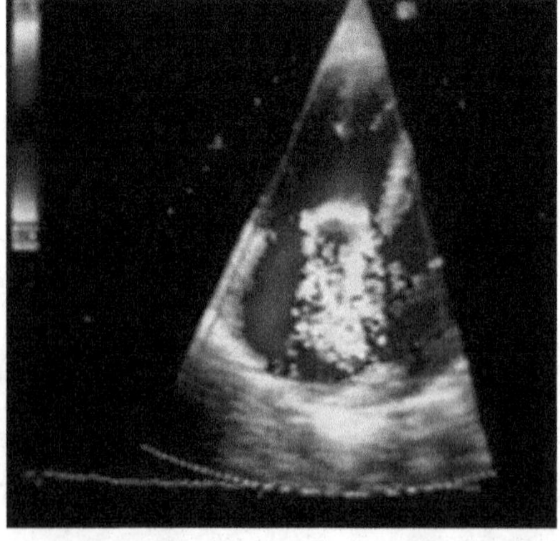

Figure 96.2 Transthoracic echocardiogram with color flow Doppler, showing severe tricuspid regurgitation.

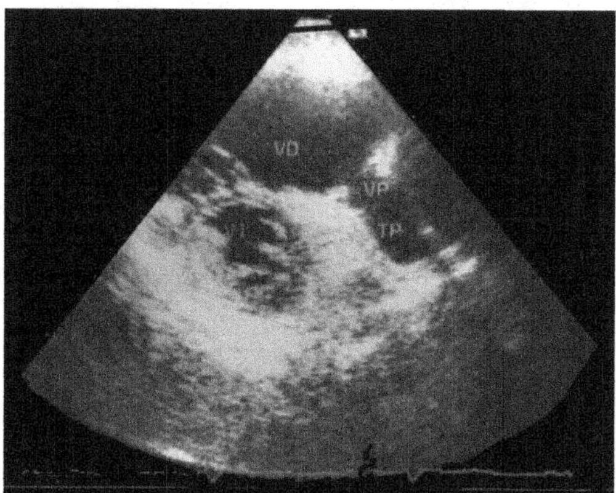

Figure 96.3 Transthoracic echocardiogram, showing the pulmonary valve (VP) with thick leaflets. VD, right ventricle; VI, left ventricle; TP, pulmonary artery.

required the administration of sublingual nitroglycerin. The urinary 5-hydroxyindoleacetic acid (5-HIAA) level was 1550 mmol/24 h (normal 0–6 mmol/24 h). She had low blood pressure after standing up.

Treatment with somatostatin was initiated to control the symptoms, and a Carpentier–Edwards bioprosthesis was implanted over the native tricuspid valve in advance of liver surgery, due to the risk of hepatic hemorrhage induced by the elevated right-sided pressures.

Forty days after the operation, the patient died due to intractable right heart failure.

Comment

Carcinoid tumors are a rare type of neoplasm that contain a high concentration of 5-hydroxytryptamine (serotonin). These tumors most commonly arise in the gastrointestinal tract, but they can also develop in the bronchus, biliary tract, pancreas, testis, and ovary.

The malignant carcinoid syndrome usually results from metastases to the liver or, rarely, from primary carcinoids alone [1]. The syndrome is produced by the secretion of tumor products into the systemic circulation, resulting in vasomotor changes, cutaneous flushing, intestinal hypermobility, diarrhea, bronchospasm, and hypotension that can lead to syncope or presyncope. In the heart, products of the tumor produce a distinctive intracardiac and valvular pathological pattern, commonly in the right side of the heart. Carcinoid heart disease has been recognized in more than half of patients with carcinoid syndrome. Coronary artery spasm has also been reported [2].

A diagnosis of carcinoid syndrome is usually suspected on the basis of the clinical features and is confirmed by increased urinary excretion of the byproduct of serotonin metabolism, 5-HIAA [1]. However, it is appropriate to carry out echocardiographic evaluation in patients with carcinoid syndrome in order to assess whether there is cardiac valvular involvement [3]. In the present case, the symptoms of right-sided heart failure, in addition to the syncopal episode, led to an echocardiographic examination before the diagnosis of carcinoid syndrome was suspected.

The echocardiographic features of advanced carcinoid heart disease are pathognomonic and include thickening and retraction of immobile tricuspid valve leaflets with associated tricuspid regurgitation, which is severe in 90% of patients. Less commonly, tricuspid valve stenosis is noted. Pulmonary valve involvement usually coexists with tricuspid valve disease, and the major finding on echocardiography is immobility of the pulmonary valve leaflets [4].

The main therapeutic modality in such patients consists of symptom control, usually with a somatostatin analog (octreotide or lanreotide). Tumor removal is of limited value, since patients with carcinoid syndrome typically have metastatic disease, and chemotherapy has shown little success. Cardiac surgery is the only effective treatment for carcinoid heart disease and should be considered for symptomatic patients whose metastatic carcinoid disease and symptoms of carcinoid syndrome are well controlled [5].

References

1 Maton PN. The carcinoid syndrome. *J Am Med Assoc* 1988; **260**: 1602–5.

2 Topol EJ, Fortuin NJ. Coronary artery spasm and cardiac arrest in carcinoid heart disease. *Am J Med* 1984; 77: 950–2.

3 Denney WD, Kemp WE Jr, Anthony LB, Oates JA, Byrd BF 3rd. Echocardiographic and biochemical evaluation of the development and progression of carcinoid heart disease. *J Am Coll Cardiol* 1998; **32**: 1017–22.

4 Pellikka PA, Tajik AJ, Khanderia BK, *et al.* Carcinoid heart disease: clinical and echocardiographic spectrum in 74 patients. *Circulation* 1993; **87**: 1188–96.

5 Connolly HM, Shaff H, Nishimura RA, Smith HC, Pellikka PA, Mullany CJ, Kvols LK. Outcome of cardiac surgery for carcinoid heart disease. *J Am Coll Cardiol* 1995; **25**: 410–6.

CASE 97

Syncope and myotonic dystrophy

J.L. Merino, R. Peinado, M. Gnoatto, M. González Vasserot

Case report

A 28-year-old man had a 2-year history of chest pain and syncopal episodes. He also had a history of maternal rubella, bilateral cataracts, clubfoot, and hypercholesterolemia, but no other cardiovascular risk factors. Sublingual nitroglycerin had been administered in an emergency department during one of the clinical episodes, followed by syncope with prompt recovery of consciousness and without residual chest pain. He was diagnosed with ischemic heart disease and had been referred to his local cardiologist, who reported an unremarkable cardiac examination and sinus rhythm, PR interval prolongation, and left bundle-branch block on the baseline electrocardiogram (ECG) (Fig. 97.1A). Routine biochemical and hematological analysis, chest radiography, transthoracic echocardiography, exercise testing, and positron-emission tomography had shown no significant alterations. He was put on aspirin treatment and followed up in the outpatient clinic.

The patient developed another recurrence of chest

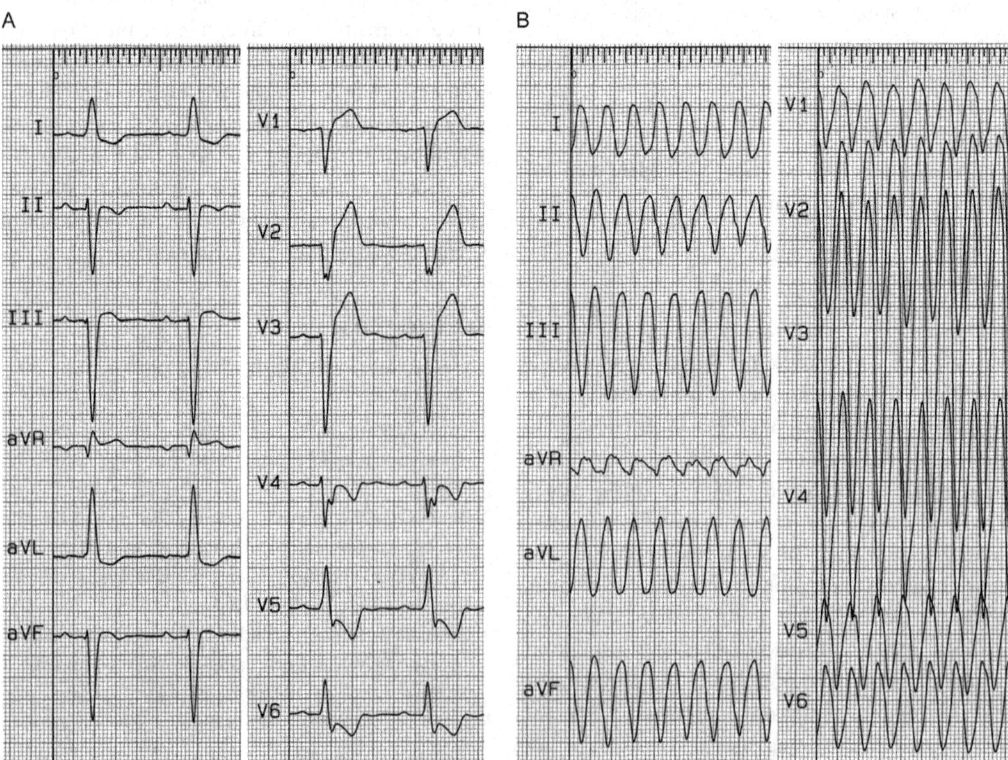

Figure 97.1 Electrocardiography tracings at baseline (A) and during tachycardia (B).

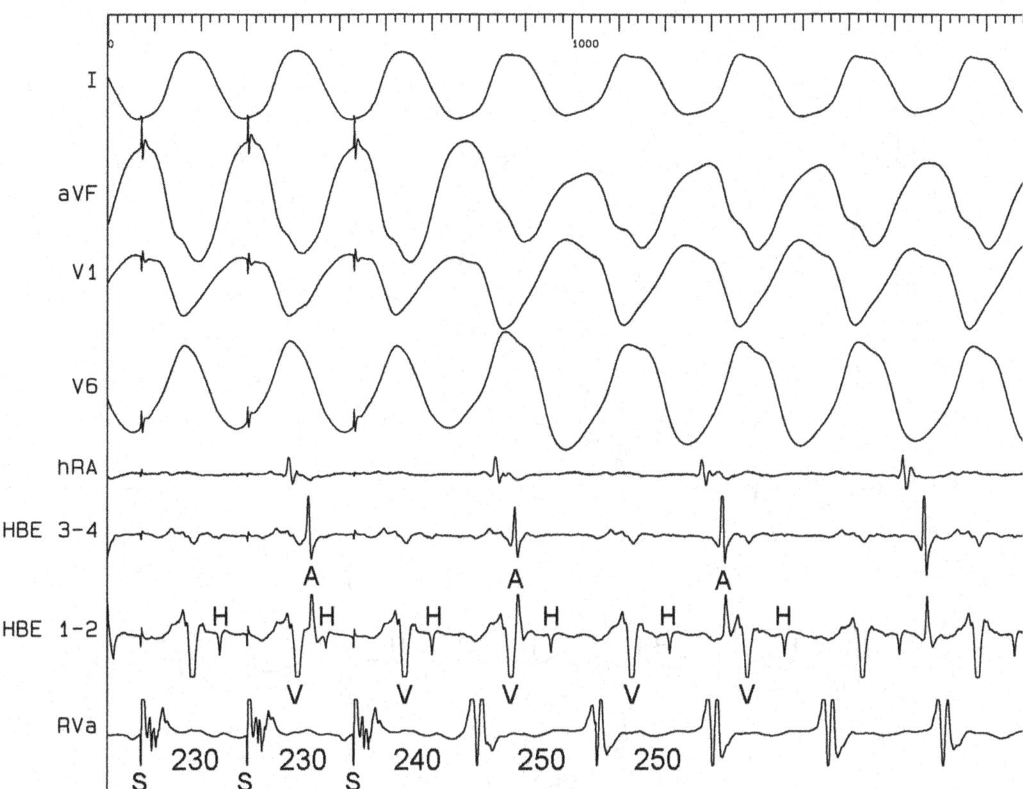

Figure 97.2 Tachycardia entrainment by right ventricular stimulation. The simultaneous 100 mm/s tracings, from top to bottom, are 20-ms time lines, with surface electrocardiogram leads I, aVF, V_1, and V_6, and bipolar intracardiac recordings from the high right atrium (hRA), His bundle area (HBE), and right ventricular apex (RVa). Pertinent intervals are labeled in milliseconds (ms). The atrioventricular dissociation should be noted; a His bundle electrogram (H) precedes each QRS complex, with spontaneous changes in the His–His interval preceding those of the ventriculogram–ventriculogram interval. The postpacing interval, slightly shorter than the tachycardia cycle length, should also be noted.

pain and dizziness and was admitted to our center. The ECG showed wide QRS complex tachycardia, with a similar QRS complex morphology to that recorded during sinus rhythm, terminating after procainamide infusion (Fig. 97.1B). The patient had a characteristic phenotype of frontal baldness and distal and parietal muscle atrophy and had myotonia and distal muscular weakness. A diagnosis of myotonic dystrophy was confirmed on electromyography, with pathological expansion of the nucleotide triplet CTG at locus 19q13.3 in the genetic study. No apparent heart disease was revealed by chest radiography, echocardiography, or coronary and left ventricle angiography.

Bundle-branch reentry was considered the most likely mechanism for the tachycardia, and an electrophysiological evaluation was scheduled. Three catheters were introduced through the right femoral vein and placed in the high right atrium, His bundle area, and right ventricular apex. The HV interval was prolonged to 80 ms. The clinical tachycardia with a cycle length of 250 ms was induced reproducibly with a single extrastimulus following a basic pacing train from the right ventricular apex. This tachycardia showed atrioventricular (AV) dissociation and a stable His electrogram before each ventricular activation during tachycardia, with an HV interval (90 ms) longer than that recorded during sinus rhythm (Fig. 97.2). Tachycardia entrainment by pacing from the right ventricular apex resulted in a postpacing interval 10 ms shorter than the tachycardia cycle length, suggesting a bundle-branch reentry mechanism (Fig. 97.2).

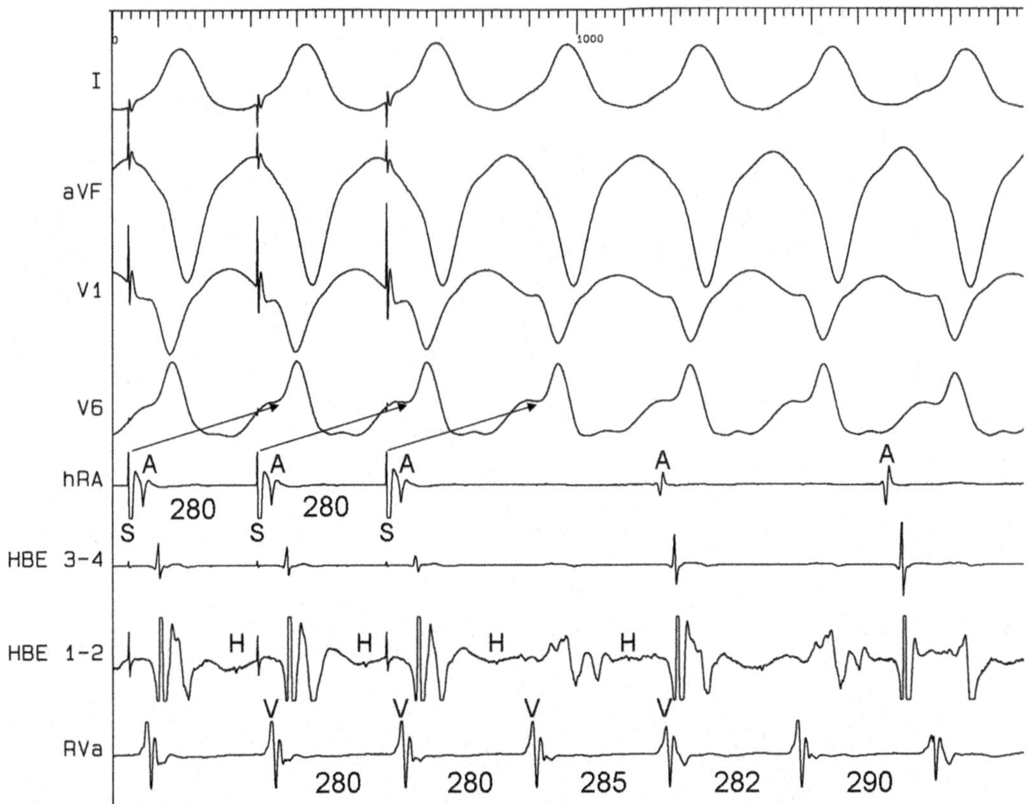

Figure 97.3 Tachycardia entrainment by atrial stimulation. The acceleration of all of the tachycardia components to the pacing cycle length, the preservation of the QRS morphology, and the resumption of the tachycardia at the end of pacing should be noted. hRA, high right atrium; HBE, His bundle area.

The QRS complex showed manifest fusion during tachycardia entrainment by ventricular stimulation, which ruled out an AV nodal reentrant mechanism. Tachycardia entrainment by atrial stimulation accelerated the tachycardia without a change in the QRS complex morphology (orthodromically concealed fusion), excluding ventricular myocardium reentry as the tachycardia mechanism (Fig. 97.3).

Bundle-branch reentry was established as the tachycardia mechanism, and ablation of the right bundle branch was achieved by a single radiofrequency application (Fig. 97.4). After bundle-branch ablation, the patient developed right bundle-branch block and HV prolongation (90 ms) and had persistent 1 : 1 AV conduction. Tachycardia was not inducible. The patient underwent permanent VVD pacemaker implantation, which was programmed to VVI mode at 50 beats/min. After a 5-year follow-up period, the patient has had no chest pain or recurrent syncope, and his ECG shows sinus rhythm, a long PR interval, a right bundle-branch block and 1 : 1 AV conduction.

The acceleration of all of the tachycardia components to the pacing cycle length, the preservation of the QRS complex morphology, and the resumption of the tachycardia after the cessation of pacing should be noted.

Comment

Myotonic dystrophy (MD), also known as myotonia atrophica and Steinert's disease, is a progressive multisystem disorder with autosomal-dominant inheritance. In its most common form, the disease is caused by an unstable expansion mutation of the cytosine–thymine–guanine (CTG) trinucleotide repeat situated in the 3′ noncoding exon of a gene that encodes a serine–threonine protein kinase (*DMPK*) [1]. In the

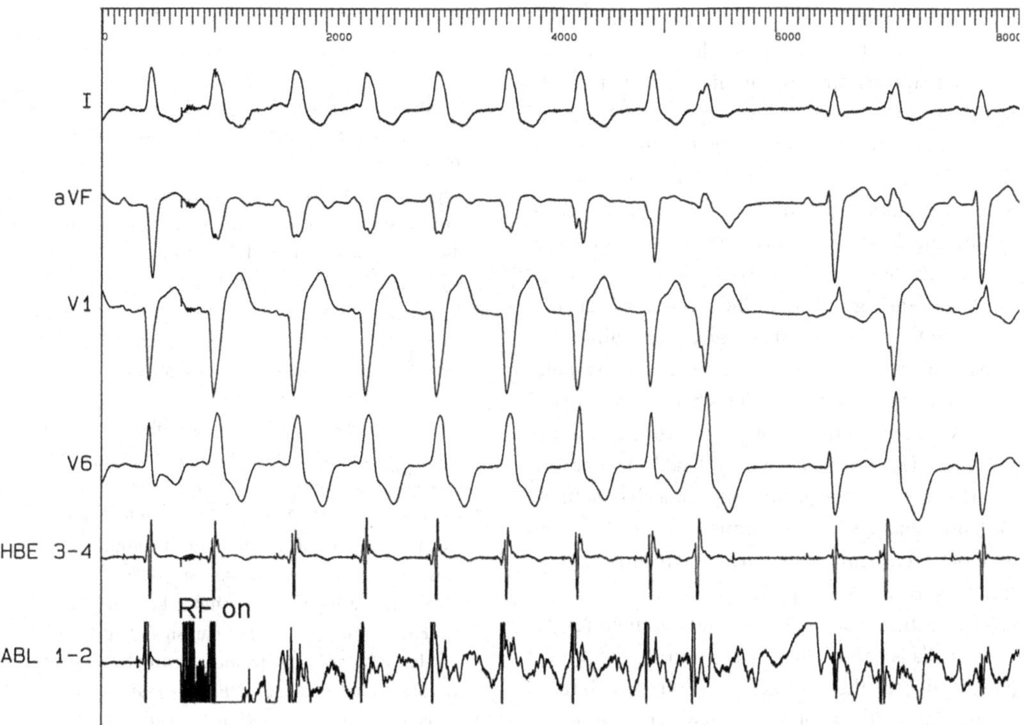

Figure 97.4 Right bundle-branch ablation. The change to a right bundle-branch QRS complex configuration, with preserved atrioventricular conduction, should be noted on the right side. HBE, His bundle area; ABL, ablation; RF, radiofrequency.

classical form of the disease, symptoms become evident between the second and fourth decades of life, showing a slow progression over time. However, a severe form of the disease, present at birth or developing during the first year of life, has also been described.

Myotonia, characterized by delayed relaxation after muscular contraction, usually begins in the muscles of the hands, feet, neck, or face and causes progressive general weakness. A wide variety of organs and systems can also be involved, including the eye (cataract), the endocrine system (diabetes, thyroid dysfunction, hypogonadism), the central nervous system (cognitive impairment, mental retardation), the gastrointestinal system (dysphagia, constipation), and the heart.

Cardiac involvement in MD includes nonspecific changes such as interstitial fibrosis or fatty infiltration of myocardium, but the most selective and common finding is extensive replacement of the His–Purkinje system by fatty and fibrous tissue [1–3]. Cardiac manifestations of Steinert's disease are ECG abnormalities [4], intraventricular conduction disorders [5,6], AV block [7,8], and ventricular arrhythmias [8,9], which generally appear in patients without apparent structural heart disease. These arrhythmias can be symptomatic and manifest in the form of palpitations, presyncope, or syncope. There is also a high incidence of sudden death that has been attributed to AV block or ventricular arrhythmia.

Prolongation of the HV interval is common in patients with MD [5,6,8], and ventricular tachycardia can be induced during electrophysiological testing [6]. Recently, Merino *et al.* [9] have shown that bundle-branch reentry is the main mechanism of sustained monomorphic ventricular tachycardia in patients with MD. His–Purkinje conduction delay in these patients represents an ideal substrate for this type of reentry. Bundle-branch reentry tachycardia should therefore be suspected in patients with MD who present with palpitations, syncope, or wide QRS complex tachycardia, and MD should be considered in patients with sustained ventricular tachycardia without apparent heart disease [9].

In the electrophysiological diagnosis of bundle-branch reentry tachycardia, the hallmark feature is that spontaneous variations in the cycle length of the tachycardia are preceded by variations in the HH intervals with a similar cycle length [10]. However, this criterion may not be applicable in certain patients, due to difficulties in maintaining His bundle recordings during the tachycardia, an absence of cycle length oscillations, or because the oscillations are produced in the descending instead of the ascending branch of the circuit [11,12]. In these cases, entraining the tachycardia from the right ventricular apex (a point close to the tachycardia circuit) is helpful in the diagnosis, showing a return cycle similar (difference < 30 ms) to the tachycardia cycle [11]. Finally, tachycardia entrainment by atrial pacing without a change in the QRS morphology (orthodromic concealed fusion) excludes ventricular myocardium reentry as the tachycardia mechanism [12].

The treatment of choice in bundle-branch reentry tachycardia is bundle-branch ablation. In the present patient, due to the presence of a long HV interval (90 ms) after the ablation and concerns regarding progression of the conduction defects during the further course of the disease, a prophylactic pacemaker was also implanted.

References

1 Pelargonio G, Dello Ruso A, Sanna T, De Martino G, Bellocci F. Myotonic dystrophy and the heart. *Heart* 2002; **88**: 665–70.

2 Phillips MF, Harper PS. Cardiac disease in myotonic dystrophy. *Cardiovasc Res* 1997; **33**: 13–22.

3 Hawley RJ, Milner MR, Gottdiener JS, Cohen A. Myotonic heart disease: a clinical follow-up. *Neurology* 1991; **41**: 259–62.

4 Oloffson B, Forsberg H, Andersson S, *et al.* Electrocardiographic findings in myotonic dystrophy. *Br Heart J* 1988; **59**: 47–52.

5 Prystowsky EN, Prichett EL, Gallagher J. The natural history of conduction system disease in myotonic muscular dystrophy as determined by serial electrophysiologic studies. *Circulation* 1979; **60**: 1360–4.

6 Lazarus A, Varin J, Ounnoughene Z, *et al.* Relationship among electrophysiological findings and clinical status, heart function and extent of DNA mutation in myotonic dystrophy. *Circulation* 1999; **99**: 1041–6.

7 Bache RJ, Sarosi GA. Myotonia atrophica: diagnosis in a patient with complete heart block and the Stokes–Adams syncope. *Arch Intern Med* 1968; **121**: 369–72.

8 Lazarus A, Varin J, Duboc D. Final results of the French diagnostic pacemaker study in myotonic dystrophy [abstract]. *Pacing Clin Electrophysiol* 2002; **25**: 599.

9 Merino JL, Carmona JR, Fernández-Lozano I, Peinado R, Basterra N, Sobrino JA. Mechanisms of sustained ventricular tachycardia in myotonic dystrophy: implications for catheter ablation. *Circulation* 1998; **98**: 541–6.

10 Caceres J, Jazayeri M, McKinnie J, *et al.* Sustained bundle branch block reentry as a mechanism of clinical tachycardia. *Circulation* 1989; **79**: 256–70.

11 Merino JL, Peinado R, Fernandez-Lozano I, *et al.* Bundle-branch reentry and the postpacing interval after entrainment by ventricular apex stimulation. *Circulation* 2001; **103**: 1102–8.

12 Merino JL, Peinado R, Fernandez-Lozano I, Sobrino N, Sobrino JA. Transient entrainment of bundle-branch reentry by atrial and ventricular stimulation: elucidation of the tachycardia mechanism though analysis of the surface ECG. *Circulation* 1999; **100**: 1784–90.

CASE 98

Syncope in a patient with Kearns–Sayre syndrome

L. García Riesco, A. Pedrote Martínez, E. Arana, G. Barón Esquivias, F. Errázquin Sáenz de Tejada

Case report

A 17-year-old girl was examined in the neurology department due to bilateral hearing loss, limb weakness, bilateral progressive palpebral ptosis, and difficulty in swallowing and writing. She had been diagnosed with diabetes mellitus at the age of seven. The physical examination showed growth deficiency, ataxia, and dysmetria. She also had external ophthalmoplegia and abnormal bilateral retinal pigmentation. Computed tomography of the brain was normal. A skeletal muscle biopsy showed ragged red fibers and an increase in oxidative activity in the peripheral muscle fibers.

The cardiac evaluation, including chest radiography and two-dimensional echocardiography, was normal. Her resting electrocardiogram (ECG) showed sinus rhythm at 70 beats/min, a PR interval of 140 ms, and a QRS duration of 120 ms, with a bifascicular block (incomplete right bundle-branch block and left axis deviation) (Fig. 98.1A). The laboratory tests were normal, with the exception of basal hyperglycemia.

Two months later, the patient suffered three syncopal episodes without prodromal symptoms within a short time, with a high-grade heart block being found on the ECG (Fig. 98.1B). It was decided to implant a bicameral pacemaker (DDD). The patient is currently asymptomatic.

Comment

In 1958, Kearns and Sayre described a syndrome of pigmentary retinitis, progressive external ophthalmoplegia, and complete heart block [1]. This syndrome is now included in the group of mitochondrial

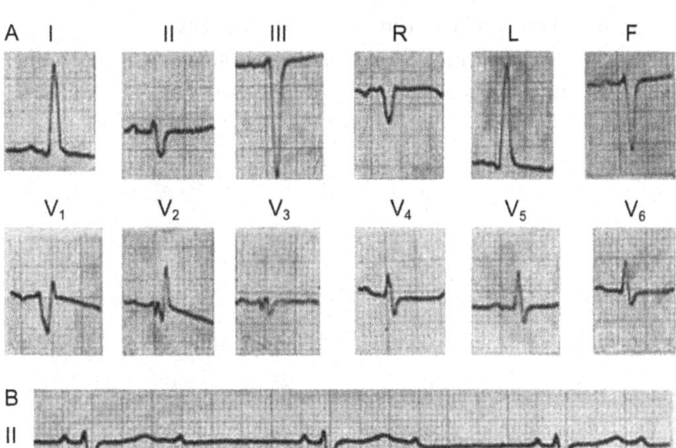

Figure 98.1 A. Electrocardiogram in sinus rhythm, with right bundle-branch block and left axis deviation. **B.** High-grade atrioventricular block.

encephalomyopathies, characterized by morphological and functional disorders in the mitochondria, with typical ragged red fibers on muscle biopsy [2]. The syndrome is a multisystem mitochondrial disorder characterized by an invariable triad of onset before the age of 20, progressive external ophthalmoplegia, and pigmentary retinal degeneration, plus at least one of the following: complete (or incomplete) heart block, cerebral dysfunction, and a cerebrospinal fluid protein level above 100 mg/dL [3]. It is also associated with hormonal disorders, dilated cardiomyopathy, and mitral valve prolapse.

The prognosis in the disease can be assessed by heart conduction system defects. Approximately 20% of patients with Kearns–Sayre syndrome have cardiac involvement, and most usually suffer conduction defects causing progressive heart blockage. Electrocardiographic abnormalities in Kearns–Sayre syndrome include first-degree atrioventricular block, fascicular block, and complete heart block, as well as nonspecific ST–T segment changes. Electrophysiological studies may reveal prolongation of the HV interval, confirming the infrahisian location of the conduction abnormalities [4]. Autopsy usually reveals muscle fibers vacuolated and substituted by fatty tissue in the distal portion of the His bundle. In genetic studies, these patients have been found to have large heterogeneous deletions in the mitochondrial genome, $tRNA^{leu(UUR)}$3243 being the most common [5].

Prophylactic pacemaker therapy is advisable in such patients because of the potential progression of the conduction abnormalities and the risk of sudden death. In the series reported by Roberts *et al.* [6], seven of 17 patients developed a high-degree heart block requiring cardiac pacing. Atrioventricular block constitutes a class I indication for permanent pacemaker placement in patients with Kearns–Sayre syndrome, according to the American College of Cardiology guidelines [7]. However, the prophylactic indication is still a matter of controversy. It has been suggested that patients with intraventricular conduction disturbances and normal atrioventricular conduction should be candidates for pacemaker implantation [4].

References

1 Kearns TP, Sayre GP. Retinitis pigmentosa, external ophthalmoplegia and complete heart block: unusual syndrome with histologic study in one of two cases. *Arch Ophthalmol* 1958; **60**: 280–9.

2 Egger J, Lake BD, Wilson J. Mitochondrial cytopathy: a multisystem disorder with ragged red fibers on muscle biopsy. *Arch Dis Child* 1981; **56**: 741–52.

3 Katsanos KH, Pappas CJ, Patsouras D. Alarming atrioventricular block and mitral valve prolapse in the Kearns–Sayre syndrome. *Int J Cardiol* 2002; **83**: 179–81.

4 Pedrote A, Varela JM, Sanchez A, *et al.* [Atrioventricular block in Kearns–Sayre syndrome; in Spanish.] *Rev Esp Cardiol* 1990; **43**: 192–4.

5 Tveskov C, Angelo-Nielsen K. Kearns–Sayre syndrome and dilated cardiomyopathy. *Neurology* 1990; **40**: 553–4.

6 Roberts NK, Perloff JK, Kark RA. Cardiac conduction in the Kearns–Sayre syndrome (a neuromuscular disorder associated with progressive external ophthalmoplegia and pigmentary retinopathy): report of 2 cases and review of 17 published cases. *Am J Cardiol* 1979; **44**: 1396–400.

7 Gregoratos G, Abrams J, Epstein AE, *et al.* ACC/AHA/NASPE 2002 guideline update for implantation of cardiac pacemakers and antiarrhythmia devices—summary article: a report of the American College of Cardiology/American Heart Association Task Force on Practice Guidelines (ACC/AHA/NASPE Committee to Update the 1998 Pacemaker Guidelines). *J Cardiovasc Electrophysiol* 2002; **13**: 1183–99; *J Am Coll Cardiol* 2002; **40**: 1703–19; *Circulation* 2002; **106**: 2145–61.

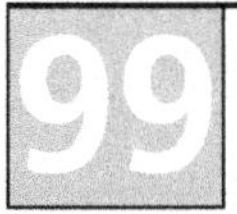

CASE 99

Syncope in aortic stenosis

P. Tornos

Case report

A 50-year-old male butcher was referred to the outpatient cardiology department for evaluation of a cardiac murmur. He was a nonsmoking and normotensive man with normal lipid levels who denied having experienced any cardiac symptoms. He had no family history of cardiac disease, and his only previous health problem had been a history of seizures diagnosed as epilepsy, which was being treated medically; he had been asymptomatic for the previous 5 years.

On examination, he appeared to be fit and athletic. His blood pressure was 130/70 mmHg, the carotid pulse was slow and mild (parvus), peripheral pulses were normal, and there was a 3/6 systolic murmur in the aortic region radiating to the carotid artery. There were no signs of heart failure, and the remainder of the physical examination was normal. The electrocardiogram (Fig. 99.1) showed sinus rhythm, with a PR of 0.24 ms and a left ventricular strain pattern. The chest radiograph showed mild enlargement of the ascending aorta, a normal-sized heart, and normal lung fields.

The Doppler ultrasound examination was consistent with severe aortic stenosis and mild regurgitation with a peak velocity of 5.7 m/s, a maximum aortic gradient of 128 mmHg, and a mean aortic gradient of 84 mmHg (Fig. 99.2), with a preserved left ventricular ejection fraction. The patient was diagnosed as having a severe asymptomatic aortic stenosis, and close follow-up was advised, as well as early reporting of any symptoms.

Two months later, the patient reported having suffered a syncopal attack. He was walking to work and suddenly collapsed. He denied noticing any premonitory symptoms and recovered immediately, without any seizures or confusional state.

It was considered that aortic stenosis was the cause of the syncope, and after a coronary angiogram showing normal coronary arteries, aortic valve replacement was carried out.

After surgery, the patient has been followed up for 10 years and has remained asymptomatic, with no further episodes of syncope.

Comment

Syncope is one of the clinical manifestations of severe aortic stenosis, along with dyspnea and angina [1].

The mechanism of syncope in these patients is not well understood, but it has been accepted that, in addition to restricted cardiac output due to left ventricular obstruction, an inappropriate neurally mediated reflex, probably triggered by increased pressure in the left myocardial wall, may play a role in the etiology of the syncope [2].

The presence of any one of the symptoms mentioned in a patient with severe aortic stenosis suggests a bad prognosis, with an increased risk of mortality during the short-term follow-up period [3]. It is well established that the presence of syncope in a patient with severe aortic stenosis is a clear indication for surgical valve replacement [4]. It has been considered that the presence of severe aortic stenosis, demonstrated on echocardiography, in a patient with syncope with no other apparent cause is a diagnostic finding [5]. In these patients, surgical valve replacement not only prevents recurrent syncope but also improves the prognosis and survival [6].

This case illustrates a typical situation in a patient with a severe aortic stenosis, which was initially asymptomatic. During the follow-up, he suffered a sudden episode of syncope. Due to the presence of symptoms, surgical valve replacement was indicated without any other additional diagnostic tests for the syncope.

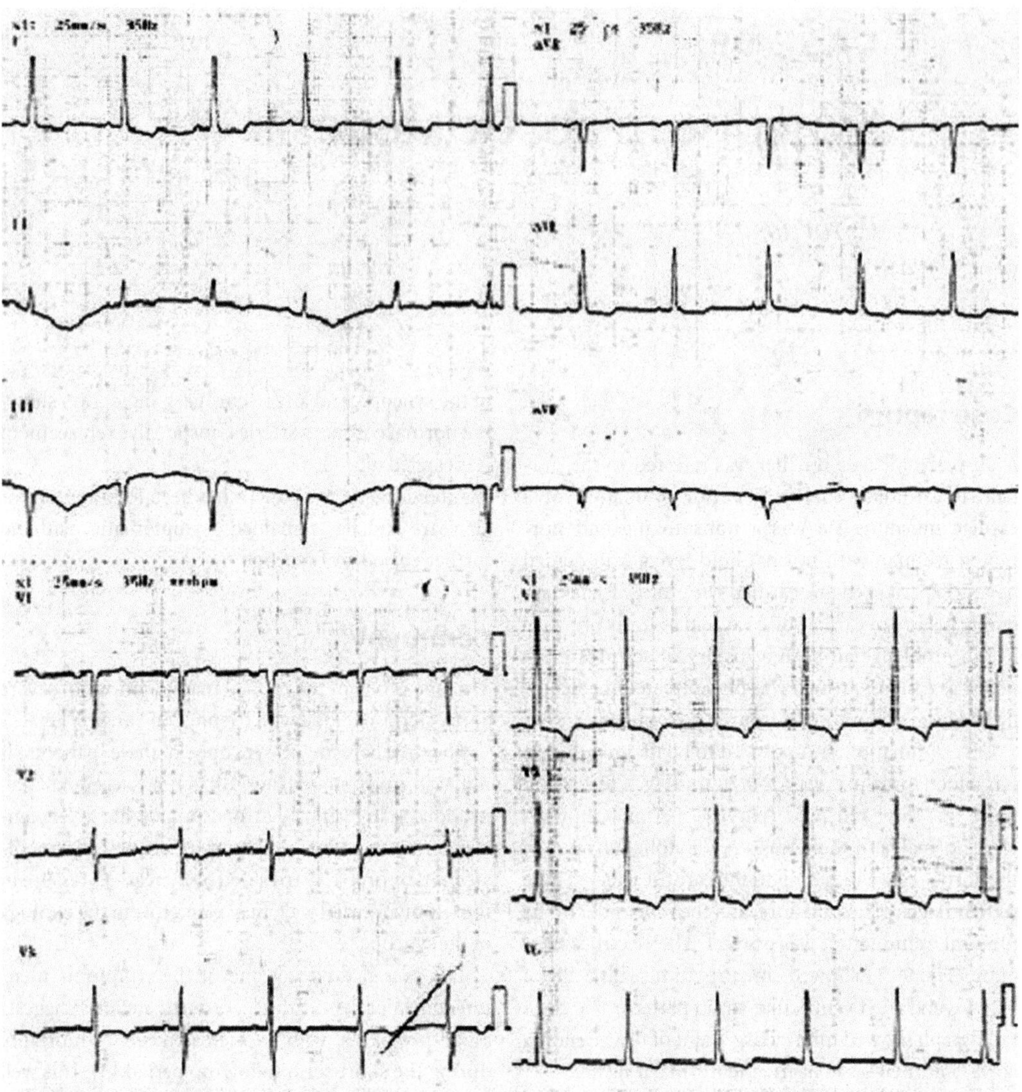

Figure 99.1 The baseline electrocardiogram. There is a normal sinus rhythm at 85 beats/min, with a prolonged PR interval (0.24 ms), and a QRS with a characteristic picture of left ventricular strain.

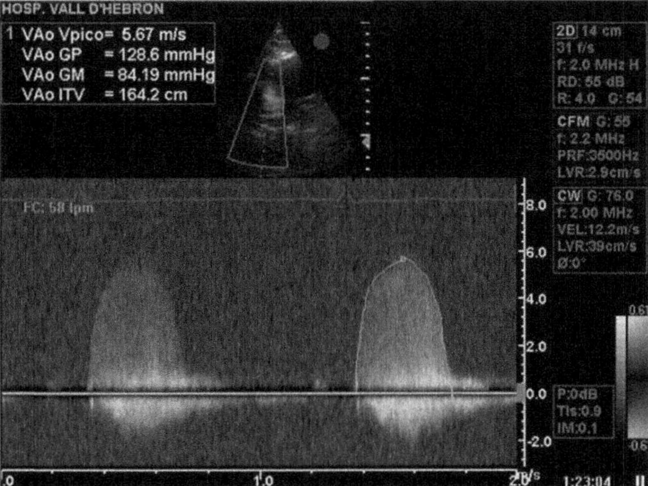

Figure 99.2 Doppler ultrasound image showing a peak velocity (VAo Vpico) of 5.67 m/s, a maximum aortic gradient (VAo GP) of 128.6 mmHg, and a mean gradient (VAo GM) of 84.19 mmHg.

The clinical follow-up, for a period of more than 10 years, shows that the patient had good survival with no further symptoms and no recurrent episodes of syncope.

References

1 Ross J Jr, Braunwald E. Aortic stenosis. *Circulation* 1968; **38** (Suppl 1): 61–7.

2 Johnson AM. Aortic stenosis, sudden death, and the left ventricular baroreceptors. *Br Heart J* 1971; **33**: 1–5.

3 Frank S, Johnson A, Ross J Jr. Natural history of valvular aortic stenosis. *Br Heart J* 1973; **35**: 41–4.

4 Azpitarte J, Alonso AM, García Gallego F, González Santos JM, Paré C, Tello A. Guías de práctica clínica de la Sociedad Española de Cardiología en valvulopatías. *Rev Esp Cardiol* 2000; **53**: 1209–78.

5 Brignole M, Alboni P, Benditt DG, *et al.* Guidelines on management (diagnosis and treatment) of syncope: update 2004. *Eur Heart J* 2004; **6**: 467–537.

6 Schwarz F, Baumann P, Manthey J. The effect of aortic valve replacement on survival. *Circulation* 1982; **66**: 1105–10.

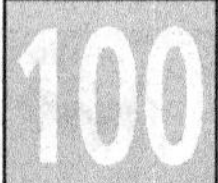

CASE 100

Syncope after aortic valve replacement

G. Gusi, I. Anguera, M. Cazorla, S. Galán, A. Martínez Rubio

Case report

A 53-year-old man was admitted to hospital due to an episode of hemoptysis and chronic dyspnea. He had a history of pulmonary tuberculosis in his youth. He was an ex-smoker and met the criteria for chronic obstructive pulmonary disease; he had been diagnosed with systemic hypertension (well controlled with angiotensin-converting enzyme inhibitors) and had suffered severe thoracic trauma in an accident 4 years before admission.

During the assessment for the episode of hemoptysis, dilation of the aorta was found on the chest radiograph. The echocardiogram showed a slightly dilated left ventricle (left ventricular end-diastolic diameter 60 mm), hypertrophy (interventricular septum of 14 mm, posterior wall 13 mm), with preserved global contractile function (ejection fraction 59%). He also had dilation of the aortic root (50 mm) and from the ascending aorta (58 mm) to the arch (42 mm), with a normal size in the descending aorta. The aortic valve was morphologically normal, but the Doppler signals showed severe regurgitation. The angiographic study demonstrated the presence of normal coronary arteries, aneurysmal dilation of the ascending aorta (> 6 cm), and confirmed severe aortic regurgitation (Fig. 100.1).

Surgery was carried out to implant a mechanical aortic valve, with interposition of a 30-mm Dacron prosthesis in the ascending aorta. There were no notable findings in the early period after surgery, apart from the appearance of a transient complete left bundle-branch block.

Approximately 1 year after the heart operation, the patient started to have episodes of loss of consciousness (four incidents lasting 1–4 s), preceded by a brief sensation of dizziness and with nonsevere trauma during two of the episodes. Echocardiography showed normal functioning of the prosthetic valve. The Holter recording showed no significant changes in cardiac rhythm. An electrophysiological study was then carried out, with no abnormal findings.

A head-up tilt-table test was carried out with beat-to-beat electrocardiography (ECG) and noninvasive blood-pressure monitoring using the Task Force monitor (CNSystems Medizintechnik Ltd., Graz, Austria). In baseline conditions, 60° tilting was accompanied by no significant changes in cardiac frequency or arterial

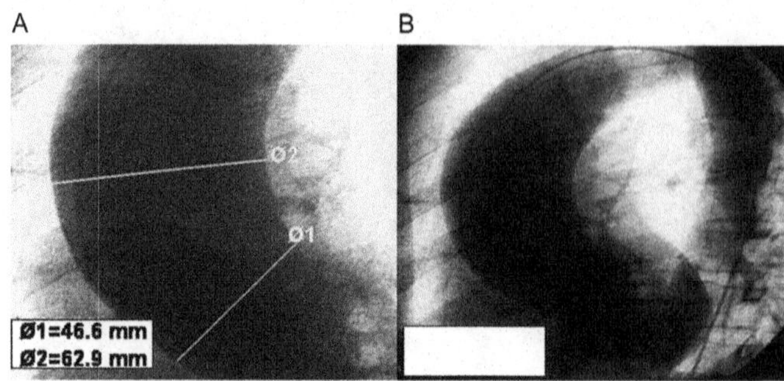

Figure 100.1 Angiography of the aorta, showing aneurysmal dilation (A) and aortic regurgitation (B).

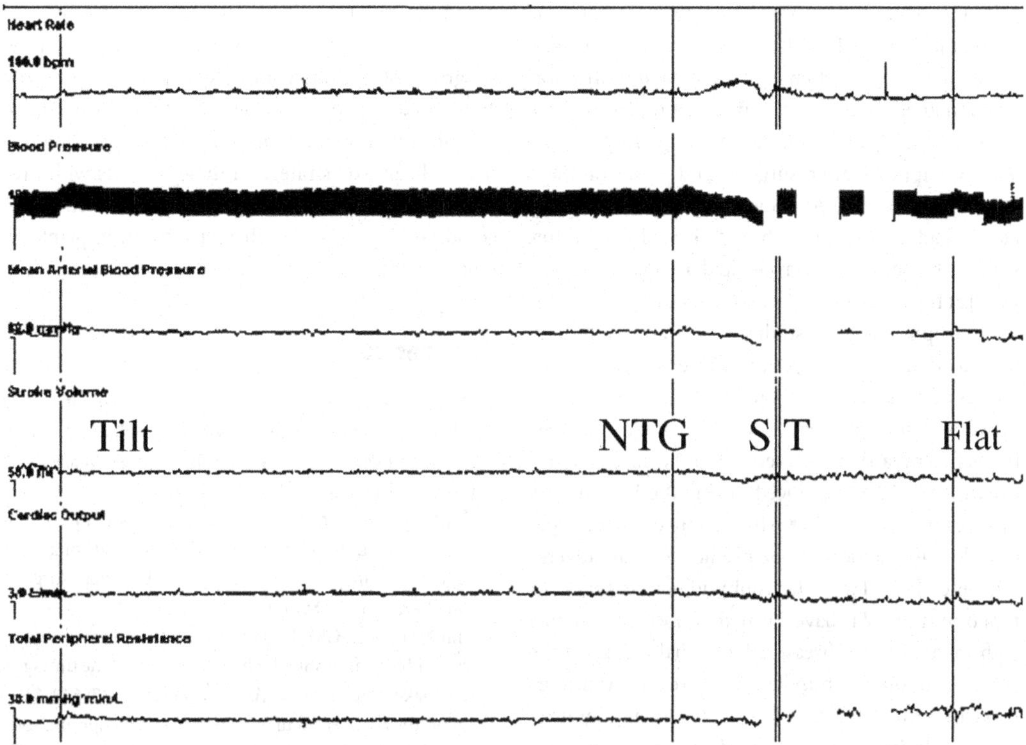

Figure 100.2 The head-up tilt-table test. NTG, moment of administration of nitroglycerin; S, syncope; T, Trendelenburg position.

pressure. Two minutes after sublingual nitroglycerin administration (0.4 mg), a progressive drop in blood pressure was observed, followed by the development of a typical syncopal episode. During the episode, a discrete reduction in heart rate was observed (Figs. 100.2, 100.3).

The various therapeutic options (invasive/noninvasive) and their risks and potential benefits were discussed in detailed conversations with the patient. The final decision was to use a conservative approach, which included providing the patient with information about how to prevent situations that could facilitate vasovagal syncope. The maneuvers of crossing the legs and increasing muscular tone in the lower limbs were also explained to the patient. During a follow-up period of more than 1 year, the patient has not experienced any further syncopal episodes.

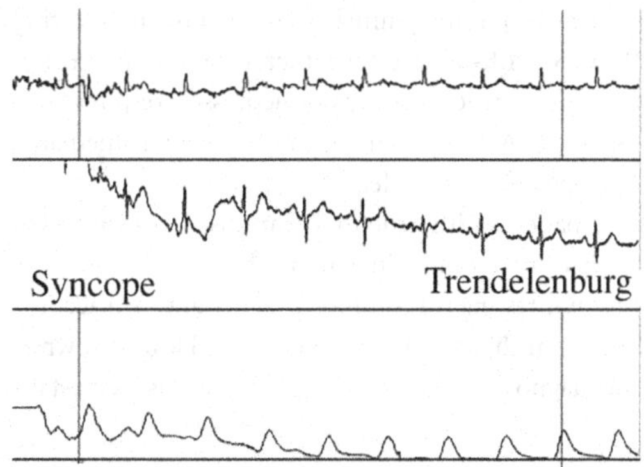

Figure 100.3 Electrocardiography and blood pressure during the syncopal episode.

Comment

Syncope after aortic valve replacement can be due to multiple causes. Syncope is rare as a manifestation of prosthesis dysfunction [1] (not present in this case), but atrioventricular conduction anomalies and ventricular arrhythmias are more common and would be considered initially in the diagnostic work-up.

Often, a complete atrioventricular block (AVB) is a transient complication of valvular heart surgery, but permanent pacing is necessary in up to 5% of cases

[2,3]. Complete AVB appears to occur immediately or within the first few days after valve surgery, and persistence for more than 48 h is considered an indication for permanent pacemaker implantation [2]. In other cases, a bundle-branch block is either present beforehand or appears after surgery, and some of these patients can develop AVB over time [4]. The present patient had a transient left bundle-branch block after surgery, but normal intraventricular conduction was noted at the time of the syncopal episodes.

Electrophysiological studies (EPS) are commonly used to detect an arrhythmic cause of syncope. In a series of 97 patients with valvular heart disease (with or without surgical correction) presenting with ventricular tachycardia (VT), ventricular fibrillation (VF), or syncope, VT was induced during the EPS in 39% of cases and VF in 20%. Induction of these types of arrhythmia appears to be predictive of an adverse outcome [5]. Two electrophysiological types of monomorphic VT have been described in patients with valvular heart disease. Myocardial reentry is the more common, but bundle-branch reentry ventricular tachycardia (BBR VT) is capable of being induced during EPS in almost one-third of the patients [6]. Interestingly, BBR VT is often related to valve replacement surgery.

In the present patient, neither conduction disturbances nor arrhythmias were documented during the EPS. A tilt-table test was therefore carried out, and a positive, predominantly vasodepressor, response was obtained. A presumed diagnosis of neuromediated syncope was then made.

In patients with structural heart disease or suspected cardiac arrhythmia in whom the EPS is negative, tilt-table testing is a common practice and is in accordance with the current guidelines [7]. However, while the diagnostic yield of the tilt-table test is well established in patients with no structural heart disease and with a normal ECG, the value of the test in the subgroup of patients with heart disease or suspected arrhythmic syncope and negative EPS has not been demonstrated with a long-term follow-up. An alternative diagnostic strategy in these patients with preserved ventricular function (as in the present case) could be long-term monitoring with an implantable loop recorder.

References

1 Frankl WS. The special problems of the patient with a valvular prosthesis. In: Frank WS, Brest AN, eds. *Valvular Heart Disease: Comprehensive Evaluation and Management.* Davis, Philadelphia, 1986: 415–25.

2 Glickson M, Dearni JA, Hyberger LK, Schaff HV, Hamill SC, Hayes DL. Indications, effectiveness, and long-term dependency in permanent pacing after cardiac surgery. *Am J Cardiol* 1997; **80**: 1309–13.

3 Kim MH, Deeb GM, Eagle KA, *et al.* Complete atrioventricular block after valvular heart surgery and the timing of pacemaker implantation. *Am J Cardiol* 2001; **87**: 649–51.

4 Kulbertus HE. Ventricular arrhythmias, syncope and sudden death in aortic stenosis. *Eur Heart J* 1998; **9** (Suppl E): 51–2.

5 Martínez-Rubio A, Schwammenthal Y, Schwammenthal E, *et al.* Patients with valvular heart disease presenting with sustained ventricular tachyarrhythmias or syncope: results of programmed ventricular stimulation and long-term follow-up. *Circulation* 1997; **96**: 500–8.

6 Narasimhan C, Jazayeri MR, Sra J, *et al.* Ventricular tachycardia in valvular heart disease: facilitation of bundle branch reentry by valve surgery. *Circulation* 1997; **96**: 4307–13.

7 Menozzi C, Brignole M, García-Civera R, *et al.* Mechanisms of syncope in patients with heart disease and negative electrophysiologic test. *Circulation* 2002; **105**: 2741–5.

CASE 101

Syncope in a patient with aortic valve prosthesis and wide QRS tachycardia

J. García Sacristán, J. Enero, R. Ceres

Case report

A man who had suffered rheumatic fever in childhood and had severe aortic insufficiency underwent surgery at the age of 41, with implantation of an aortic valve prosthesis (Hall–Kaster no. 25). During the subsequent course, the patient developed episodes of paroxysmal atrial fibrillation and mild arterial hypertension. He was in New York Heart Association (NYHA) grade II and was receiving treatment with digoxin, furosemide, enalapril, simvastatin, and acenocoumarin. At the age of 57, he was admitted to the emergency department due to a syncopal episode preceded by palpitations, an oppressive sensation in the chest, and dyspnea. The electrocardiogram (ECG) showed regular tachycardia at 200 beats/min, with a wide QRS complex and an appearance resembling that of a right bundle-branch block. The tachycardia was terminated with a synchronized direct-current shock, and the patient was admitted to the hospital for cardiological evaluation.

The ECG in sinus rhythm showed left axis deviation in the frontal plane and a QRS duration of 100 ms. A Doppler ultrasound examination showed a dilated left atrium (51 mm), an end-diastolic left ventricular diameter of 60 mm, and a left ejection fraction of 40%. The aortic prosthesis was functioning normally, and a mild stenosis/insufficiency of the mitral valve was noted.

An electrophysiological study was carried out. The baseline conduction intervals were AH 80 ms and HV 70 ms. With programmed stimulation in the apex of the right ventricle at a basic cycle length of 500 ms and with the introduction of extrastimuli, two types of ventricular tachycardia (VT) were induced:

- With one extrastimulus, monomorphic sustained VT was induced, with a QRS similar to that of left bundle-branch block, atrioventricular (AV) dissociation, and His bundle deflexion preceding the onset of ventricular depolarization, with an HV interval longer than the HV in sinus rhythm. At the beginning of the tachycardia, spontaneous variations in the VV intervals were preceded by similar changes in the HH intervals (Fig. 101.1).
- With the introduction of two extrastimuli, a second type of monomorphic sustained VT was induced (Fig. 101.2). This tachycardia had a cycle length similar to that of the previous one, and showed AV dissociation and a QRS morphology similar to that of a right bundle-branch block (identical to the clinical tachycardia). As in the other tachycardia, His bundle deflexion preceded the onset of ventricular depolarization, with an HV interval longer than the HV in sinus rhythm. Entrainment of the tachycardia was obtained with stimulation at the apex of the right ventricle. With suppression of the stimulation, the difference between the return cycle and the tachycardia cycle was less than 30 ms.

A final diagnosis of bundle-branch reentry ventricular tachycardia (BBR VT) (orthodromic and antidromic types) was made, and ablation of the right bundle was carried out (Fig. 101.3). After the ablation, no further tachycardia was inducible basally or after isoproterenol infusion. During a 3-year follow-up period, the patient has remained free of tachycardia and syncope.

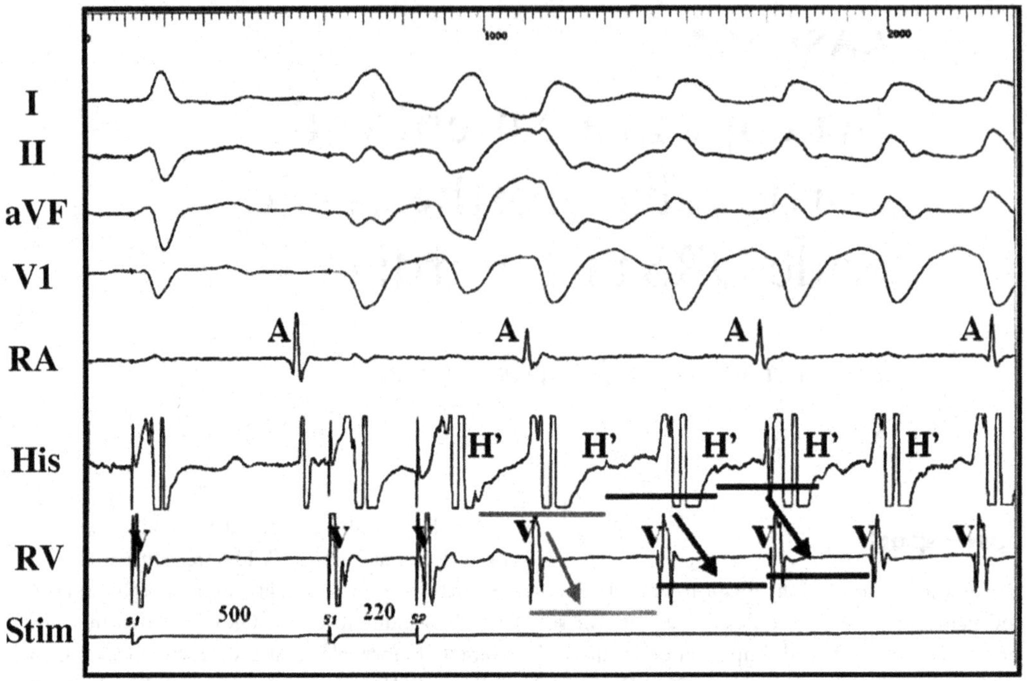

Figure 101.1 Induction of ventricular tachycardia with a QRS morphology resembling a left bundle-branch block. Changes in the HH cycle lengths precede similar changes in the VV cycle lengths.

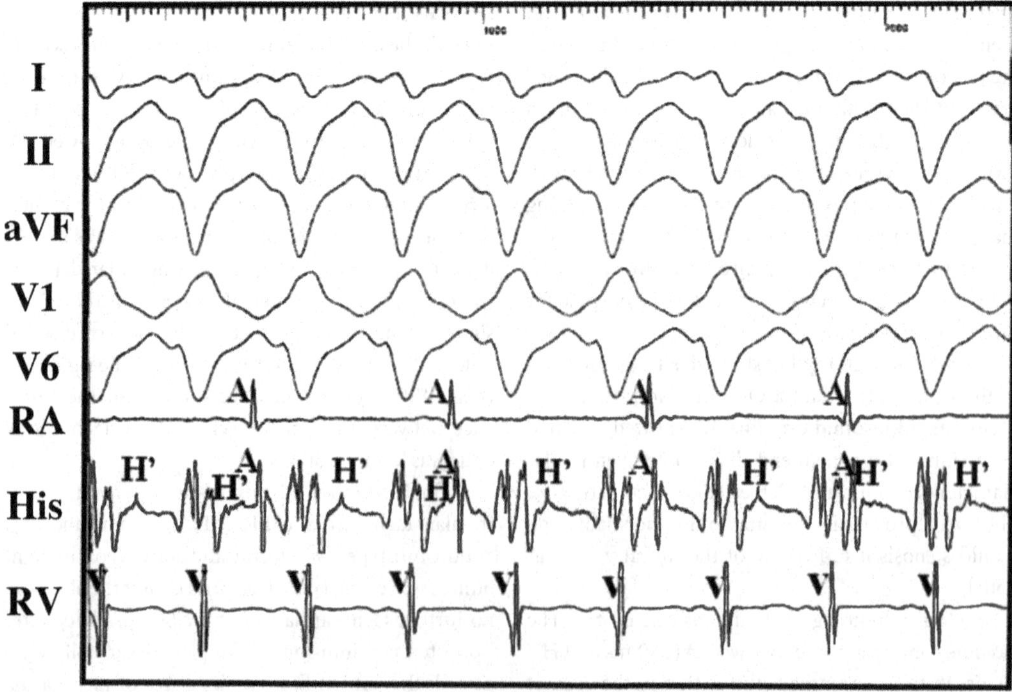

Figure 101.2 Ventricular tachycardia with a QRS morphology resembling a right bundle-branch block.

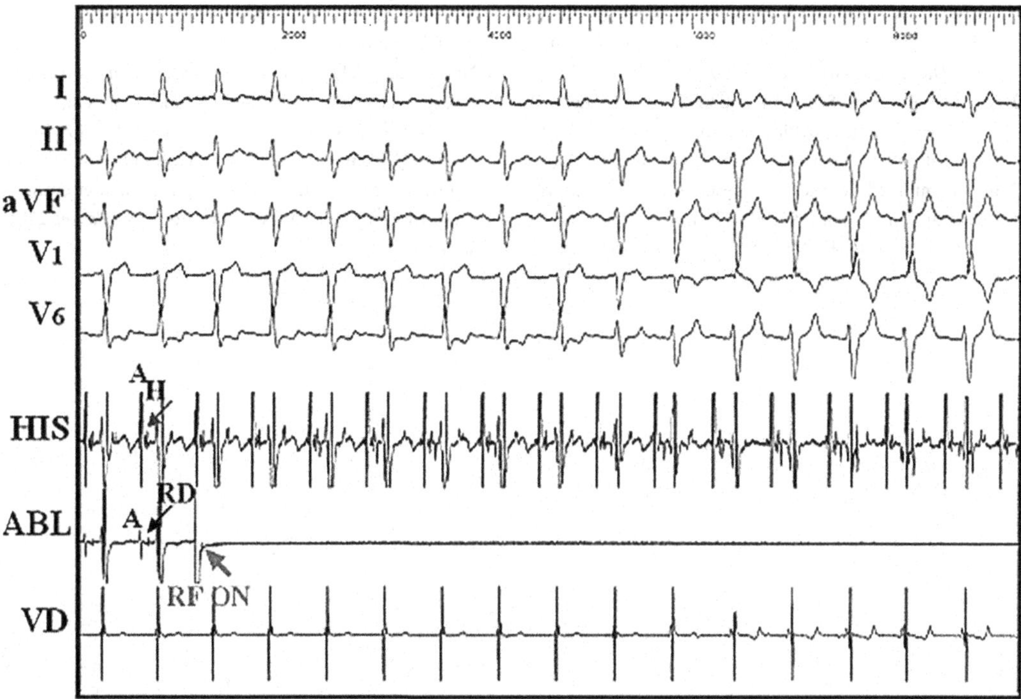

Figure 101.3 Radiofrequency ablation of the right bundle branch.

Comment

Patients with aortic valve disease can present with VT before and after aortic valve replacement [1–3]. Two electrophysiological mechanisms for sustained VT have been described in these patients [4]: myocardial reentry tachycardia and BBR VT.

Myocardial reentry tachycardia is the most common mechanism after aortic valve surgery, being responsible for 70% of all inducible VTs. In this type of VT, there is no temporal relationship between the onset of the tachycardia and the valve surgery. Frequently, the patients have associated coronary artery disease or poor ventricular function [5].

Bundle-branch reentry produces VT via a macroreentry circuit involving the His–Purkinje system. Usually, there is antegrade conduction over the right bundle branch and retrograde conduction over the left bundle branch, giving place to a QRS configuration that resembles a left bundle-branch block during the tachycardia (the orthodromic type). However, the circuit can also be used in the inverse direction, producing a QRS configuration resembling a right bundle-branch block (the antidromic type). Sustained BBR VT requires a long circuit or a slow conduction. Ventricular dilation or impaired conduction in the His–Purkinje system can therefore facilitate BBR VT. In patients with aortic valve disease, BBR VT represents 30% of all inducible VTs and typically occurs early after valve replacement [5].

A hallmark feature of BBR VT is that spontaneous variations in the tachycardia cycle length are preceded by similar cycle-length variations in the HH intervals [4]. Equally, entrainment of the tachycardia from the right ventricular apex (a point close to the tachycardia circuit) is helpful in the diagnosis [6].

In the present patient, both orthodromic and antidromic forms of BBR VT were demonstrated during the electrophysiological study, and subsequent ablation of the right bundle allowed complete control of the arrhythmia.

References

1 Von Olshausen KV, Schwartz F, Apfelbach J, Rohring N, Kramer B, Kubler W. Determinants of the incidence and severity of ventricular arrhythmias in aortic valve disease. *Am J Cardiol* 1983; **51**: 1103–9.

2 Michel PL, Mandagout O, Vahanian A, *et al.* Ventricular arrhythmias in aortic valve disease before and after surgery. *J Heart Valve Dis* 1992; **1**: 72–9.
3 Martínez-Rubio A, Schwammenthal Y, Schwammenthal E, *et al.* Patients with valvular heart disease presenting with sustained ventricular tachyarrhythmias or syncope: results of programmed ventricular stimulation and long-term follow-up. *Circulation* 1997; **96**: 500–8.
4 Caceres J, Jazayeri M, McKinnie J, *et al.* Sustained bundle branch block reentry as a mechanism of clinical tachycardia. *Circulation* 1989; **79**: 256–70.
5 Narasimhan C, Jazayeri MR, Sra J, *et al.* Ventricular tachycardia in valvular heart disease: facilitation of bundle branch reentry by valve surgery. *Circulation* 1997; **96**: 4307–13.
6 Merino JL, Peinado R, Fernandez-Lozano I, *et al.* Bundle-branch reentry and the postpacing interval after entrainment by ventricular apex stimulation. *Circulation* 2001; **103**: 1102–8.

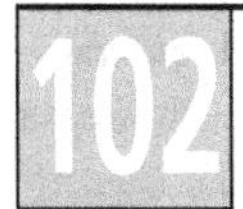

CASE 102

Presyncope due to left atrial myxoma

B. Vaquerizo, A. Peláez González, V. Montagud Balaguer, M.T. Tuzón Segarra, M.D. Orriach

Case report

A 71-year-old woman was referred for cardiological evaluation due to presyncopal episodes and permanent atrial fibrillation. She had a history of high blood pressure but was not receiving pharmacological treatment. The patient reported having exercise-induced presyncopal episodes during the previous 3 months, which were not preceded by palpitations, chest pain, or dizziness. The physical examination showed a blood pressure of 180/90 mmHg, a holosystolic murmur in the apex radiating to the axilla, a normal second sound, normal central and peripheral pulses, an absence of edema, and a normal neurological examination.

The 12-lead electrocardiogram (Fig. 102.1) showed atrial fibrillation with an irregular ventricular response around 80 beats/min, a QRS complex with left axis deviation in the frontal plane, and normal repolarization. Biochemical determinations and chest radiography were normal.

Transthoracic echocardiography (Fig. 102.2) showed dilated left atria with a large, mobile mass inside. The mass had a plain border and a heterogeneous density, with calcified areas. Its attachment in the atrial wall was elusive. Echocardiography detected mild mitral and aortic regurgitation, as well as mild tricuspid regurgitation, allowing estimation of the systolic pulmonary pressure as 45 mmHg.

For better characterization of the mass, transesophageal echocardiography was carried out, which identified a wide attachment of the mass in the atrial septum. It had a diameter of 6 cm and very limited mobility. Its acoustic density was similar to that of the myocardium (Fig. 102.3). The left atrial appendage was free of thrombi.

With a diagnosis of giant left atrial myxoma, the patient was referred for cardiac surgery. Left

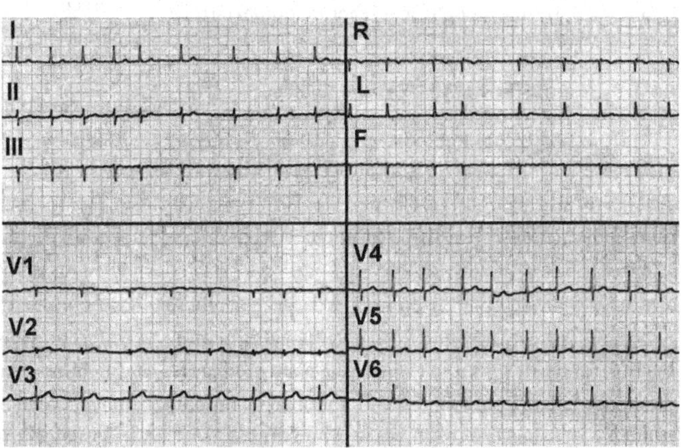

Figure 102.1 The baseline electrocardiogram.

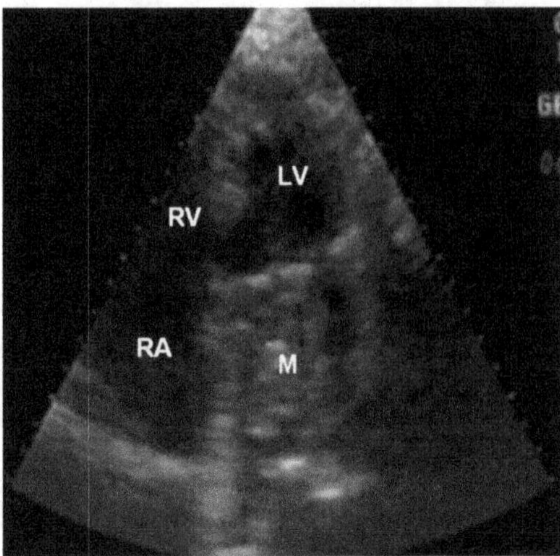

Figure 102.2 The transthoracic echocardiogram. LV, left ventricle; RV, right ventricle; RA, right atrium; M, myxoma.

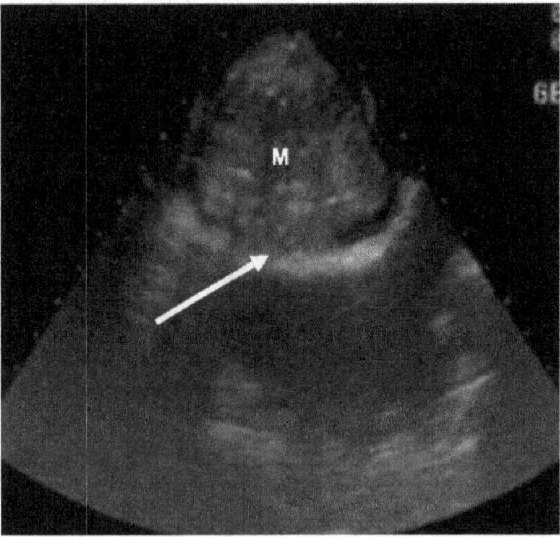

Figure 102.3 The transesophageal echocardiogram (arrow: pedicle). M, myxoma.

atriotomy uncovered a myxomatous mass occupying the entire left atrial cavity and attached to the interatrial septum through a 4-cm pedicle. The mass was removed and sent to the pathology department. Macroscopic evaluation showed a nodular lobulated tumor 7 × 5 × 4 cm in size, with a large pedicle, a gelatinous appearance, and both calcified and hemorrhagic areas. Microscopic examination showed small mesenchymal myxomatous cells surrounded by mucoid connective tissue. The diagnosis was myxoma.

No postoperative complications appeared, and transthoracic echocardiography 1 month later showed a dilated left atrium without any mass inside.

Comment

Primary heart tumors are rare; 75% of heart tumors are benign, and 50% of these are myxomas. The myxoma is a tumor of endocardial origin, usually pediculate and located in the left atrium in 75% of cases [1]. Myxomas are usually found as sporadic cases, but there are also cases of familial occurrence. Familial cases can form part of what is known as the Carney complex (an association of cardiac myxomas, cutaneous myxomas, lentiginosis, Cushing syndrome, and acromegaly) [2].

The clinical manifestations of atrial myxomas mimic many cardiovascular diseases, and a high index of suspicion is therefore important for early and correct diagnosis. The classic triad of myxoma presentation [3] consists of:

- Symptoms of mitral valve obstruction (auscultation, pulmonary congestion, and syncope).
- Embolism.
- Constitutional symptoms (fever, weight loss, or symptoms resembling connective-tissue disease).

Syncope is relatively infrequent. Some 15–25% of patients with myxomas present with syncope [3,4]. In these cases, syncope is caused by obstruction of the mitral, tricuspid, or pulmonary valves. Occasionally, the syncope is triggered by some postural change. In the present case, presyncope was triggered by effort, suggesting that, during the effort, the size of the tumor limited the increase in pulmonary venous return to the left atrium or flux across the mitral valve.

According to Goswami *et al.* [4], large atrial myxomas are closely related to constitutional symptoms, congestive heart failure, syncope, and auscultatory findings suggestive of mitral-valve disease, whereas smaller myxomas and an irregular surface are associated with embolization.

The primary diagnostic method for myxoma is echocardiography (transthoracic or transesophageal). This makes it possible to assess the location of the tumor and its size and attachment [4,5]. However, differentiating between atrial myxoma and atrial thrombus can be difficult in some cases [5]. Other methods such as computed tomography and magnetic resonance imaging can be helpful in the diagnosis.

Cardiac myxoma is an indication for urgent surgery, owing to the risk of thromboembolism or sudden death due to valvular obstruction. The results of the intervention are generally good, leading to complete cure in the majority of cases [6,7]. However, a strong tendency toward relapse has been reported in cases of familial occurrence [7].

References

1 Reynen K. Cardiac myxomas. *N Engl J Med* 1995; **333**: 1610–7.

2 Carney JA, Hruska LS, Beauchamp GD, *et al.* Dominant inheritance of the complex of myxomas, spotty pigmentation, and endocrine overactivity. *Mayo Clin Proc* 1986; **61**: 165–72.

3 Pineda L, Duhaut P, Loire R. Clinical presentation of left atrial cardiac myxoma: a series of 112 consecutive cases. *Medicine (Baltimore)* 2001; **80**: 159–72.

4 Goswami KC, Shrivastaba S, Bahl VK, Saxena A, Manchanda SC, Wasir HS. Cardiac myxomas: clinical and echocardiographic profile. *Int J Cardiol* 1998; **28**: 251–9.

5 Otto CM. *Textbook of Clinical Echocardiography.* Saunders, Philadelphia, 2000: 351–72.

6 Lijoi A, Scoti P, Faveto C, *et al.* Surgical management of intracardiac myxomas: a 16-year experience. *Tex Heart Inst J* 1993; **20**: 231–4.

7 Bhan A, Mehrota R, Choudhary SK, *et al.* Surgical experience with intracardiac myxomas: long-term follow-up. *Ann Thorac Surg* 1998; **66**: 810–3.

CASE 103

Syncope due to left atrial thrombus

F. López Pardo, G. Barón Esquivias, A. Pedrote Martínez, M. Fernández Quero, F. Errázquin Sáenz de Tejada

Case report

A 76-year-old woman was admitted to hospital after an episode of syncope, which resolved without consequences. The patient had a previous clinical history of arterial hypertension and long-standing palpitations, and had experienced frequent presyncopal attacks during the previous month. The patient was fully conscious and oriented during the physical examination, which showed a blood pressure of 180/100 mmHg, arrhythmic heart sounds, a heart rate of 110 beats/min, holosystolic murmur grade 2/4 at the apex, isolated bibasilar rales, and edema in the lower limbs. The hematological and biochemical tests were normal.

The electrocardiogram revealed atrial fibrillation (mean ventricular rate 110 beats/min) and left anterior hemiblock. Chest radiography showed a normal cardiothoracic index, bilateral hilar alveolar infiltrates, and scissural effusion. Transthoracic echocardiography disclosed a free-floating mass 3.5 cm in diameter in the left atrium, partly obstructing the mitral valve (Fig. 103.1). No wall attachment was observed. The mitral valve was normal, with mild insufficiency but no signs of stenosis. The left atrium showed slight enlargement (45 mm), but the left ventricle showed no enlargement or hypertrophy, and the left ejection fraction was normal. A mild tricuspid insufficiency was noted, with a gradient of 45 mmHg and an estimated systolic pulmonary pressure of 55 mmHg.

Transesophageal echocardiography confirmed the transthoracic echocardiographic findings and disclosed a free-floating mass in the left atrium. The mass was smooth, homogeneous, and without calcifications or attachment to the atrial wall (Fig. 103.2A). The mass was causing intermittent obstruction of the mitral valve (Fig. 103.2B). Echocardiography also showed small dense masses in the left atrial appendage, suggestive of thrombi.

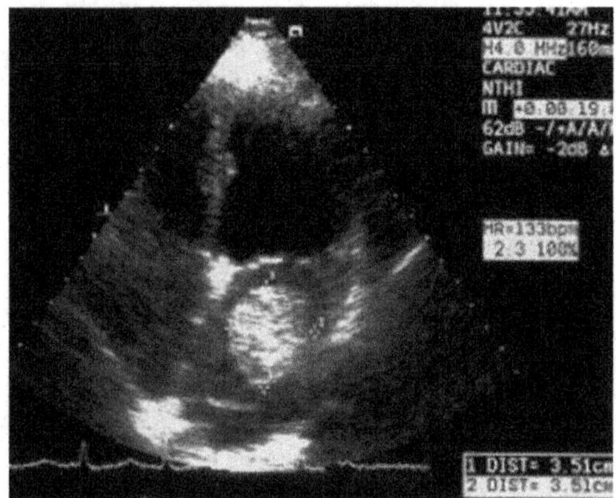

Figure 103.1 Apical four-chamber transthoracic echocardiogram, showing a mobile ball thrombus in the left atrium.

Differential diagnosis was initially carried out between an atrial myxoma and (as the more probable alternative) a free-floating thrombus, in view of the patient's history of atrial fibrillation and the images observed in the left atrial appendage. The patient received anticoagulant therapy with intravenous sodium heparin for 72 h, with no modifications being observed in the echocardiogram. The patient was then urgently scheduled for surgery. An elastic, whitish-grayish mass of the size suggested in the echocardiography was removed. The left atrial cavity was revised and the thrombi in the left atrial appendage were aspirated. No complications occurred after surgery. The patient recovered a normal heart rhythm and was discharged with oral anticoagulant therapy (dicumarol) and amiodarone. Histological examination of the material from the mass confirmed that it was a thrombus.

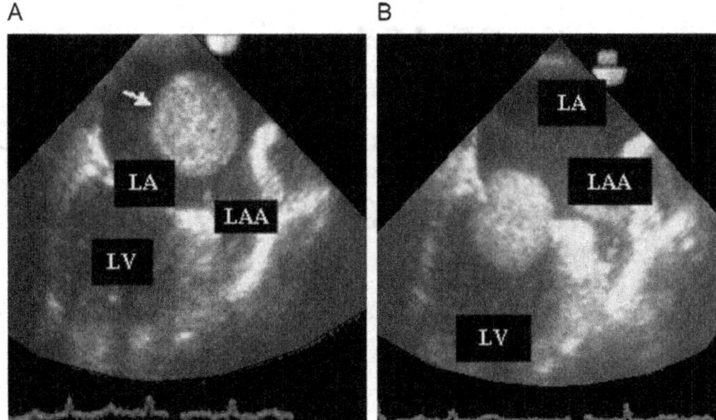

Figure 103.2 The transesophageal longitudinal plane, showing a free-floating ball thrombus (arrow in A) that is intermittently protruding through the mitral valve (B). LA, left atrium; LAA, left atrial appendage; LV, left ventricle.

Comment

Free-floating thrombus in the left atrium is a rare clinical syndrome, which may have a fatal outcome if adequate diagnosis is not achieved [1]. It usually affects patients with mitral valve disease [2], but has also been reported in patients with hypertrophic cardiomyopathy [3] and less frequently in patients without mitral valve disease [4].

Thrombus may be detected on routine echocardiography in asymptomatic patients [5]. However, the patients usually have clinical symptoms, which can include peripheral embolic events resulting from fragmentation of the thrombus, and symptoms related to intermittent total or partial occlusion of the mitral valve orifice, such as dyspnea, pulmonary congestion, syncope, and even sudden death [1,4]. Patients with left atrial thrombus who do not receive adequate therapy have a negative prognosis. Anticoagulant therapy may be an effective option in the case of partly attached thrombi less than 1 cm in diameter [6], but regular echocardiographic monitoring is required in order to check on the development of the thrombus. However, in view of the unpredictable results and the high risk of embolism resulting from anticoagulant therapy and thrombolysis, surgical removal of the thrombus appears to be the most appropriate therapeutic option [1,5].

References

1 Wrisley D, Giambartolomei A, Lee I, Brownlee W. Left atrial ball thrombus: review of clinical echocardiographic manifestations with suggestions for management. *Am Heart J* 1991; **121**: 1784–90.

2 Misumi T, Kudo M, Ito T, Matsubara T, Kumamaru H. Floating ball thrombus in the left atrium with mitral stenosis. *Jpn J Thorac Cardiovasc Surg* 2003; **51**: 387–9.

3 Tekten T, Onbasili OA, Ceylan C, Ercan E. Left atrial free floating ball thrombus in hypertrophic cardiomyopathy: a case report. *J Am Soc Echocardiogr* 2002; **15**: 1018–20.

4 Yoshida K, Fujii G, Suzuki S, Shimomura T, Miyahara K, Matsuura A. A report of a surgical case of the left atrial free floating ball thrombus in the absence of mitral disease. *Ann Thorac Cardiovasc Surg* 2002; **8**: 316–8.

5 Vitale M, Agnino A, Serena D, *et al.* Asymptomatic large left-atrial ball thrombus secondary to mitral stenosis. *Tex Heart Inst J* 1997; **24**: 376–8.

6 Nagaraja KV, Jaishankar S, Venkateswara C, *et al.* Free-floating ball thrombus in left atrium. *Echocardiography* 1998; **15**: 377–80.

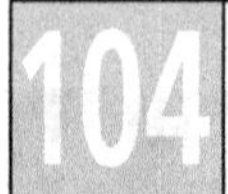

CASE 104

Cardiac tamponade presenting as syncope

J. Sagristá

Case report

A 56-year-old woman presented to the emergency department due to an episode of loss of consciousness. Her medical history included mild hypertension and chronic spondylitis, for which she was receiving treatment with methotrexate and corticosteroids. She reported having had no previous episodes of syncope. She had been in good general condition until 7 days before admission, when she had started to complain of fever and anterior chest pain radiating to both shoulders. The pain increased with inspiration and when she was in the supine position. In addition, she had had progressive dyspnea on exertion during the previous 3 days. On the day of hospital admission, while staying at home and immediately after standing up from a chair, she had sudden weakness, light-headedness, and blurred vision, followed by fainting and loss of consciousness. A witness found her lying on the ground with pallor and with a few clonic jerks in the limbs and face. Sphincter control was maintained. She recovered consciousness shortly afterwards, but when she got up she experienced weakness and blurred vision again, which improved after she had lain down again.

On admission to hospital, the patient was conscious, and the examination showed fever (38 °C), tachypnea (26 respirations/min), and tachycardia (110 beats/min). Her blood pressure was 107/81 mmHg, with an inspiratory fall in systolic arterial pressure of 22 mmHg. Jugular venous distension was present, and brisk jugular venous pulsations were apparent in the neck. A pericardial friction rub was heard over the left external border. An enlarged liver was palpated below the right costal border, but no leg edema was found. The electrocardiogram (ECG) showed sinus tachycardia, low QRS voltage, and mild ST-segment elevation in nearly all leads, with upright T waves (Fig. 104.1). The chest film showed an enlarged cardiac silhouette, clear lungs, and a small left pleural effusion (Fig. 104.2).

Echocardiography showed a large pericardial effusion with an anterior echo-free space 15 mm in size and posterior echo-free spaces of 18 mm, diastolic compression in the right atrial and right ventricular walls, with a marked decrease in mitral and aortic flow during inspiration (Fig. 104.3). A diagnosis of acute pericarditis with cardiac tamponade was made. Pericardiocentesis with hemodynamic monitoring was carried out in the catheterization laboratory. Intrapericardial pressure was raised to 17 mmHg and equalized with the diastolic right ventricular and diastolic left ventricular pressures and with the mean right atrial pressure; cardiac output was reduced (cardiac index 1.8 L/min/m^2). After 720 mL of serosanguineous pericardial fluid had been removed, the intrapericardial pressure approached zero and the cardiac index increased to 3.1 L/min/m^2 (Fig. 104.4). The patient's subsequent hospital course was uneventful, and she was discharged 6 days after admission in good general condition, with a small residual pericardial effusion evident on echocardiography. No further episodes of syncope occurred during a 3-month follow-up period.

Comment

This case shows that pericardial tamponade can be an uncommon cause of syncope [1]. Cardiac tamponade can be defined as compression of the heart caused by a

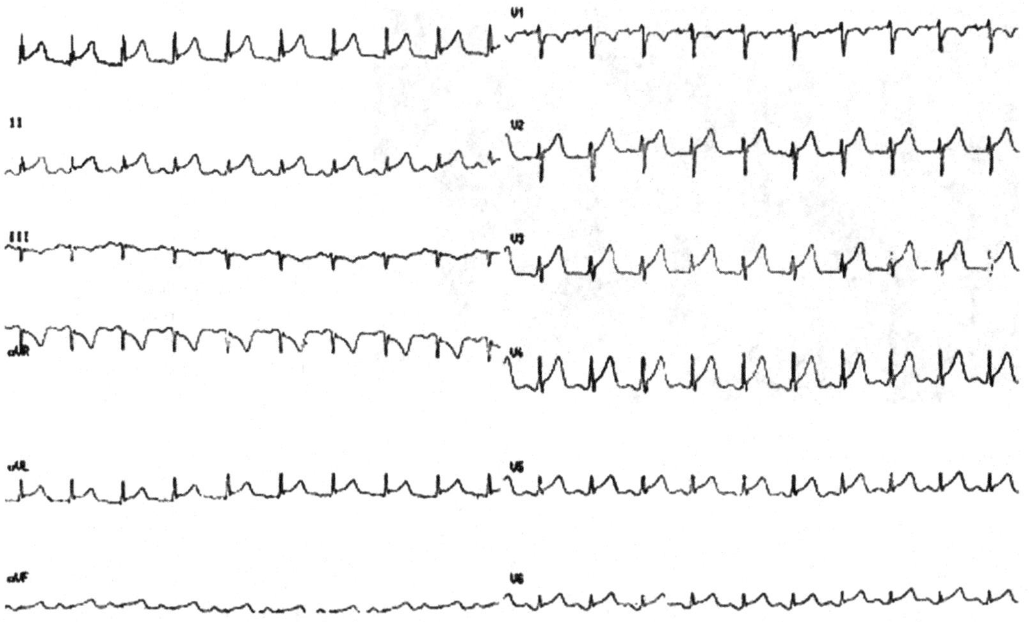

Figure 104.1 The baseline electrocardiogram, showing sinus rhythm at a heart rate of 120 beats/min, with a slight decrease in QRS voltage and ST-segment elevation in all leads.

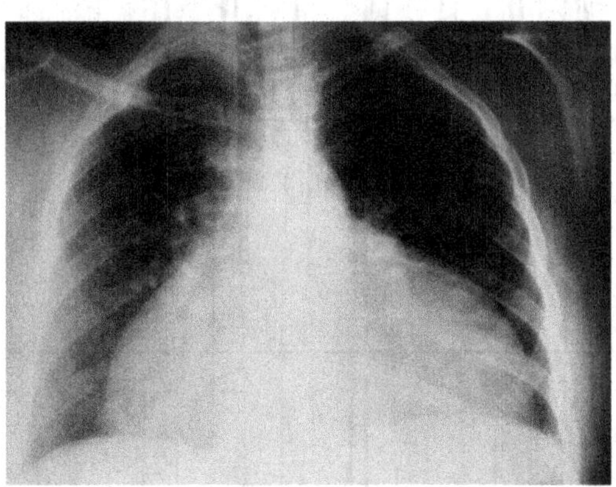

Figure 104.2 Chest radiograph. Marked enlargement of the cardiac silhouette can be seen, with no signs of left heart failure.

pericardial fluid accumulation [2]. Pericardial effusion can appear as a consequence of different situations, such as acute pericarditis, chest trauma, cardiac surgery, heart failure, tuberculosis [3], renal failure, or neoplasia.

The hemodynamic consequences of pericardial effusion depend not only on the amount of fluid, but also on the rate at which it appears. With slow accumulation of fluid, larger amounts can accumulate without hemodynamic consequences, but when pericardial fluid collects rapidly, small amounts of fluid can lead to a dramatic increase in intrapericardial pressure. The clinical presentation of pericardial tamponade can vary from mild symptoms to life-threatening cardiogenic shock. Syncope can be one of the clinical manifestations and is usually caused by transient severe compression and collapse of the right cardiac chambers [2].

This case underlines the fact that the initial clinical evaluation, consisting of careful history-taking and a physical examination, is crucial in the diagnosis [1,4]. In this patient, syncope appeared after several days of symptoms such as dyspnea, fever, and characteristic pleuritic pain. In addition, the physical examination showed signs suggestive of pericardial tamponade, such as tachycardia, tachypnea, paradoxical pulse [5], jugular venous distension, an enlarged hepatic border, and pericardial friction rub. Additional tests such as chest radiography and a baseline ECG were highly suggestive of pericardial effusion. When pericardial effusion with tamponade is suspected, echocardiography should be carried out to confirm the presence of pericardial fluid as well as signs of

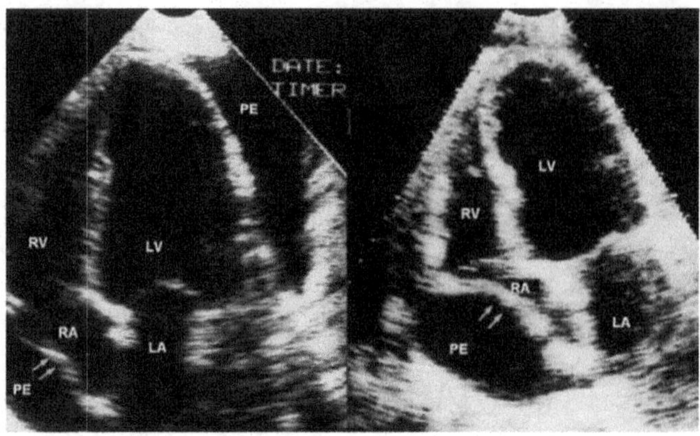

Figure 104.3 Echocardiography, showing marked pericardial effusion, with collapse of the right atrium during inspiration. LA, left atrium; LV, left ventricle; PE, pericardial effusion; RA, right atrium; RV, right ventricle.

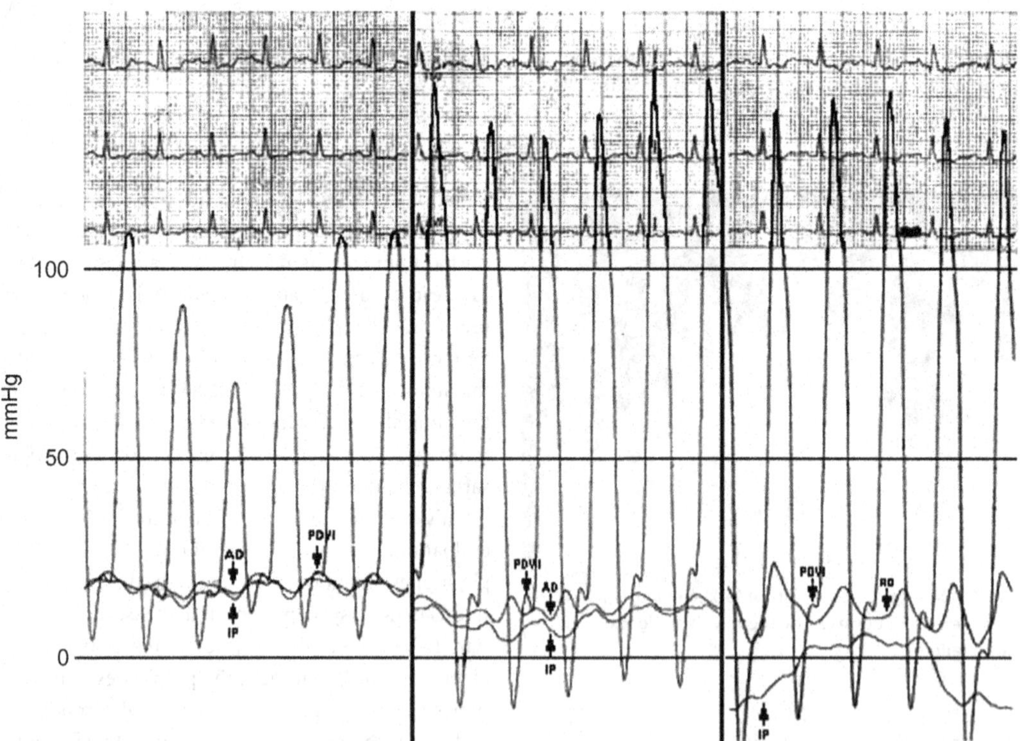

Figure 104.4 Intracardiac and intrapericardial pressures before (*left*), during (*center*) and at the end (*right*) of pericardial drainage. As can be seen, initially (*left*), pressure in the right atrium (AD), end-diastolic pressure in the left ventricle (PDVI), and intrapericardial pressure (IP) are elevated (20 mmHg) and equalized. It is also evident that there is a marked change in systolic left ventricular pressure that alters with respiratory movement, up to 30 mmHg (paradoxical pulse). After the removal of 720 mL of pericardial fluid, there is a decrease in intrapericardial pressure, which changes with respiration, and a decrease in right atrial and end-systolic left ventricular pressure. In addition, there is a marked increase in systolic left ventricular pressure, with disappearance of the paradoxical pulse.

tamponade [6]. In this case, as is seen in Fig. 104.3, echocardiography demonstrated severe pericardial effusion, with collapse of the right atrium at inspiration, confirming the diagnosis of pericardial tamponade.

When cardiac tamponade is present with hemodynamic compromise, pericardial fluid has to be drained, usually using needle pericardiocentesis. In this case, Fig. 104.4 illustrates the hemodynamic behavior of cardiac tamponade as well as its improvement after pericardiocentesis. The intrapericardial pressure is elevated (Fig. 104.4, left) and equals the right atrial pressure as well as the end-diastolic left ventricular pressure. The figure also shows that the systolic left ventricular pressure is low, with marked variation with respiratory movements (paradoxical pulse). After drainage of 720 mL of pericardial fluid (Fig. 104.4, right), the intrapericardial pressure and right atrial pressure drop, and there is an increase in systolic left ventricular pressure and disappearance of the paradoxical pulse.

References

1 Brignole M, Alboni P, Benditt D, *et al.* Guidelines on management (diagnosis and treatment) of syncope. *Eur Heart J* 2001; **22:** 1256–306.

2 Spodick DH. Acute cardiac tamponade. *N Engl J Med* 2003; **349:** 684–90.

3 Sagrista-Sauleda J, Permanyer-Miralda G, Soler-Soler J. Tuberculous pericarditis: ten year experience with a prospective protocol for diagnosis and treatment. *J Am Coll Cardiol* 1988; **11:** 724–8.

4 Sagrista-Sauleda J, Angel J, Permanyer-Miralda G, Soler-Soler J. Long-term follow-up of idiopathic chronic pericardial effusion. *N Engl J Med* 1999; **341:** 2054–9.

5 Curtiss EI, Reddy PS, Uretsky BF, Cecchetti AA. Pulsus paradoxus: definition and relation to the severity of cardiac tamponade. *Am Heart J* 1988; **115:** 391–8.

6 Merce J, Sagrista-Sauleda J, Permanyer-Miralda G, Evangelista A, Soler-Soler J. Correlation between clinical and Doppler echocardiographic findings in patients with moderate and large pericardial effusion: implications for the diagnosis of cardiac tamponade. *Am Heart J* 1999; **138:** 759–64.

105

CASE 105

Syncope in acute aortic dissection

R. Sanjuán Mañez, M.L. Blasco, J. Martínez León, R. Ruiz Granell

Case report

A 68-year-old woman, with a history of arterial hypertension and hypercholesterolemia, was referred to the hospital due to sudden-onset chest and back pain. When she reached the emergency room and before monitoring was started, she developed a syncopal attack with myoclonic jerks and urinary and fecal incontinence. The loss of consciousness was brief. When she recovered, without neurological sequelae, chest and back pain persisted.

The physical examination in the emergency room showed an anxious and dyspneic woman with feeble pulses and a blood pressure of 100/60 mmHg. Routine 12-lead electrocardiography (ECG) monitoring (Fig. 105.1) showed atrial fibrillation with an irregular ventricular response (65–80 beats/min) and a right bundle-branch block. Chest radiography showed an abnormally widened aortic contour, without pleural effusion. The transthoracic echocardiography findings suggested aortic root dissection due to aortic dilation, an intimal flap, and mild aortic regurgitation. Pericardial effusion was excluded.

Computed tomography (Fig. 105.2) confirmed an intimal flap in the ascending aorta and brachiocephalic trunk (aortic dissection type A in the Stanford classification). The dissection progressed through the abdominal aorta up to the iliac bifurcation. During the evaluation, the patient remained hypotensive, and laboratory studies showed a progressive fall in hematocrit from 35% to 21% and a drop in hemoglobin from 12.0 to 7.5 g/dL.

The patient underwent urgent surgical treatment without further complications. Because of the fragility

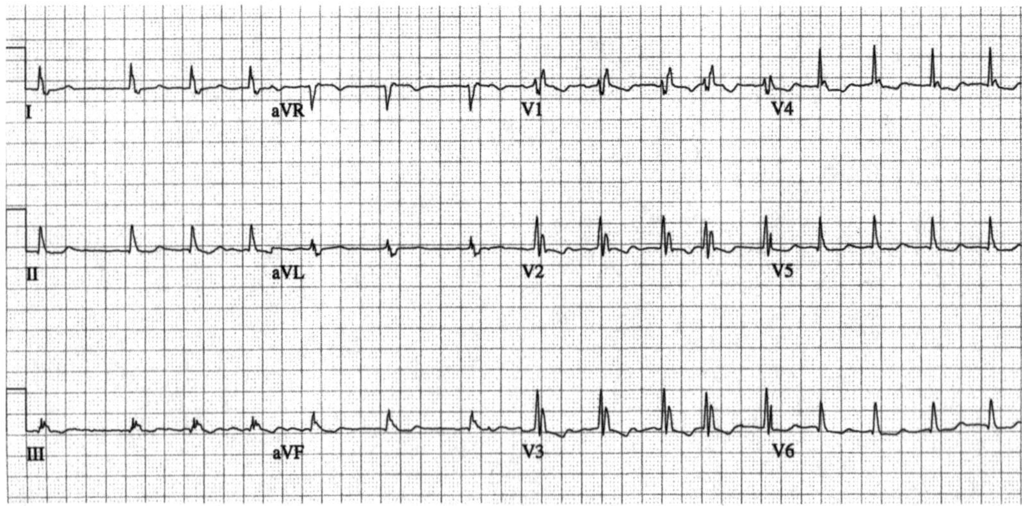

Figure 105.1 The electrocardiogram at admission.

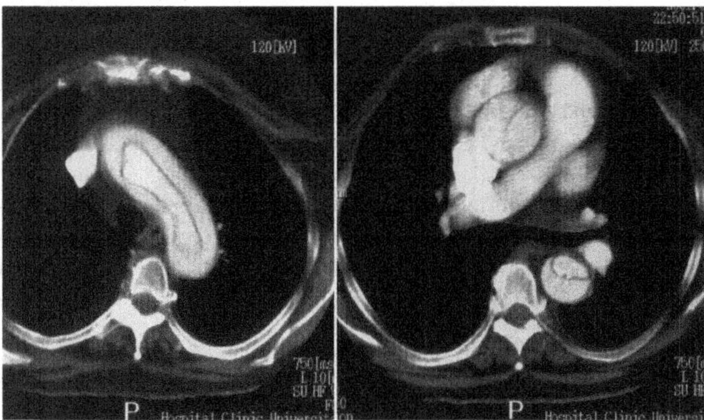

Figure 105.2 Contrast-enhanced computed tomography, showing an intimal flap separating the contrast-filled true lumen from the false lumen of the dissected aorta.

of the proximal aorta, a Bentall procedure was performed. With this technique, a composite prosthetic graft (prosthetic aortic valve sewn onto the end of a 30-mm Dacron tube graft) facilitates replacement of both the ascending aorta and aortic valve together. The patient was discharged from hospital 9 days after the surgical procedure. After 1 year of follow-up, she is alive in good general condition.

Comment

Acute aortic dissection occurs when blood seeps through a tear in the aorta, separating the outer and middle layers of the vascular wall. In the Stanford classification [1], proximal (or type A) dissections involve the ascending aorta, and distal (or type B) dissections are confined to the descending aorta, distal to the left subclavian artery ostium.

Death from acute dissection occurs most often as a result of disruption of the outer wall of the false channel. Rupture of the proximal dissection therefore produces hemopericardium and cardiac tamponade or hemorrhage into the mediastinum or pleural space. Other complications include aortic valve insufficiency and occlusion of the cerebral, spinal, renal, splanchnic, or iliac arteries [2].

Most patients with acute aortic dissection arrive in the emergency department suffering from chest pain or upper back pain, and fewer than 10–20% present with atypical symptoms [3]. Some patients may experience syncope as an early manifestation of acute aortic dissection. Syncope is generally associated with chest or back pain, but there are cases of painless aortic dissection presenting as syncope [4,5].

In the International Registry of Aortic Dissection (IRAD), 13% of 728 patients had syncope, with 3% of them having no symptoms of chest or back pain. Patients with proximal dissections had syncope more often than those with distal dissections (19% versus 3%). The in-hospital mortality rate was higher in patients with syncope than in patients without syncope (34% versus 23%). Cardiac tamponade was also more frequent in patients with syncope than in those without (28% versus 8%). Other complications, such as stroke or other neurological deficits, are also more common in patients with syncope than in those without syncope. However, nearly half of these patients do not have any of these complications to explain their loss of consciousness [6]. When patients with complications were excluded, syncope alone did not increase the risk of death.

Several mechanisms may be responsible for syncope in patients with acute aortic dissection. Syncope can be a manifestation of cardiac tamponade, acute hypotension secondary to the rupture of the outer wall, or obstruction of the aortic arch arteries. On the other hand, neuromediated mechanisms triggered by pain or direct stretching of baroreceptors in the aortic wall can also produce syncope. The significance of syncope can therefore vary in complicated or uncomplicated cases.

The present patient had a type A aortic dissection, presenting with chest pain and syncope. In the diagnostic work-up, transthoracic echocardiography suggested the presence of aortic dissection and ruled out cardiac tamponade or severe aortic insufficiency. Aortic dissection was subsequently confirmed on computed tomography. In the absence of significant complications, the syncope did not have an ominous prognosis in this case.

References

1 Nienaber CA, Eagle KA. Aortic dissection: new frontiers in diagnosis and management, 1: from etiology to diagnostic strategies. *Circulation* 2003; **108**: 628–35.

2 Lindsay J, DeBakey ME, Beall AC. Diagnosis and treatment of the diseases of the aorta. In: Schlant RC, Alexander RW, eds. *Hurst's The Heart, Arteries, and Veins*, 8th ed. McGraw-Hill, New York, 1994: 2163–80.

3 Vech RJ, Besterman EMM, Bromley LL, Eascott HHG, Kenyon JR. Acute aortic dissection: historical perspectives and current management. *Am Heart J* 1981; **102**: 1087–9.

4 Kulhmann SI, Powers RD. Painless aortic dissection: an unusual cause of syncope. *Ann Emerg Med* 1984; **13**: 549–51.

5 Young J, Herd AM. Painless aortic dissection and rupture presenting as syncope. *J Emerg Med* 2002; **22**: 171–4.

6 Nallamothu BK, Mehta RH, Saint S, *et al.* Syncope in acute aortic dissection: diagnostic, prognostic, and clinical implications. *Am J Med* 2002; **113**: 468–71.

CASE 106

Pulmonary embolism presenting as syncope

V. Montagud Balaguer, A. Peláez González, P. Aguar Carrascosa, M.T. Tuzón Segarra, A. Salvador Sanz

Case report

An 86-year-old woman was admitted to the emergency room due to two episodes of syncope and presyncope that had occurred when she was at home during the previous 24 h. Both episodes were associated with sweating and nausea, and began when she was standing up. She had had another syncopal fall 45 days before, which had resulted in a fractured arm. She had also had an episode of pulmonary embolism 5 years before, and breast cancer treated with surgery and radiotherapy.

The physical examination was normal. Serum troponin T levels were elevated (0.20 mg/dL) and D-dimer was also raised (2.833 ng/dL). The chest radiograph was normal. The 12-lead electrocardiogram (ECG) showed sinus rhythm at 100 beats/min, with a PR interval of 0.18 s and a right bundle-branch block with an $S_1Q_3T_3$ pattern (Fig. 106.1).

Doppler echocardiography documented normal cardiac chambers and preserved ventricular function (with a left ventricular ejection fraction of 65%). A septal posterior diastolic movement was visualized, which was more accentuated during inspiration. A systolic pulmonary artery pressure of 70 mmHg was estimated, with a slight tricuspid regurgitation.

On the basis of suspected pulmonary embolism, spiral computed tomography (CT) with intravenous contrast administration was carried out, and embolisms were found in both principal pulmonary arteries and all of the lobar and segmental arteries (Fig. 106.2).

Comment

Pulmonary embolism (PE) is a common and potentially fatal disorder, with clinical presentations that range widely, from those classically described (e.g., acute cor pulmonale, pulmonary infarction, or sudden and unexplained dyspnea) to silent cases. The mortality rate in untreated patients with PE is approximately 30%, but it can be reduced to 2–8% with adequate treatment [1]. Unfortunately, the diagnosis is often difficult to reach and is frequently missed, as PE presents with nonspecific signs and symptoms.

Syncope can be one form of presentation of PE [2–5]. In 1880, Luzzatto [2] wrote, "The most important initial neural manifestation of PE is undoubtedly loss of consciousness, which is far from uncommon." The reported prevalence of syncope among patients with PE has varied in different series. In a recent literature review, Morpurgo and Zonzin [5] found that the prevalence ranged from 2.2% to 40%, with an average of 15%. By contrast, two reports found that PE was the cause of syncope in 0.8% and 1.3%, respectively, of patients with syncope admitted to the emergency department [6,7].

The exact mechanism of syncope in patients with PE is not well understood and may be multifactorial. Three main mechanisms (obstructive, reflex, and metabolic) have been postulated. Obstruction of the pulmonary arteries in massive embolism leads to hemodynamic derangement, with acute right ventricular failure, reduced stroke volume and cardiac output, and systemic hypotension. However, only

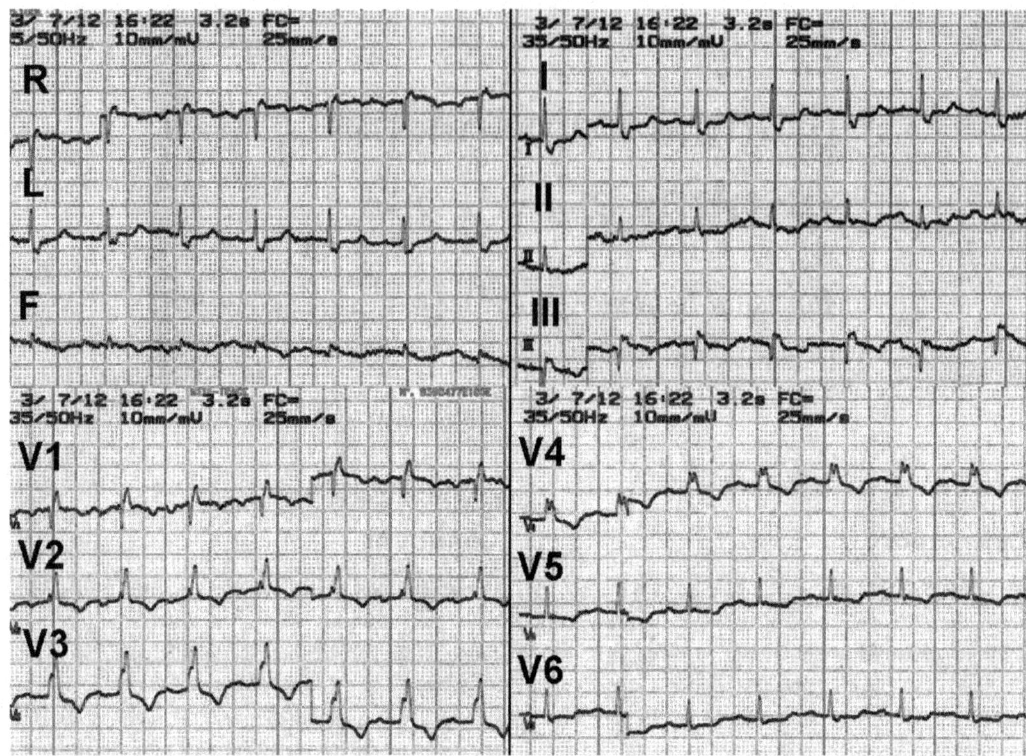

Figure 106.1 The electrocardiogram at admission.

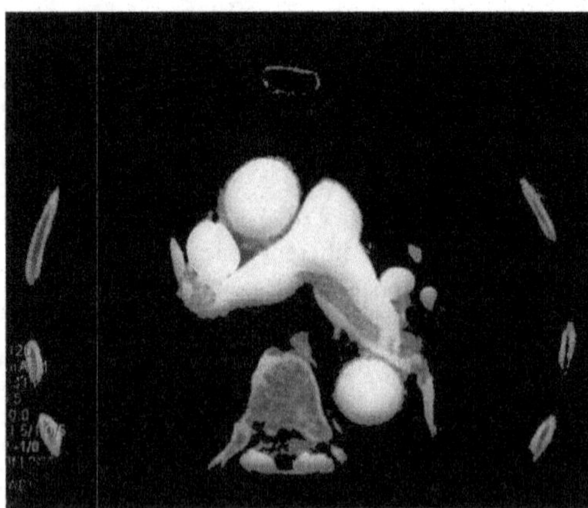

Figure 106.2 Spiral computed-tomographic angiogram, showing thrombus in the principal pulmonary arteries and lobar and segmental pulmonary branches.

13% of PE patients with syncope included in the International Cooperative Pulmonary Embolism Registry (ICOPER) were hypotensive [8]. Reflex neuromediated mechanisms have been postulated to explain cases of syncope associated with bradyarrhythmias [9,10] or syncope in the setting of non-massive PE [11]. Finally, metabolic factors such as hypocapnia caused by hyperventilation and hypoxemia can play a role in the loss of consciousness in PE patients [5].

Syncope is more frequently associated with massive PE [11–13], and the presence of syncope is thus a sign of a poor prognosis. In the ICOPER [8], the 3-month mortality among syncopal patients was 26.8%, in comparison with an overall mortality rate of 17%.

A discussion of the diagnostic strategies and the value of various techniques in patients with suspected PE is beyond the scope of this comment. A complete review of the subject can be found in the guidelines on the diagnosis and management of acute pulmonary embolism published by the European Cardiac Society [1]. In the present case, the history of PE, the syncopal episodes, the $S_1Q_3T_3$ pattern on the ECG, and the elevated level of D-dimer strongly suggest PE. The raised serum troponin level has no value in the differential diagnosis from myocardial infarction, as more than one-third of patients with PE have elevated troponin levels [14]. The echocardiographic estimates of pulmonary pressure also suggest PE, which was ultimately confirmed with spiral CT angiography.

References

1 Task Force on Pulmonary Embolism, European Society of Cardiology. Guidelines on diagnosis and management of acute pulmonary embolism. *Eur Heart J* 2000; **21**: 1301–36.

2 Luzzatto B. *L'Embolia dell'Arteria Polmonale.* Fratelli Richidei, Milan, 1880: 413–4.

3 Thames MD, Alpert JS, Dalen JE. Syncope in patients with pulmonary embolism. *J Am Med Assoc* 1977; **238**: 2509–11.

4 Koutkia P, Wachtel TJ. Pulmonary embolism presenting as syncope: case report and review of the literature. *Heart Lung* 1999; **28**: 342–7.

5 Morpurgo M, Zonzin P. Syncope in acute pulmonary embolism. *Ital Heart J* 2004; **5**: 3–5.

6 Blanc JJ, L'Her C, Touiza A, Garo B, L'Her E, Mansourati J. Prospective evaluation and outcome of patients admitted for syncope over a 1 year period. *Eur Heart J* 2002; **23**: 815–20.

7 Sarasin FP, Lois-Simonet M, Carballo D, *et al.* Prospective evaluation of patients with syncope: a population-based study. *Am J Med* 2001; **111**: 177–84.

8 Goldhaber SZ, Visani L, De Rosa M. Acute pulmonary embolism: clinical outcomes in the International Cooperative Pulmonary Embolism Registry (ICOPER). *Lancet* 1999; **353**: 1386–9.

9 Simpson RJ, Podolack R, Mangano CA, Foster JR, Dalldorf FG. Vagal syncope during recurrent pulmonary embolism. *J Am Med Assoc* 1983; **249**: 390–3.

10 Akinboboye OO, Brown EJ Jr, Queirroz R, *et al.* Recurrent pulmonary embolism with second-degree atrioventricular block and near syncope. *Am Heart J* 1993; **126**: 731–2.

11 Castelli R, Tarsia P, Tantardini C, Pantaleo G, Guariglia A, Porro F. Syncope in patients with pulmonary embolism: comparison between patients with syncope as the presenting symptom of pulmonary embolism and patients with pulmonary embolism without syncope. *Vasc Med* 2003; **8**: 257–61.

12 Toda R, Vidal F, Bernet A, Blavia R, Garcia V, Richard C. Síncope como forma de presentación de tromboembolismo pulmonar. Estudio de 15 casos. *Med Clin (Barc)* 1992; **98**: 561–4.

13 Kasper W, Konstantinides S, Geibel A, *et al.* Management strategies and determinants of outcome in acute major pulmonary embolism: results of a multicenter registry. *J Am Coll Cardiol* 1997; **30**: 1165–71.

14 Meyer T, Binder L, Hruska N, Luthe H, Buchwald AB. Cardiac troponin I elevation in acute pulmonary embolism is associated with right ventricular dysfunction. *J Am Coll Cardiol* 2000; **36**: 1632–6.

CASE 107

Subclavian steal syndrome as a cause of syncope

J. Martínez León, I. Martín González, M. Juez López

Case report

A 56-year-old man who was a truck driver was evaluated after suffering two recent episodes of syncope while repairing a ceiling at the weekend. He had a history of heavy smoking (more than 20 cigarettes a day), was not diabetic, and also reported nonlateralizing ischemic attacks (dizziness and vertigo) when doing physical activities involving the upper extremities.

At the physical examination, the radial pulse was palpable and normal in the right upper extremity but was absent in the left arm. His blood pressure was 150/90 mmHg in the right arm and 75 mmHg in the left arm, as determined by Doppler sounds. Bruits were not audible either in the arm or in the supraclavicular space. Electrocardiography (ECG), chest radiography, and blood tests were normal. No cervical rib was observed.

Duplex scanning showed a normal triphasic waveform at all levels in the right arm and a monophasic waveform with loss of the reverse-flow component in the left arm. All of the extracranial carotid arteries had normal flow patterns. Cerebral computed tomography (CT) was normal.

An aortic arteriography was indicated and was carried out via the right femoral approach. The initial image showed the entire aortic arch, with a normal appearance in the innominate artery and common left carotid artery. The left subclavian artery was absent and a small stump was present at its origin (Fig. 107.1A). Later frames showed filling of a distal left subclavian artery via retrograde flow through the vertebral artery (Fig. 107.1B), establishing the diagnosis of subclavian steal syndrome secondary to total occlusion of the left subclavian artery.

Angioplasty was not considered to be indicated for this chronically obstructed artery, and surgery was suggested and accepted by the patient. The primary objectives of surgery in this situation are to prevent a major neurological event, to prevent complications secondary to episodes of cerebral ischemia, and to relieve symptoms. Carotid–subclavian artery bypass grafting was carried out without complications (Fig. 107.2), and the patient has remained asymptomatic since then.

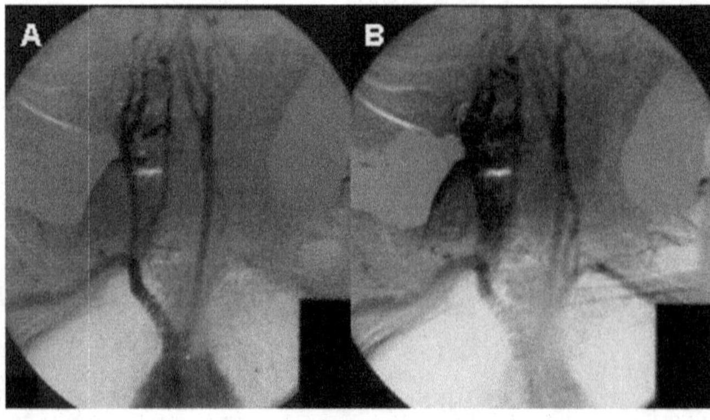

Figure 107.1 **A.** Early phase of the aortic arch angiography, showing the absence of the left subclavian artery. **B.** Late phase of the angiography, showing the left subclavian artery filled up via collateral circulation from the ipsilateral vertebral artery.

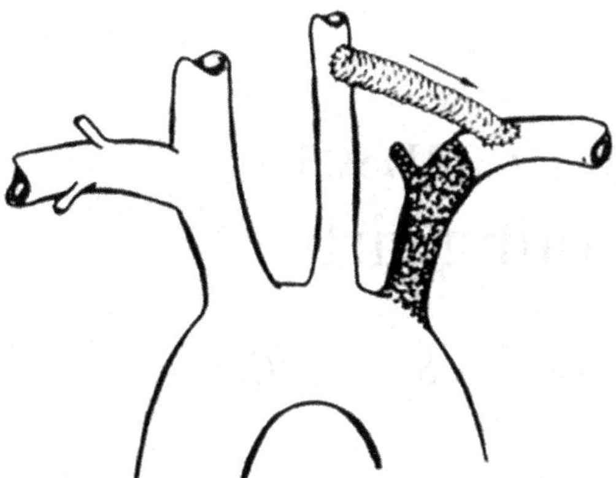

Figure 107.2 Diagram illustrating the carotid–subclavian bypass procedure. The operation can be carried out with a supraclavicular approach, using a synthetic or autologous vein graft.

Comment

Subclavian steal syndrome is a rare cause of syncope [1]. The anatomical findings were first observed in 1960 by the Italian radiologist Contorni [2], and the clinical syndrome was subsequently described by Reivitch *et al.* [3]. Subclavian steal syndrome is caused by occlusion or stenosis of the proximal subclavian artery, with subsequent retrograde filling of the artery via the ipsilateral vertebral artery. Blood flow is therefore stolen from the vertebrobasilar circulation, resulting in symptoms of vertebrobasilar insufficiency that can include presyncope or syncope.

Subclavian occlusion or stenosis is produced in most cases by atherosclerotic plaques located in the initial portion of the subclavian artery. Obstruction involves the left subclavian artery more often than the right one, and associated arterial lesions are found in more than 80% of cases [4]. Other causes of subclavian obstruction and subclavian steal include Takayasu arteritis [5] and congenital anomalies of the aortic arch [6].

Patients with subclavian steal syndrome may present with symptoms related to vertebrobasilar insufficiency: vertigo, diplopia, blurred vision, and cranial nerve dysfunction, as well as syncope or drop attacks. Strictly speaking, loss of consciousness resulting from subclavian steal should not be considered as syncope, as it is not due to global but to regional cerebral hypoperfusion, affecting the vertebrobasilar system [7].

The present patient, a 56-year-old man, presented with syncope that was triggered when he raised his arms over his head. In addition, the physical examination disclosed significant differences in blood pressure between the two arms. The clinical picture therefore strongly suggests a subclavian steal syndrome. The diagnosis can be confirmed by carotid duplex ultrasonography and magnetic resonance angiography, or aortic arch aortography.

Symptomatic patients require surgical intervention, such as a carotid–subclavian bypass or percutaneous transluminal angioplasty of the subclavian artery, with stent placement.

References

1 Chan-Tack KM. Subclavian steal syndrome: a rare but important cause of syncope. *South Med J* 2001; **94**: 445–7.

2 Contorni L. Il circolo collaterale vertebro-vertebralle nella obliterazione dell'arteria subclavia alla suo origine. *Minerva Chir* 1960; **15**: 268–71.

3 Reivitch M, Holling HE, Roberts B, Toole JF. Reversal of blood flow through the vertebral artery and its effect on cerebral circulation. *N Engl J Med* 1961; **265**: 878–85.

4 Fields WS, Lemack NA. Joint study of extracranial arterial occlusion, 7: subclavian steal—a review of 168 cases. *J Am Med Assoc* 1972; **222**: 1139–43.

5 Moncada G, Kobayashi Y, Kaneko E, Nishiwaki Y, Kishi Y, Numano E. Subclavian steal syndrome secondary to Takayasu arteritis. *Int J Cardiol* 1998; **66** (Suppl 1): S231–6.

6 Engelman DA, Mortazavi A. Congenital subclavian steal syndrome. *Tex Heart Inst J* 1998; **25**: 216–7.

7 van Dijk JG. Conditions that mimic syncope. In: Benditt D, Blanc JJ, Brignole M, Sutton R, eds. *The Evaluation and Treatment of Syncope.* Futura-Blackwell, Elmsford, New York, 2003: 184–200.

108

CASE 108

Multiple malignant causes of syncope in a young girl

R. Ruiz Granell, F. Nuñez, J.I. Muñoz, S. Morell Cabedo, A. Roselló, R. García Civera

Case report

A 14-year-old girl was referred to hospital for evaluation of a syncopal episode. On the day of admission, she had been asleep in bed and her sister noticed that she did not get up when the alarm clock went off. As it was difficult to wake her up, the patient was transferred to a local hospital in an ambulance, where she arrived conscious and alert; however, a complete atrioventricular (AV) block was documented on the 12-lead electrocardiogram (ECG), and she was transferred to our hospital for further evaluation.

She was an apparently normally developed girl without growth problems, who had been menstruating since she was 13 and had no personal or familial history of significant diseases, syncope, AV block, or sudden death. The physical examination showed bradycardia, but was otherwise normal. The ECG showed a complete AV block (Fig. 108.1) with a narrow QRS escape rhythm at 52 beats/min and with a corrected QT interval of 440 ms. Chest radiography, echocardiography, and laboratory tests were completely normal. Due to the atypical clinical presentation, an electrophysiological study was performed, during which the AV block was found to be located in the AV node and no ventricular arrhythmias were induced with programmed ventricular pacing (two sites, two cycle lengths, up to three extrastimuli,

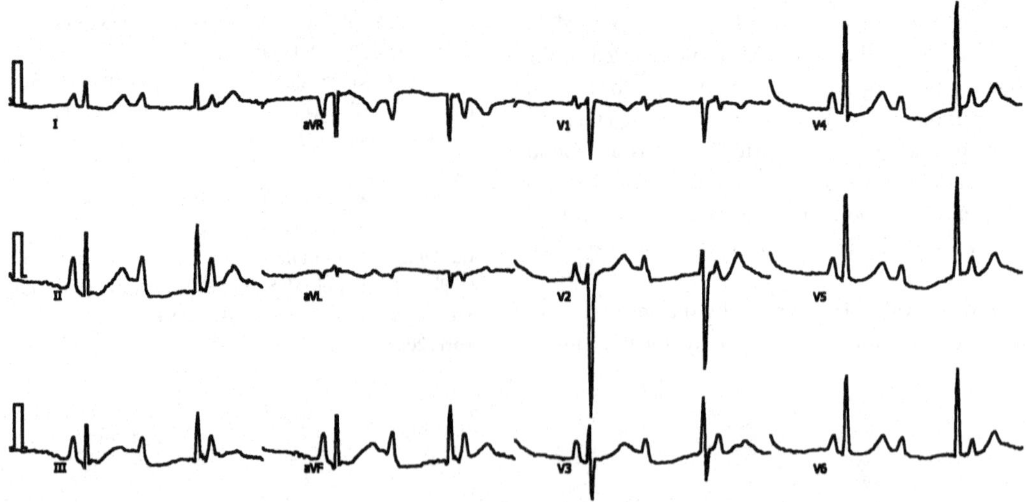

Figure 108.1 The 12-lead electrocardiogram obtained at the patient's first admission to the hospital, showing a complete atrioventricular block.

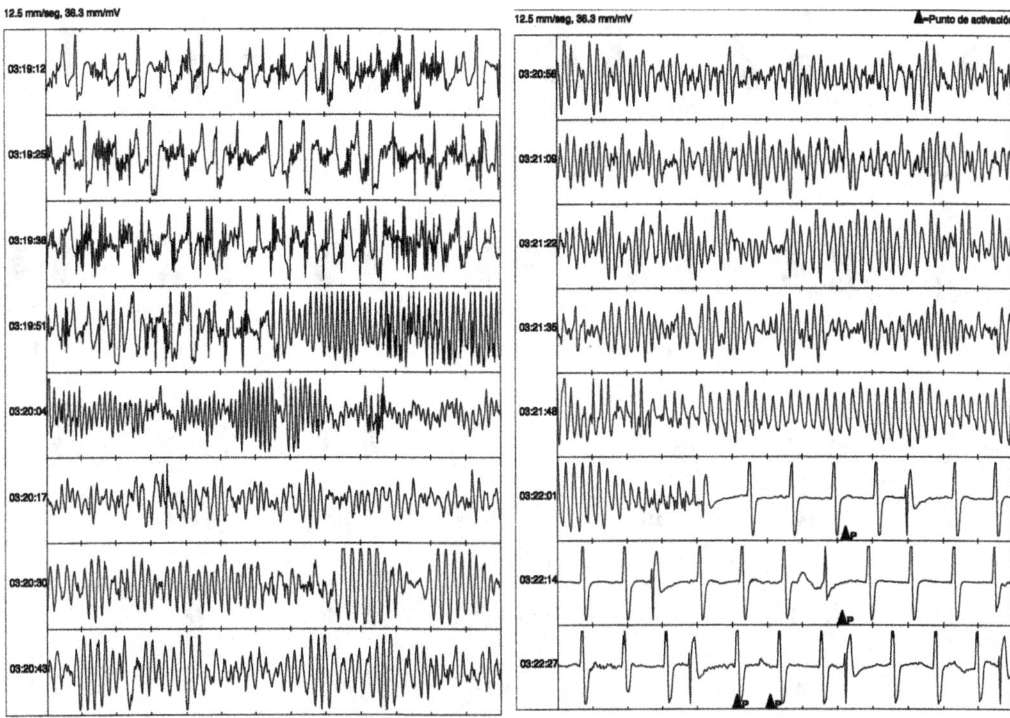

Figure 108.2 The implantable loop recorder tracing retrieved after the syncopal episode, showing long-lasting polymorphic ventricular tachycardia.

short–long–short sequences, and burst pacing). The diagnosis was syncope due to a presumably congenital AV block, and a single-lead VDD permanent pacemaker was implanted uneventfully.

Two months later, the patient was referred to our center again after suffering a recurrent episode of syncope in a swimming pool, with near-drowning that required medical assistance. The patient said she had eaten badly that day and had been standing up for a long time in the sun, and when she dived into the water she felt very dizzy. The physical examination, ECG, echocardiogram, chest radiograph, laboratory tests, tilt test, and evaluation of pacemaker function did not reveal any abnormalities. In view of the unexplained nature of the relapse, placement of an implantable loop recorder (ILR) (Reveal, Medtronic, Inc., Minneapolis, Minnesota, USA) was suggested and accepted by the family.

Five weeks later the patient had another relapse while she was at a party, with loss of consciousness for more than 3 min. The ILR was activated, and the recorded arrhythmia proved to be a long-lasting, self-limited polymorphic ventricular tachycardia (Fig. 108.2). The pacemaker was then removed, and a dual-chamber implantable cardioverter-defibrillator (ICD) was implanted.

One month after discharge, the patient was referred to our hospital again with a new loss of consciousness, during which neither jerks nor activation of the ICD were noticed by the family. She was again evaluated at a local hospital, where she was admitted; mental confusion and hypotension were noticed on admission, the laboratory tests showed discrete anemia, and mild pleural and pericardial effusions were noticed on chest radiography and echocardiography. She was transferred to our hospital and admitted to the pediatric intensive-care unit (ICU), presenting with a new loss of consciousness with deep and sustained hypotension that did not resolve with the usual pharmacological management. Urgent echocardiography showed severe pericardial effusion with signs of cardiac tamponade. Urgent pericardiocentesis was carried out, with blood being obtained from the pericardium with a temporary rise in blood pressure, but with immediate worsening

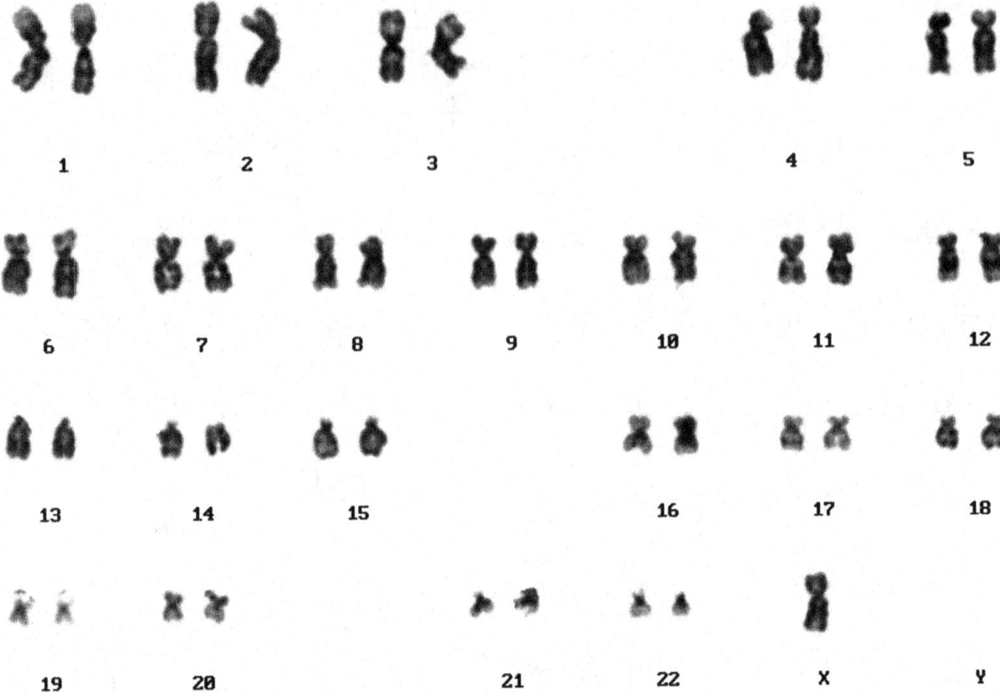

Figure 108.3 Karyotyping, showing a single X chromosome (45,XO).

of the condition. As a last resort, a medial thoracotomy was carried out in the ICU, which led to the discovery of severe hemopericardium due to a 1-cm long rupture in the posterior wall of the ascending aorta. No perforations related to the ICD leads or the cannula used for pericardiocentesis were seen. After the rupture had been sutured, the patient was stabilized and transferred to the cardiac surgery room, where meticulous visual inspection did not disclose any anomalies in the aortic wall (apart from the rupture) or any other cause of intrapericardiac bleeding. Intraoperative transesophageal echocardiography did not identify any anomalies either. Her postoperative recovery was slow and difficult but complete, with no neurological sequelae. The vascular computed tomography findings were normal. Karyotyping disclosed mosaicism (12% of the cells) for Turner's syndrome (Fig. 108.3).

The patient was discharged 3 months after the episode and has remained free of syncope during a 1-year follow-up period. The complete AV block has persisted and no ventricular arrhythmias have been recorded by the ICD.

Comment

Syncope is a symptom that can be provoked by multiple causes; patients can therefore experience syncopal episodes due to different etiologies, making the diagnosis difficult. This situation is not unusual in elderly people, probably due to the comorbidities in this population. Vasovagal or neurocardiogenic syncope is more frequent as a unique cause of syncope in young people without overt heart disease and therefore has to be suspected first.

Syncope is seldom seen in congenital AV block, but its presentation must lead to consideration of pacemaker implantation, particularly if, as in this case, syncope appears when the patient is in the recumbent position or sleeping. Given the atypical clinical presentation, the authors carried out an electrophysiological study in the patient, and, as it was negative, implanted a pacemaker. The subsequent course was strikingly convoluted, with relapses due to ventricular arrhythmia and to aortic rupture.

Turner's syndrome is a disorder characterized by the absence of all or part of a normal second sex chromosome. The syndrome occurs in one in 2500 to one in 3000 live-born girls. Approximately half have X monosomy (45,X), 5–10% have a duplication (isochromosome) of the long arm of one X, and most of the remainder have mosaicism for 45,X [1]. The prevalence of congenital heart disease ranges from 17% to 45%, with coarctation of the aorta and a bicuspid aortic valve being the most common malformations [1,2]. Although conduction defects and other arrhythmias have been described in Turner's syndrome, there is no established relationship between the syndrome and AV block or ventricular polymorphic tachycardia.

Aortic dissection has frequently been reported in patients with Turner's syndrome [1–3], associated with aortic coarctation, a bicuspid aortic valve, hypertension, or combinations of these in 93% of cases. Isolated dissection and isolated perforation of the aorta are thus atypical modes of presentation of cardiovascular complications in Turner's syndrome. Cystic medial necrosis, similar to the findings in aortic dissection in Marfan's syndrome, has also been reported in Turner's syndrome, and some observations support the notion that aortic dilation may represent or be similar to an inherited disorder of connective tissue [3].

The case presented here illustrates the difficulties one has to face when trying to diagnose the cause of syncope in complex, atypical, rare—and frequently serious—cases.

References

1 Sybert VP, McCauley E. Turner's syndrome. *N Engl J Med* 2004; **351**: 1227–38.

2 Sybert VP. Cardiovascular malformations and complications in Turner syndrome. *Pediatrics* 1998; **101**: 11–7.

3 Lin AE, Lippe B, Rosenfeld RG. Further delineation of aortic dilation, dissection, and rupture in patients with Turner syndrome. *Pediatrics* 1998; **102**: 12–20.

Index

9 781405 151092